D1483376

Schizotypal personality disorder was first introduced as a diagnostic entity in 1980 and has been the subject of increasing interest and study since that time. Attention has focused not only on diagnostic and treatment issues but also on the etiological relationship of schizotypal disorder to schizophrenia.

This is the first book devoted to schizotypal personality. It provides a comprehensive overview of current knowledge from some of the world's leading researchers in the field and includes reviews of genetics, neurodevelopment, assessment, psychophysiology, neuropsychology, and brain imaging. A central theme is the exploration of categorical and dimensional approaches to the understanding of schizotypal personality disorder. Introductory and concluding chapters set in context the sometimes divergent opinions and findings presented by the book's contributors, and there are reviews of methodological issues and assessment schedules for the benefit of researchers in the field.

In setting out to answer, from phenomenological, psychological, and neurobiological perspectives, the fundamental question – What is schizotypal personality disorder? – and to develop coherent etiological models, this book will serve as an authoritative resource for clinicians and researchers interested in this major personality disorder.

SCHIZOTYPAL PERSONALITY

SCHIZOTYPAL PERSONALITY

Edited by

ADRIAN RAINE
University of Southern California

TODD LENCZ
University of Southern California

SARNOFF A. MEDNICK
University of Southern California

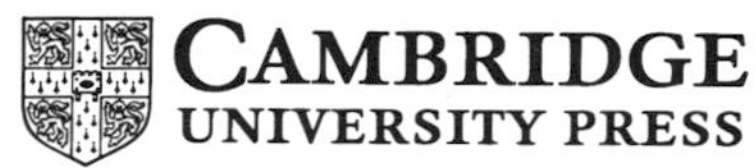

Published by the Press Syndicate of the University of Cambridge
The Pitt Building, Trumpington Street, Cambridge CB2 1RP
40 West 20th Street, New York, NY 10011-4211, USA
10 Stamford Road, Oakleigh, Melbourne 3166, Australia

First published 1995

Printed in the United States of America

Library of Congress Cataloging-in-Publication Data

Schizotypal personality / edited by Adrian Raine, Todd Lencz, Sarnoff A. Mednick.

p. cm.

Includes bibliographic references and indexes.

ISBN 0-521-45422-0 (hc)

1. Schizotypal personality disorder – Congresses. I. Raine, Adrian. II. Lencz, Todd. III. Mednick, Sarnoff A.
[DNLM: 1. Schizotypal Personality Disorder – congresses. WM 203 S33988 1995]
RC569.5.S35S35 1995
616.89′82 – dc20
DNLM/DLC
for Library of Congress 94-26903
CIP

A catalog record for this book is available from the British Library.

ISBN 0-521-45422-0 Hardback

Contents

Contributors

Nancy C. Andreasen
University of Iowa Hospitals and Clinics
Department of Psychiatry Administration, #2887 J.P.P.
200 Hawkins Drive
Iowa City, IA 52242

Tony Beech
Department of Experimental Psychology
Oxford University
South Parks Road
Oxford OX1 3UD
U.K.

Deana S. Benishay
Department of Psychology
S.G.M. Building
University of Southern California
Los Angeles, CA 90089-1061

Laura Bird
Department of Psychology
S.G.M. Building
University of Southern California
Los Angeles, CA 90089-1061

Tyrone D. Cannon
Department of Psychology
University of Pennsylvania
3815 Walnut Street
Philadelphia, PA 19104

Jean P. Chapman
Department of Psychology
W.J. Brogden Building
University of Wisconsin – Madison
1202 West Johnson Street
Madison, Wisconsin 53706-1611

Loren J. Chapman
Department of Psychology
W.J. Brogden Building
University of Wisconsin – Madison
1202 West Johnson Street
Madison, Wisconsin 53706-1611

Gordon Claridge
Department of Experimental Psychology
Oxford University
South Parks Road
Oxford OX1 3UD
U.K.

Michael Coleman
Department of Psychology
Harvard University
33 Kirkland Street
Cambridge, MA 02138

Michael E. Dawson
Department of Psychology
S.G.M. Building
University of Southern California
Los Angeles, CA 90089-1061

Diane L. Filion
Department of Psychology
S.G.M. Building
University of Southern California
Los Angeles, CA 90089-1061

Michael A. Flaum, M.D.
University of Iowa Hospitals and Clinics
Department of Psychiatry Administration, #2887 J.P.P.
200 Hawkins Drive
Iowa City, IA 52242

Susan Gale
Department of Psychology
Emory University
Atlanta, Georgia 30322

John Gruzelier
Department of Psychiatry
Charing Cross and Westminster Medical School
University of London
St. Dunstan's Road
London W6 8RF
U.K.

Raquel E. Gur
Brain–Behavior Laboratory
Neuropsychiatry Section
Department of Psychiatry
University of Pennsylvania,
Philadelphia, PA 19104-4283

Ruben C. Gur
Brain–Behavior Laboratory
Neuropsychiatry Section
Department of Psychiatry
University of Pennsylvania
Philadelphia, PA 19104-4283

Nicholas Haslam
Department of Psychology
University of Pennsylvania
3815 Walnut Street
Philadelphia, PA 19104

Erin A. Hazlett
Department of Psychiatry
Box 1505
Mount Sinai School of Medicine
One Gustave L. Levy Place
New York, NY 10029-6574

Philip S. Holzman
Department of Psychology
Harvard University
33 Kirkland Street
Cambridge, MA 02138

Matti O. Huttunen
Department of Psychiatry
University of Helsinki
Lapinlahdentie, SF 00180
Helsinki 18
Finland

Loring J. Ingraham
Laboratory of Psychology and Psychopathology
NIMH/NIH
Building 10, Room 4C116
Bethesda, Maryland 20892

Lauren Korfine
Department of Psychology
Harvard University
William James Hall
33 Kirkland Street
Cambridge, MA 02138

Thomas R. Kwapil
Department of Psychology
University of Wisconsin–Madison
1202 West Johnson Street
Madison, Wisconsin 53706

José LaFosse
Center for Longitudinal Studies
Social Science Research Institute
Denney Research Building
University of Southern California
Los Angeles, CA 90089-1111

Todd Lencz
Department of Psychology
S.G.M. Building
University of Southern California
Los Angeles, CA 90089-1061

Mark Lenzenweger
Psychopathology Area
Cornell University
Van Rensselaer Hall
Ithaca, New York 14853-4401

Deborah L. Levy
McLean Hospital
115 Mill Street
Belmont, MA 02178

Ricardo A. Machón
Center for Longitudinal Studies
Social Science Research Institute
Denney Research Building
University of Southern California
Los Angeles, CA 90089-1111

Steven Matthysse
McLean Hospital
115 Mill Street
Belmont, MA 02178

Sarnoff A. Mednick
Center for Longitudinal Studies
Social Science Research Institute
Denney Research Building
University of Southern California
Los Angeles, CA 90089-1111

Shari Mills
Department of Psychology
S.G.M. Building
University of Southern California
Los Angeles, CA 90089-1061

Keith H. Nuechterlein
Department of Psychiatry and Biobehavioral Science
300 UCLA Medical Plaza, Suite 2200
UCLA
Los Angeles, Ca 90024-6968

Gillian O'Driscoll
Department of Psychology
Harvard University
33 Kirkland Street
Cambridge, MA 02138

Sohee Park
Department of Psychology
Harvard University
33 Kirkland Street
Cambridge, MA 02138

Adrian Raine
Department of Psychology
S.G.M. Building
University of Southern California
Los Angeles, CA 90089-1061

Anne M. Schell
Department of Psychology
Occidental College
1600 Campus Road
Los Angeles, CA 90041

Larry J. Siever, M.D.
Department of Psychiatry
Bronx VA Medical Center
130 West Kingsbridge Road, Rm. 116A
East Bronx, NY 10468

Audrey R. Tyrka
Department of Psychology
University of Pennsylvania
3815 Walnut Street
Philadelphia, PA 19104

Peter H. Venables
Department of Psychology
University of York
Heslington
York YO1 5DD
U.K.

Elaine F. Walker
Department of Psychology
Emory University
Atlanta, Georgia 30322

Preface

This is the first book of any kind to be published on schizotypal personality. Such a book has long been overdue. Although the concept of schizotypal personality has been in existence for many years, it was 1980 before it was formalized in DSM-III-R. The past 15 years have witnessed a steady increase in research on schizotypal personality and recognition of its importance as a major personality disorder that has the potential for contributing to our understanding of schizophrenia. We hope, therefore, that this first book will fill a significant and pressing gap in the current literature.

The importance of understanding schizotypal personality cannot be overemphasized. At a clinical level, schizotypal personality disorder is defined as a lifelong personality disorder characterized by nine traits: ideas of reference, excessive social anxiety, magical thinking, unusual perceptual experiences, eccentric behavior or appearance, no close friends or confidants, odd speech, constricted affect, and suspiciousness. This syndrome can be socially and occupationally debilitating, but because schizotypals are socially avoidant, they rarely present themselves for treatment. It is becoming increasingly important, therefore, to understand this personality disorder in order ultimately to help people afflicted with schizotypal personality disorder. In nonclinical populations, research on schizotypy can help us to understand the normal variations that exist in the general population of schizotypal traits and perhaps give some insight into the more advantageous features of schizotypy, such as increased creativity. In addition, the research described in this book can prove informative for those seeking to understand the biological bases of normal personality processes.

Understanding schizotypy is also important for a different reason. It is thought that schizotypal personality disorder is genetically related to schizophrenia, and some researchers suspect that schizotypy may even represent the primary disorder, with schizophrenia being an offshoot or complication of schizotypy. Recently, increasing numbers of schizophrenia researchers have turned to examining schizotypal personality as a crucial complement to more traditional research. This trend promises to open up new and exciting vistas into the origins of schizophrenia, particularly because schizotypals tend to be free of the institutionalization and medication confounds that impede schizophrenia research.

The main aim of this book is to provide comprehensive overviews of our current knowledge in the main fields of schizotypal personality research. A second aim is to provide researchers in this area with a solid basis upon which to proceed by outlining directives for further research and highlighting important conceptual, theoretical, and methodological issues that need to be tackled head-on before genuine advances can be made in this field. A third aim is to place schizotypal research in the wider context of schizophrenia research (where relevant), because we feel such a juxtaposition of findings can be mutually informative. A fourth aim is to represent the two main approaches taken to understanding schizotypal personality: the categorical approach, which focuses on clinical manifestations of schizotypal personality *disorder* (most commonly pursued by psychiatrists), and the dimensional or personality approach, which focuses on *individual differences* in schizotypy in the general population (most commonly pursued by experimental psychopathologists). We believe that both approaches are critical to helping us more fully understand the manifestation of schizotypy in all its forms.

Important theoretical and conceptual issues facing this field of research are described in the introduction. The bulk of the chapters are divided into six main areas: genetics and neurodevelopment, assessment, the categorical versus dimensional approach to schizotypy, psychophysiology and psychopharmacology, neuropsychology, and brain imaging. The last chapter attempts to provide an overview and synthesis, together with future directives.

We are aware that there are other areas of potential importance that we have not devoted chapters to, such as treatment, EEG and event-related potentials, and creativity; coverage of other areas, such as psychopharmacology, is not extensive. Some areas are not included (e.g., event-related potentials) in some instances because excellent reviews already exist, but in most cases because findings to date are too sparse to warrant an extensive review. We hope that in a future book these areas can be incorporated. Conversely, we have devoted two chapters to the field of brain imaging, even though empirical findings are sparse. The reason is that we believe structural and functional brain imaging hold the promise of an exponential increase in our knowledge on the neurophysiology of schizotypy, and consequently, we wanted to lay the groundwork here for encouraging such research.

This book is intended largely for an academic audience made up of research scientists, advanced graduate students, and clinicians, including psychiatrists, psychologists, social workers, and neuroscientists. We expect this book to be of value to researchers interested in schizotypal personality, schizophrenia, schizophrenia-spectrum disorders, and personality disorders, as well as personality and psychopathology in general. We sincerely hope that the contents of this book will make some contribution to stimulating this research community into devoting even more time and resources to pursuing the causes and prevention of this enigmatic disorder.

Acknowledgments

This book is a direct outcome of the first-ever conference on schizotypal personality, held at Il Ciocco, Castelvechio Pascoli, Tuscany, Italy, from May 31 to June 4, 1993. Funding for this international conference was made possible by NATO's Advanced Research Workshop program, which allowed us to bring together most of the world's leading researchers on schizotypal personality for one week. In addition to thanking NATO for its generous support, we wish to thank Peter Venables and Fini Schulsinger for acting as international codirectors of the conference. We are deeply indebted to Susan Stack, our conference coorganizer, for her incredible organizational skills and marvelous sense of humor, both of which contributed greatly to the success of the conference. We are also grateful to Deana Benishay and Karen Dykes for their technical help throughout the conference. Finally, we wish to thank our editor, Richard Barling, for encouraging us to develop this book and for his enthusiasm, advice, and good counsel.

PART I
Introduction

1

Conceptual and theoretical issues in schizotypal personality research

ADRIAN RAINE and TODD LENCZ

Many researchers argue that research into schizotypal personality is important not only in furthering our understanding of this personality disorder, but also in providing key insights into our understanding of schizophrenia. For example, several studies have indicated that schizotypal personality disorder (SPD) is a disturbance that may be genetically related to schizophrenia, insofar as it is prevalent among first-degree biological relatives of schizophrenics. It is also argued that SPD research is of key importance in overcoming methodological weaknesses of schizophrenia research. Psychotic symptoms may mask and blur the more subtle cognitive impairments underlying the schizophrenia spectrum, and they also create difficulty in ensuring that schizophrenics fully understand and comply with the experimental protocol. In addition, effects of neuroleptics and lengthy hospitalization create further confounds in interpreting research on schizophrenic subjects. Thus, research in SPD has become increasingly important as a means of studying biological and cognitive markers of the schizophrenia spectrum without the confound of severe clinical symptoms.

Research since the 1980s has provided grounds for this optimistic view. Schizotypals have been shown to display a number of the biological/neuropsychological markers for schizophrenia, such as eye-tracking impairment, abnormalities on evoked potentials, and attentional deficits. In schizophrenics, these deficits have been linked to damage at brain sites such as the frontal lobes, temporal lobes, and subcortical areas. Examination of these markers is one of the central paradigms in schizophrenia research, and extension of these methods to those afflicted with SPD represents a significant test of the biological and neuropsychological processes thought to underlie schizophrenia. Such research in SPD may also identify those intact cognitive abilities that serve as "protective factors," protecting some schizotypals from developing schizophrenia.

Nevertheless, research on schizotypal personality (relative to other conditions) is still in its infancy, and there are important conceptual and theoretical issues that need to be addressed head-on in the next decade of research in order that genuine advances be made in this area. The aim of this chapter is to outline some of these issues in the hope that this may be of help in directing future research along productive lines. Some of these issues will be addressed in chapters that follow; other issues have yet to be addressed. These issues are grouped under the five headings that follow, namely, diagnostic issues, phenomenological and assessment issues, methodological issues, mechanisms and etiology, and clinical issues.

Diagnostic issues

Axis I or Axis II?

SPD is currently viewed as an Axis II disorder alongside other personality disorders, but the issue of moving it into Axis I alongside schizophrenia was raised during discussions on changes to be made for DSM-IV. Such a move has not occurred but it raises the question of whether SPD is best construed as a deviation representing an exaggeration of an ostensibly normal personality process which places subjects at risk for schizophrenia, or a major disorder that is much more integrally related to schizophrenia itself. The question that needs to be considered in the next decade is what type of research can help address this issue for the future DSM-V. This issue also relates to the issue of dimensional versus categorical conceptualizations of schizotypy, in that retention as an Axis II disorder debatably argues more in favor of a dimensional conceptualization of schizotypy.

Changes in diagnostic content

Should there be changes in the diagnostic content of SPD? Virtually no change was made in the revision for DSM-IV, but there are a number of important issues that require further resolution over the next few years. For example, should anhedonia, which has frequently been viewed as central to schizophrenia, be included as a key feature of SPD? Conversely, social anxiety is a broad-based symptom that does not so cleanly "map on" to other schizophrenia prodromal symptoms as do other features, such as unusual perceptual experiences or paranoid ideation. Recent findings by Chapman and Chapman (1992, and Chapter 5, this volume) on the extent to which different schizotypal personality features predict breakdown for later psychosis represent the type of future research that can help address such questions.

A related issue concerns which of the nine features of schizotypal personality disorder share a common genetic loading with schizophrenia. Answers to such questions can help refine the way in which SPD is conceptualized in DSM-IV, and further promote research on its etiology.

Boundary between SPD and schizophrenia

Where is the boundary between SPD and schizophrenia, and how may this boundary be best defined or conceptualized? The problem of deciding where the defining line between disorder and normality lies has created considerable debate (e.g., Braff et al., 1992). Central to this issue lies the question of whether there is *any* boundary between the two conditions. The possibility must also be faced that our approach to how we answer this question may in part be biased by pragmatic issues and our research experiences. For example, researchers who have regular access to large populations of undergraduates may be biased more to an individual difference / dimensional approach (no discrete boundary), whereas hospital-based researchers who have ready access to clinical schizotypals may be biased more to a categorical (relatively clear boundary) approach.

Late-onset SPD

Are we correct in stipulating that SPD must be lifelong for a diagnosis to be given? In our clinical work we have come across cases where SPD has become manifest relatively later in life (e.g., mid-thirties). Given that we have the concept of late-onset schizophrenia, is it conceivable that late-onset SPD is also a meaningful concept? And if so, can it shed light on the etiology of late-onset schizophrenia, and does it present differently from SPD with onset in early adulthood?

Phenomenological and assessment issues

Categories versus dimensions

Perhaps the most important conceptual issue concerns whether schizotypal personality is best construed as a category or a dimension. This will be reflected in some of the chapters that follow. A number of possibilities come to mind. First, can this issue be addressed using statistical techniques such as MAXCOV-HITMAX (see Lenzenweger & Korfine, Chapter 7, this volume)? Alternatively, can the issue of categories versus dimensions best be addressed by pursuing both approaches (i.e., the clinical approach and the individual difference approach) and assessing which research approach produces the strongest set of findings?

How many dimensions/factors?

An important issue that needs to be addressed concerns the number of factors or dimensions that underlie schizotypal personality, and the implications for our conceptualization of both SPD and schizophrenia. If schizophrenia and SPD are closely linked phenomenologically, factors of SPD should reflect factors of schizophrenia. To date there has been relatively little factorial validity research on SPD, though this is crucial to helping us confirm or reject syndrome models of SPD.

"Schizophrenias" and "schizotypes"

Given that we often refer to the "schizophrenias," should we also talk about the "schizotypes"? We do this in part by referring to positive and negative schizotypal processes, but to what extent is this dichotomy overly simplistic? Is it more accurate to talk about cognitive–perceptual and interpersonal deficit subtypes of SPD? Whereas the paranoid–nonparanoid division is frequently made in schizophrenia research, this has not to date been applied to SPD research.

Family history of SPD

The question of whether SPD with a family history of schizophrenia differs from SPD without such a history is a potentially very important one, but to date there has been very little research on this issue (although see Condray & Steinhauer, 1992). Important questions that need to be addressed in this area are: (1) Are there major phenomenological differences in terms of presenting symptoms between these two groups? (2) Are there fundamentally different mechanisms underlying these two SPD "types"? (3) Do these differences reflect those found in schizophrenics with and without a family history of schizophrenia?

Psychosis proneness versus schizotypal personality

In what ways does the concept of self-report psychosis-proneness map onto concepts of self-report and clinical schizotypal personality? There is a tendency in the literature to assume that research on psychosis proneness is of automatic relevance to SPD research, but to what extent are these only partially overlapping processes? For example, some psychosis proneness scales such as Psychoticism, Physical Anhedonia, Social Anhedonia, and Schizoidia do not directly reflect schizotypal features, at least as defined by DSM-III-R and DSM-IV. Whereas on the one hand findings from research on such scales may be of less relevance to SPD as defined in DSM-III-R, on the other hand they may yield valuable information on ways in which such psychiatric definitions of SPD may require extension and revision.

Mechanisms and etiology

Same or different causal mechanisms?

There is an assumption that mechanisms underlying individual differences in schizotypal personality are the same ones underlying schizophrenic symptomatology and that therefore such research yields important insights into schizophrenia. Is this assumption justified? Although schizotypal features appear to reflect milder versions of schizophrenic symptoms, this does not guarantee that the causes of schizophrenia are an exaggeration of the dysfunctional mechanisms that cause SPD. Just as there can be many different causes of what ostensibly presents as the same symptom (e.g., cough, which may be caused by smoking, food lodging in throat, anxiety and nervous habits, air pollution, infection of mucous membranes of nose/throat, inflammation of bronchial tubes via a viral infection), so too may very different mechanisms underlie, for example, thought disorder in schizophrenia and its analogue in SPD, odd speech. Is it even possible that further understanding of the mechanisms underlying SPD actually misinforms us about processes involved in schizophrenia?

Protective factors

We currently know very little about what factors may protect against the development of schizophrenia. Can an elaboration of the differences between SPD and schizophrenia give us important leads into understanding what these factors may be? Presumably, schizotypals who do not go on to develop schizophrenia may possess some characteristic that shields them from a full breakdown (although it is also possible that they lack an important risk factor, such as birth complications). Conversely, do differences between schizophrenics and SPDs merely indicate that SPD is not really a good model for understanding schizophrenia?

SPD as the basic disorder

The extensive amount of research conducted on schizophrenia leads one to assume that schizophrenia is obviously the fundamental disorder that needs to be explained, but is this assumption really justified? May not SPD instead represent the fundamental disorder, with schizophrenia arising as a complication of this more fundamental process through the presence of some additional risk factor? If the latter is true, what factors, when present in schizotypals, lead to eventual breakdown for schizophrenia?

Single or multiple vulnerability factors?

Although there is growing evidence for multiple vulnerability factors for SPD, several authors conceptualize SPD as the product of one fundamental vulnerability factor (e.g., Grove et al., 1991). Although there may be a number of identifiable etiological mechanisms underlying SPD (e.g., eye tracking abnormalities, sustained attention deficits, negative priming), these deficits may be interrelated rather than independent, thus reflecting the operation of a relatively unitary dysfunction. Research needs to go beyond the establishment of individual correlates and move toward a more integrative framework for understanding SPD.

New processes or neurodegenerative processes?

We need to know more about the way in which SPDs eventually break down for schizophrenia. Are there discrete new processes that come to act as triggers that transform a schizotypal into a schizophrenic (e.g., psychosocial stress or a new physiological process) and that are additional to some other more static predisposition? Alternatively, does schizophrenia largely develop with the passage of time, allowing an existing neurodegenerative process to develop fully? The latter scenario might suggest that SPD is merely the clinical manifestation of some midpoint in this slowly evolving process and that the rate and extent to which the neurodegenerative process develops determine whether a schizotypal eventually is transformed into a schizophrenic.

Is schizophrenia a good model for understanding SPD?

There are probably many causes of schizophrenia, just as there are many causes of mental retardation. If we use mental retardation as an analogy, we might consider that having a borderline IQ of 75 is to mental retardation (IQ below 70) as SPD is to schizophrenia. Just as there are many relatively discrete causes of mental retardation, there may be many more (normal as well as pathological) processes that play a role in determining borderline IQ. By analogy, there may be many more processes that play a role in determining SPD which we never assess because our strategy in SPD research is invariably to take a correlate of schizophrenia and see if it is found in SPD. If such a correlate successfully extrapolates from schizophrenia to SPD, we take this to support the notion that it is a true vulnerability factor for schizophrenia. But if not, we often argue for methodological/conceptual problems (e.g., small *N* or inappropriateness of SPD as a model for schizophrenia) as explanations for null findings. This approach, however, may lead to a misunderstanding of SPD, because SPD may in reality be a broader clinical concept than schizophrenia, involving many more processes and mechanisms. If understanding schizophrenia requires a full understanding of SPD, and if researchers never step outside schizophrenia research to select alternative potentially relevant processes to help explain SPD, will we inevitably fail to understand schizophrenia fully? One question therefore concerns whether there are any other alternative models to schizophrenia that we can utilize to help study SPD. In this context, research on more "normal" personality processes related to SPD traits may provide one important lead.

Mechanisms and etiology

Clinical versus individual difference approach

Perhaps the clearest differentiator among researchers of schizotypal personality concerns whether a clinical or an individual difference approach is taken. This bifurcation is paralleled by a preference for the use of either (1) psychiatric diagnostic instruments to assess clinical manifestations of SPD or (2) more psychologically based self-report questionnaires to assess degrees of schizotypy. An obvious question concerns which approach is more likely in the long term to result in greater advances in our understanding of SPD. Alternatively, will the greatest advances be made by a combination of these two approaches? Currently there are very few empirical data that can help address this issue. This is important, because it is likely to be the first and most fundamental question to which any new researcher in this area requires an answer.

Cause–effect relationships

Teasing out causality is one of the major challenges for the next generation of SPD research. The conceptual issue concerns the fact that although it is not explicitly stated, we tend to make assumptions of causality in interpreting findings from SPD research; for example, if cognitive deficits are found in schizotypals, it is implicitly assumed that such deficits are in some way causally related to SPD. Yet are schizotypal symptoms a result of the proposed pathophysiological process, or is the pathological process caused by the symptoms? For example, does poor or inappropriate resource allocation (e.g., as indexed by the P300 event-related potential or the skin conductance orienting response) result in unusual perceptual experiences, or do perceptual aberrations interfere with resource allocation and produce the observed attentional deficits? Alternatively, is a reiterative process involved whereby both causal processes make up a deleterious feedback loop, exacerbation of which may result in perceptual aberrations being upgraded to hallucinations? One way of teasing out such cause–effect relationships may be by looking at a subgroup that possesses the deficit in question and then showing that members of the subgroup can be differentiated in meaningful ways from those without the deficit on an unrelated variable/process (e.g., family history of schizophrenia, being winter-born, possession of minor physical anomalies) that cannot easily be viewed as an artifact of the symptomatology in question (e.g., unusual perceptual experiences). Such a pattern of results would lend support to the notion that the deficit is a meaningful one and is not purely an artifact of the symptoms it correlates with. A second alternative is to make use of the longitudinal prospective design in the hope of demonstrating that the deficit in question precedes the onset of the symptoms.

Comorbidity

The issue of comorbidity has not seriously impinged on published research on SPD to date. The reason is probably that the state of such research is largely still at the initial level of establishing correlates of SPD. Nevertheless, future research – that is, both clinical research and individual difference research – needs to deal seriously with the issue of the potential confound of comorbidity. Affective disturbance is common among clinical schizotypals, and we have recently found in our own research on community schizotypals that alcohol abuse, drug use, and antisocial behavior are common in SPDs within the community. Consequently, we need to establish that correlates of SPD that we believe are of etiological significance are independent of coexisting psychiatric conditions. On the other hand, there is a danger that researchers will correct for comorbid conditions, such as depression, that may turn out to be an essential, core feature of SPD. The pressing conceptual question therefore concerns how future research should best ride between these competing concerns.

The importance of normal personality processes

Do we have to turn much more to understanding normal processes in order to understand pathological processes? For example, in order to understand more fully what it means for SPDs to show abnormalities in brain structure and function, we need to map in greater detail just exactly what constitutes "normal" brain processes in order to both define and understand deviations from normality. Just as we use SPD as a tool to understand schizophrenia, do we also have to understand normal personality processes in order fully to understand SPD symptomatology, and in turn schizophrenia? This process is not the same as researching individual differences in schizotypy in the normal population; rather, it refers to understanding normals who have no discernible schizotypal tendencies. For example, what are the normal processes that shape appropriate levels of social anxiety and suspiciousness?

Hospital versus community approaches

Clinical studies of SPD recruit subjects from a hospital sample; or alternatively (and less frequently), they are recruited from the community and have not previously been hospitalized. It is possible that these two sampling approaches may yield fundamentally different patterns of findings, as such populations differ in important ways. Both approaches have advantages and disadvantages. The advantage of hospital samples is that they represent relatively severe clinical cases; a potential disadvantage is that the reason for hospitalization means that subjects are likely to have a coexisting major disorder that complicates the clinical picture. The advantage of community schizotypals is that they have not been hospitalized and may be less likely to have a serious coexisting condition (though this advantage is probably more relative than absolute); the disadvantage may be that social dysfunction may be less serious, and hence it may be more difficult to establish the correlates of this relatively weaker clinical manifestation of SPD.

Expected effect sizes

Current research is largely concerned with the statistical significance of a finding, however, given the difficulty in obtaining large samples of schizotypals, the size of the effect obtained may be a more meaningful guide to assessing the "significance" of findings. This in turn raises the question, What effect sizes should one expect? One might expect stronger effect sizes in SPDs than in schizophrenics because there are no or fewer drug/institutional contaminants with SPDs. Alternatively, should one perhaps expect weaker effect sizes because SPD is a weaker version of schizophrenia? Then again, some findings for SPD may not have a parallel in schizophrenia. A related issue is that we tend to ignore or not report null findings for schizotypy; but are these findings of potential importance in indicating the presence of a protective factor against the development of schizophrenia?

Appropriate control groups

Current research, encapsulating both clinical and individual difference approaches, tends not to use control groups, which raises a problem of establishing specificity of the purported deficit for schizotypy. This is a serious problem that requires resolution, yet the resolution involves using control groups, and this in turn raises the question as to which control groups are appropriate for SPD. Such control groups in clinical research may include borderline personality disorder, which has been closely associated with SPD; or an Axis II disorder that is unrelated to schizophrenia spectrum disorders, such as self-defeating personality disorder. Alternatively, should affectives or alcoholics be used to help address the issue of comorbidity? With respect to individual difference research, should questionnaire measures of depression or borderline personality be employed?

An issue even more problematic is, How can a true "normal" control group be delineated? Cleansing such normal groups of all pathology may be unrealistic and may represent a Holy Grail that cannot in reality be attained. Cleansing "normal" control groups of schizotypal tendencies in clinical studies also precludes the possibility of relating dependent variables to such tendencies within the control group in addition to making the usual SPD–control comparison. Perhaps a stronger approach would be to allow for wide variability in schizotypal tendencies in a nonhospitalized control group and therefore allow for both individual difference and clinical approaches to be employed in the same study.

Do reciprocal methodologies result in the same conclusions?

Do symmetrical methodological approaches converge on the same answers for SPD? Some methodologies are reciprocal in nature. That is, to answer the question of whether there is a genetic link between SPD and schizophrenia, one can assess rates of SPD in the offspring of schizophrenics or, conversely, assess rates of schizophrenia spectrum disorders in relatives of SPDs. A second example of a reciprocal methodological approach would be research on biological vulnerability factors: One can assess rates of biological dysfunction in SPDs, or one can define subject groups in terms of presence/absence of a biological marker and assess rates of SPD in these groups. To date, these methodologies have resulted in findings that are not necessarily convergent (see, e.g., Ingraham, Chapter 2, this volume). The key conceptual questions here concern how any discrepancies should be interpreted, what the theoretical implications are, and which is the preferred approach for the two.

Clinical issues

Treatment of schizotypals

Should we treat individuals with SPD? On the one hand, schizotypals have symptoms that can interfere with optimal psychosocial functioning and can reduce the quality of their lives. On the other hand, they do not seek out treatment, probably do not view themselves as disturbed or in need of help, and may instead learn to value their eccentricity, oddities, and unusual experiences as individuality and insight. Schulz, Schulz, and Wilson (1988) among others have argued for treatment of schizotypals and have reviewed data from four studies showing the effectiveness of low dosages of neuroleptic medication in the treatment of schizotypals, particularly those with more positive schizotypal features. Others, such as Claridge and Beech (Chapter 9, this volume), would argue against such an approach and would instead emphasize the positive and creative features that some believe are associated with schizotypy. However, if some schizotypals self-medicate using alcohol and drugs, would more structured treatment allow such individuals to lead a more fulfilling and fully functioning life?

Symptom continuity

One question that has received very little attention to date concerns whether there is significant continuity between symptoms of SPD prior to schizophrenia breakdown and later symptoms of schizophrenia. For example, do schizotypals with predominantly cognitive–perceptual deficits develop into schizophrenics with predominantly positive symptoms? If there is symptom continuity, then studying schizotypal symptoms would be of clear importance in understanding schizophrenic symptomatology. Alternatively, if there is significant discontinuity in symptom development, this would clearly question whether SPD represents a good model for understanding schizophrenia.

Is self-report schizotypy predictive for schizophrenia?

Individual difference research using scales purporting to measure schizotypy rests on the assumption that these scales do genuinely measure schizotypal personality. One critical test of this assumption concerns whether high schizotypy scorers do manifest psychosis and schizophrenia. Furthermore, is there specificity for progression to schizophrenia as opposed to disorders such as depression or anxiety states? Alternatively, are such scales predictive of psychosis per se? To date the only long-term follow-up study (Chapman & Chapman, 1992) provides some initial support for the predictive validity of a number of psychosis proneness scales (though not of physical anhedonia). Clearly this is a critically important area that requires further attention.

The following chapters

To gain a complete understanding of schizotypal personality disorder, we need to understand SPD in its historical context; its relationship to schizophrenia in a developmental context; its manifestation in the general population; the genetic, neural, biochemical, psychophysiological, neuropsychological, and cognitive processes that mediate this disorder; and the implications of this research for biological diathesis–stress models of schizophrenia. The following chapters attempt to provide some of this essential empirical background; they also address some of the key theoretical and conceptual issues surrounding this work and make recommendations for further research.

It must inevitably be acknowledged that these chapters cannot address all of the issues raised above. Indeed, some chapters may not address any of these issues adequately, because the focus is on establishing empirical correlates at this early stage of research on schizotypy. Furthermore, this introduction has not attempted to provide answers or solutions to the conceptual, theoretical, and methodological issues raised. It is hoped, however, that with some of these issues formally stated, researchers will be more cognizant of them and will attempt to design their schizotypy research in ways that will result in genuine progress.

References

Braff, D. L., Siever, L., Freedman, R., Raine, A., Tsuang, M., Mohs, R., & Goldberg, T. (1992). Defining the boundaries of schizophrenia. *American College of Neuropsychopharmacology: Abstracts of Panels and Posters,* 44.

Chapman, J. P., & Chapman, L. J. (1992, November). *Follow-up of psychosis-prone subjects.* Paper presented at the Seventh Annual Meeting of the Society for Research in Psychopathology, Chicago.

Condray, R., & Steinhauer, S. (1992). Schizotypal personality disorder in individuals with and without schizophrenic relatives: Similarities and contrasts in neurocognitive and clinical functioning. *Schizophrenia Research, 7,* 33–41.

Grove, W. M., Lebow, B. S., Clementz, B. A., Cerri, A., Medus, C., & Iacono, W. G. (1991). Familial prevalence and coaggregation of schizotypy indicators: A multitrait family study. *Journal of Abnormal Psychology, 100,* 115–121.

Schulz, S. C., Schulz, P. M., & Wilson, W. H. (1988). Medication treatment of schizotypal personality disorder. *Journal of Personality Assessment, 2,* 1–13.

PART II
Genetics and neurodevelopment

2

Family–genetic research and schizotypal personality

LORING J. INGRAHAM

The nonpsychotic schizophrenia-like syndrome that has come to be called schizotypal personality disorder (SPD) existed before DSM-IV (American Psychiatric Association, 1993), before Meehl's classic presidential address on schizotaxia, schizotypy, and schizophrenia to the American Psychological Association in 1962 (Meehl, 1962), before the original *Diagnostic and Statistical Manual* of the American Psychiatric Association (1952). This chapter attempts to give the reader a sense of the origins of the SPD diagnosis, the course of its development as a nosological entity, and where it stands today. The role of family–genetic studies in defining SPD and its relationship to schizophrenia is emphasized throughout.

The chapter begins with a brief historical overview of early descriptions of nonpsychotic schizophrenia-like syndromes and notes that familiality has been associated with these syndromes since their initial description. Next, more recent empirical family–genetic approaches that have led to the development of the current diagnostic criteria for SPD in DSM-IV are reviewed. The chapter concludes with the results from a recent analysis of the present diagnostic criteria as an example of one approach to the continuing development of reliable and valid descriptors of SPD and suggests other contributions that future family and genetic studies may offer.

Historical background

Schizophrenia and nonpsychotic schizophrenia-like syndromes

The history of SPD begins with the history of schizophrenia. Eugen Bleuler, in his initial description of schizophrenic illness, broadened Kraepelin's construct of dementia praecox to include what Bleuler termed latent schizophrenia (*latente schizophrenie;* Bleuler, 1911), a less severe, nonpsychotic presentation of schizophrenia. Bleuler characterized latent schizophrenia as having in a nutshell all the symptoms of schizophrenia:

> There is also a latent schizophrenia, and I am convinced that this is the most frequent form, although admittedly these people hardly ever come for treatment. It is not necessary to give a detailed description of the various manifestations of latent schizophrenia. In this form, we can see *in nuce* all the symptoms and all the combinations of symptoms which are present in the manifest types of the disease. Irritable, odd, moody, withdrawn or exaggeratedly punctual people arouse, among other things, the suspicion of being schizophrenic. Often one discovers a concealed catatonic or paranoid symptom and exacerbations occurring in later life demonstrate that every form of the disease may take a latent course. (Bleuler, 1911/1950, p. 239)

Further characterization of latent schizophrenia by Bleuler described it as a disorder exhibiting schizophrenic symptoms within normal limits:

> Latent schizophrenias are very common under all conditions so that the "disease" schizophrenia has to be a much more extensive term than the pronounced psychosis of the same name. This is important for studies of heredity. At what stage of anomaly any one should be designated as only a "schizoid" psychopathic, or as a schizophrenic mentally diseased, cannot at all be decided as yet. At all events, the name latent schizophrenia will always make one think of a morbid psychopathic state, in which the schizoid peculiarities are within normal limits. (Bleuler, 1924, p. 437)

As is evident, Bleuler suggested that schizophrenia might be considered from a dimensional perspective. Elsewhere (Bleuler, 1911/1950, p. 13) he emphasized that latent schizophrenia was observed much more frequently than more severe schizophrenic illness.

The observation of a range of severity of symptoms in schizophrenia did not establish that similar symptoms reflected similar underlying etiologies for mild and severe cases. Empirical evidence that latent schizophrenia might share a common etiology with more severe schizophrenia was Bleuler's observation of a familial link between latent and chronic schizophrenia (Bleuler, 1911/1950, pp. 238–239; 1924, p. 441).

A familial, nonpsychotic syndrome in the relatives of schizophrenic individuals was also noted by Bleuler's contemporaries. Rosanoff (1911, p. 234) described the relatives of patients with dementia praecox as "cranky, stubborn; worries over nothing; religious crank, nervous, queer; restless, has phobias; suspicious of friends and relatives." Kretschmer (1925) published illustrative pedigrees demonstrating the occurrence of schizophrenia-like symptoms among the family members of schizophrenic individuals, and described in some detail the characteristics of what he called a schizoid temperament observed among some of the relatives of these patients.

During the 1930s, Kallman (1938) conducted a systematic investigation of the relatives of schizophrenic patients and described two types of schizoid personality (borderline cases and schizoid psychopaths) he observed in the families of schizophrenic patients. Both personality types had symptoms similar to those of their schizophrenic relatives; both were nonpsychotic.

Investigators noted nonpsychotic, not necessarily familial, variants of schizophrenic psychopathology. Zilboorg (1941) coined the term "ambulatory schizophrenia" to describe patients characterized by schizophrenia-like autistic thinking and absence of intimate relationships. Deutsch (1942) described the "as-if personality," characterized by lack of affective connection to work or others and by a lack of personal identity. She believed that the as-if personality was related to schizophrenia, based on the similarity of the symptoms to early symptoms of schizophrenia, and on family history, which indicated that many of her as-if personality patients had schizophrenic or psychotic relatives. Hoch and Polatin (1949) coined the term "pseudoneurotic schizophrenia" to describe their superficially neurotic patients who on closer examination revealed evidence of schizophrenia-like symptoms, particularly brief psychotic episodes. Family studies continued with the systematic investigation of twins by Slater (1953), in which paranoid traits, eccentricities, lack of feeling, reserve, and anergy were more common among the relatives of schizophrenic patients than among controls.

Initial definition of schizotypal

The coining of the term "schizotypal" for a familial nonpsychotic schizophrenia-like syndrome was the work of Rado (1953), who abbreviated the term "schizophrenic phenotype" to "schizotype," and intended it to be the description of the observable symptoms of an individual's inherited disposition to schizophrenia before (if ever) a psychosis developed. Rado proposed that schizotypal individuals suffered from an integrative pleasure deficiency, an absence of experienced pleasure that led to a deficient motivational strength and an inability to organize purposive action. From this fundamental deficiency arose the symptoms of anhedonia, fearfulness, and disorganization, exacerbation of which led to the more severe symptoms of frank schizophrenia.

Although Rado made the initial use of the term "schizotypal," Meehl's (1962, 1989) description, theoretical rationale, and development of a program of research marked the beginning of the modern study of schizotypal disorders. Meehl proposed that an integrative neural defect, which he named "schizotaxia," is inherited by some family members of schizophrenic individuals, and that the various forms of schizophrenic illness result from subsequent environmental influences interacting with this deficit.

The publication of the DSM-II (American Psychiatric Association, 1968) may have helped to further empirical work on schizophrenia-related syndromes by explicitly recognizing a nonpsychotic schizophrenia-like illness as a subtype of schizophrenia. DSM-II schizophrenia, latent type, was described as having clear symptoms of schizophrenia but no history of a psychotic episode.

Several research programs with varying perspectives were initiated in the following decades to investigate the psychopathological syndromes associated with schizophrenia and their relationship with each other (e.g., Tsuang, Kendler, & Gruenberg, 1985). The present chapter focuses on the adoptee family approach; other chapters will discuss the development of other approaches. Readers interested in a more detailed overview of the history of schizotypal personality and approaches to its study are referred to Shields, Heston, and Gottesman (1975), Kendler (1985), Ingraham and Kety (1988), or Siever, Kalus, and Keefe (1993); the early history of the development of the concept of dementia praecox is well described by Wender (1963).

Family–genetic studies and diagnostic criteria

The Danish–American adoption studies of schizophrenia

The Danish–American adoption studies of schizophrenia (Kety et al., 1968, 1975, 1994) are characterized by blind, controlled, empirical investigation of psychopathology. Starting in 1963, Kety, Rosenthal, Schulsinger, Wender, and their colleagues have used a series of adoption designs to investigate the role of genetic factors in schizophrenia and other forms of psychopathology and have demonstrated that heritable genetic factors account for the observed familiality of chronic schizophrenia.

One of the original goals of this series of studies was to elucidate which (if any) of the syndromes associated with chronic schizophrenia in the then current classification systems (ICD-7, 8: World Health Organization, 1957, 1967–1969; DSM-I, II: American Psychiatric Association, 1952, 1968) were observed more frequently among the biological relatives of schizophrenic adoptees than among the biological relatives of control adoptees.

The Copenhagen and Provincial adoptees' family studies were designed to separate the effect of shared genetic material from that of shared family environment in the genesis of schizophrenia. Five aspects of the study design helped achieve this:

1. All Danish adoptions from 1924 to 1947 (N = 14,427) were screened to identify schizophrenic adoptees; this avoided the potential problem of using subsamples that might have had selection biases. The population was divided into two samples (the city of Copenhagen sample and the Provincial, or rest of Denmark, sample), which allowed independent replication.
2. Interviews and diagnoses were made blindly without knowledge of a subject's index, control, adoptive, or biological relative status.
3. The prevalence of illness among the biological relatives of ill adoptees was compared with the prevalence among the biological relatives of well controls. This controlled design corrects for bias that would be present if prevalence were compared with adoptive relatives (adopting families may be different from parents giving up children for adoption) or with nonadoptive control families (adoptees' biological families may be different from nonadoptees' families).
4. The families of schizophrenic adoptees were studied, not the adopted children of schizophrenic parents. Bias in placement due to adoption agencies' knowledge of parental illness was thus removed as a potential artifact, as were potential complications arising from assortative mating of ill parents.
5. This design allows for the comparison of the prevalence of illness in adoptive relatives of index and control probands in order to evaluate the effect of family environment on adoptees' illness.

In brief, index probands were selected from the total register of Danish adoptees by identifying those adoptees with a history of hospitalization for a mental illness and selecting those with evidence from hospital records of chronic schizophrenia, latent schizophrenia, or acute schizophrenia. Control adoptees were selected from the pool of adoptees with no history of mental hospitalization to match index adoptees on age, gender, social class of the adopting parents, and time spent with the biological mother. Biological and adoptive relatives of the index and control adoptee probands were identified through adoption court records and population registers, and the national psychiatric register was consulted to identify those relatives who had ever been hospitalized. Subsequently, living relatives were personally interviewed, and diagnoses were made based on the interview and hospital records, if any. The interviews of the index and control probands made it possible to screen the control probands more carefully. In order to qualify as a control, the putative control probands must have been interviewed and found to be free of significant psychopathology. Further methodological details of the adoptees' family approach taken with the Copenhagen and Provincial samples are given in the original reports (Kety et al., 1968, 1975, 1994).

The schizophrenia spectrum

Results from the Copenhagen sample of the Danish–American adoption studies provided empirical support for the presence of a nonpsychotic schizophrenia-like disorder – latent schizophrenia – among the biological relatives of schizophrenic individuals. Further, since the increased prevalence of latent schizophrenia was observed among biological relatives who had not shared a family environment with the schizophrenic adoptee, the presence of illness could be attributed to shared genes, rather than a shared environment.

Chronic schizophrenia was observed more frequently among the biological relatives of chronic schizophrenic adoptees (5.6%) than among the biological relatives of control adoptees (0.9%). The nonpsychotic schizophrenia-like syndrome of latent schizophrenia was significantly concentrated among the biological relatives of the schizophrenic adoptees (14.8%), more than twice the prevalence of chronic schizophrenia in these relatives; latent schizophrenia was observed in only 0.9% of the biological relatives of controls. These results confirmed empirically E. Bleuler's description of a more common, but less severe, schizophrenia-like illness among the relatives of schizophrenic patients, and the adoption methodology used permits the conclusion that the excess of illness seen among biological relatives of schizophrenic probands was due to the influence of genes rather than family environment. On the other hand, schizoid personality was not seen in excess among the biological relatives of schizophrenic adoptees, indicating that this syndrome may not have a genetic basis in common with chronic schizophrenia, and that the expression of liability to schizophrenia-like illness may not be a continuous distribution from normalcy through psychosis.

In the initial report of the Copenhagen sample, Kety et al. (1968, p. 353) conceptually defined the schizophrenia spectrum as ranging from inadequate personality to chronic schizophrenia based on the qualitative similarities in the features that characterize them. The empirical findings, however, primarily supported commonality between chronic and latent schizophrenia and provided little support for including schizoid personality in the spectrum of syndromes genetically related to schizophrenia. As the initial report was based on hospital records alone, and as the less severe syndromes might be unlikely to have required hospitalization, subsequent interviews were expected to be informative. Results from the interview study in Copenhagen (Kety et al., 1975) confirmed the hospital results, with the diagnoses of chronic and latent schizophrenia making up an empirically defined schizophrenia spectrum. The diagnoses in the Copenhagen sample were based on the consensus of three judges. One judge individually found a significant excess of schizoid personality among the biological relatives of index probands (Rosenthal, 1975, p. 21), raising the possibility that there may be a weak association between chronic schizophrenia and schizoid personality.

The development of diagnostic criteria for SPD

As part of the development of empirically based diagnostic criteria for DSM-III (American Psychiatric Association, 1980), Spitzer, Endicott, and Gibbon (1979) worked toward developing an operational definition of the nonpsychotic schizophrenia-like syndrome demonstrated to be related to chronic schizophrenia in the Danish–American adoption studies. "Schizotypal personality was chosen ... since the term means 'like schizophrenia' " (Spitzer et al., 1979, p. 18).

To help develop diagnostic criteria, Spitzer et al. evaluated a mixed subsample of 36 cases from the Copenhagen sample with diagnoses of schizoid personality, latent schizophrenia, and cases where the diagnosis had been based on limited information; these cases represented both biological and adoptive relatives of both index and control adoptees. As part of the process of developing diagnostic criteria, Spitzer et al. developed a set of items that were relatively sensitive and specific to the 36 schizoid, latent, and uncertain cases when compared with 43 noncases. These items were then cross-validated and psychometrically evaluated after being rated by a sample of 808 members of the American Psychiatric Association as to how well they described patients with schizophrenia-like illness seen in their practices compared with control patients without psychosis or a borderline condition.

The final item set for schizotypal personality contained eight items. In descending order of their ability to separate schizotypal patients from control patients in the sample of American Psychiatric Association members' ratings, they are (Spitzer et al., 1979, p. 18):

1. Odd communication
2. Inadequate rapport in face-to-face interaction
3. Magical thinking
4. Ideas of reference
5. Suspiciousness
6. Recurrent illusions
7. Social isolation
8. Undue social anxiety or hypersensitivity to criticism

The diagnosis of SPD by DSM-III criteria required the presence of four of these items in individuals who do not meet the DSM-III criteria for schizophrenia. When the DSM-III SPD criteria were blindly applied to the interviews of the Copenhagen sample (Kendler, Gruenberg & Strauss, 1981b), SPD was significantly concentrated among the biological relatives of schizophrenic adoptees, independently replicating the original findings (Kety et al., 1975) from that sample.

Although based on interviews from the Copenhagen sample, the DSM-III items were not based exclusively on interviews of the biological relatives of schizophrenic index adoptees, but on a mixed group of biological and adoptive relatives. The criterion group also included individuals with a diagnosis of schizoid personality, which did not appear to be genetically linked to schizophrenia in the Copenhagen sample. These criteria, based on a mixed group of diagnoses and various family relationships, may be limited in what they reveal about the familiality of the disorder they describe or its relationship to chronic schizophrenia.

In a study designed to focus specifically on the characteristics of the familial nonpsychotic schizophrenia-like illness observed in the family members of schizophrenic individuals and its relationship to schizophrenia and borderline personality disorder, Gunderson, Siever, and Spaulding (1983) reanalyzed the interviews of the Copenhagen sample. The authors' analyses of specific symptoms led to the suggestion that brief psychotic experiences be deemphasized in the diagnosis of SPD and that somatization and social role dysfunction were more typical of these individuals.

DSM-III-R (American Psychiatric Association, 1987) revised the diagnostic criteria for SPD by adding a criterion for odd or eccentric behavior, and by requiring five of the now nine criteria to make a diagnosis of SPD. More recently, the DSM-IV (American Psychiatric Association, 1993) retained the nine criteria of DSM-III-R SPD with relatively minor modifications and with a reordering of the sequence of their listing; mood disorders with psychotic features and psychotic disorders were added as exclusionary diagnoses.

Recent family–genetic studies of the schizophrenia spectrum and SPD

Over the past two decades a growing body of empirical studies investigating SPD has developed and is reflected in the other chapters of the present volume. Here, the focus will be specifically on recent family–genetic studies, excluding those dimensional family–genetic studies covered elsewhere.

Following the development of DSM-III, Kendler and his colleagues applied the newly developed criteria to material from the Copenhagen sample of the Danish–American adoption study of schizophrenia to investigate which

DSM-III diagnoses selectively clustered among the biological relatives of the schizophrenic index adoptees (Kendler, Gruenberg, & Strauss, 1981a–c, 1982a,b; Kendler & Gruenberg, 1984). Using DSM-III criteria, they found SPD in 10.5% of the biological relatives of schizophrenic probands versus 1.3% of other relatives; comparison with the corresponding rates of Kety et al. (1975) – 15.9% and 4.9% – suggested that the DSM-III criteria for SPD had a greater specificity but less sensitivity. In addition to SPD, Kendler and his colleagues' reanalysis of the Copenhagen sample found a genetic link between schizophrenia and paranoid personality disorder. No such links were found between schizophrenia and anxiety disorders, paranoid psychosis, or affective disorder. This pattern of results led to Kendler and colleagues' conclusion that the empirically demonstrated schizophrenia spectrum consists of DSM-III schizophrenia, SPD, and paranoid personality disorder. Support for SPD as a discrete disorder rather than a prodromal or residual phase of chronic schizophrenia was provided by McGlashan's (1986) follow-up study of SPD which described the stability of the long-term course of SPD.

Other samples and analyses have provided evidence for familial relatedness between schizophrenia and SPD. For example, Lowing, Mirsky, and Pereira (1983) applied DSM-III diagnostic criteria to the adopted-away children of 39 matched pairs of schizophrenic and control parents, and found SPD in 6 (15.4%) of the adopted-away children of schizophrenic parents in comparison with 3 (7.7%) adopted-away children of control parents. Baron and colleagues' family study of schizophrenia (Baron et al., 1983, 1985) found schizotypal personality in 14.6% of the first-degree relatives of chronic schizophrenic probands, a rate close to that found by previous investigators. Although the Baron et al. study was conducted in a nonadoptee sample and thus cannot rule out the operation of nongenetic factors in familial risk for SPD, the similarity of the rate to that found in adoptee designs suggests that nongenetic familial factors may play a relatively minor role in the observed familiality of SPD.

Several investigators have found a lower risk of schizotypal personality in the relatives of schizophrenic probands than reported in the above studies, but still at an excess compared with the prevalence in the biological relatives of controls. Prevalence estimates are subject to variability due to uninterviewed relatives, particularly in the case of SPD, where the social withdrawal characteristic of the disorder may make identification and evaluation of SPD difficult. Kendler et al. (1984) employed a family history design using information from a family member judged to be the most knowledgeable about the family to evaluate the presence of SPD in the families of schizophrenic patients. The authors did not discriminate schizoid personality from schizotypal personality, but used a combined schizoid–schizotypal diagnostic category. Schizoid–schizotypal personality was observed at a morbid risk of 4.2% in the relatives of the schizophrenic probands, compared with no such diagnoses among the relatives of controls. Frangos et al. (1985) examined the first-degree relatives of 116 schizophrenic patients and found schizophrenia-related personality disorders at a morbid risk of 5.2%, compared with 1.7% in controls. Gershon et al. (1988) found potential schizophrenia-spectrum disorders (schizotypal, schizoid, paranoid, borderline personality disorder) in 3.1% of the first-degree relatives of 24 chronic schizophrenic probands, and in none of the relatives of control probands. Onstad et al. (1991) interviewed the parents and siblings of ill twins, 59 with schizophrenia, 20 with mood disorders, and 9 with nonaffective psychoses. Schizotypal personality disorder was found exclusively in the relatives of the probands with schizophrenia at a rate of 7.4%.

In addition to an increased risk of SPD in the families of schizophrenic individuals, significantly increased risk for schizophrenia and SPD in the family members of schizotypal individuals has also been reported. Battaglia et al. (1991) observed a morbid risk for schizophrenia of 4.6% among the first-degree relatives of 21 SPD patients, compared with 1.1% and 0.6% in relatives of psychiatric and medical controls. Thaker et al. (1993) reported an increased risk for schizophrenia, schizophrenia-related personality disorders, and unspecified functional psychoses in the families of subjects meeting criteria for schizophrenia-related personality disorders in the absence of any Axis I diagnosis. Siever and colleagues (1990) have provided evidence for increased risk of schizophrenia-related disorders in the relatives of clinically diagnosed SPD patients, indicating a specific familial association between schizophrenia-related personality disorders and SPD; the observed morbid risk for schizotypal or paranoid personality disorder in the relatives of probands with SPD was 17.9%.

Questions in the relationship between schizophrenia and SPD

Not all investigators have reported an increased prevalence of SPD in the families of schizophrenic individuals, and not all investigators have found SPD to be specific to schizophrenia. Controversy continues over the boundaries of hypothesized components of a schizophrenia spectrum, whether such a spectrum is dimensional or dichotomous (and if dimensional, whether uni- or multidimensional).

In particular, Coryell and Zimmermann (1988, 1989) failed to find an excess of SPD among the relatives of schizophrenic probands when compared with controls; likewise, chronic schizophrenia was not found in excess among the relatives of schizophrenic probands. Relatives were blindly diagnosed following personal or telephone interviews using the Structured Interview for DSM-III Personality Disorders (Stangl et al., 1985); results were not substantially changed when restricted to relatives with a personal interview (Coryell & Zimmerman, 1989, p. 498). Specifically, the age-adjusted morbid risk of SPD was 2.8% among the relatives of schizophrenic probands, and 1.9%, 5.3%, and 2.5% among the relatives of major depression (psychotic), schizoaffective disorder (depressed), and never ill probands, respectively. Coryell and Zimmerman suggest that the dissimilarity between their findings and that of other authors may be due to differing proportions of familial and nonfamilial forms of psychopathology between samples.

The set of DSM-III personality disorders that should be included in the schizophrenia spectrum continues to be investigated. Dorfman, Shields, and DeLisi (1993) examined the frequency of DSM-III-R personality disorders in the parents of 58 patients with a first admission for a schizophrenia-like psychosis, contrasted with 65 control families. Schizoid (31%), histrionic (12%), schizotypal (6%), and sadistic (5%) personality disorder were observed more frequently in the parents of patients when compared with control families (14%, 3%, 0%, 0% respectively); paranoid personality disorder was observed in 10% of both index and control families. In contrast, Fulton and Winokur's (1993) study of hospitalized patients with schizoid and paranoid personality disorder did not observe an excess of schizophrenia in the families of probands with schizoid personality, with only 2.6% of relatives so affected.

Specificity of SPD

Some investigators have raised concerns over whether SPD, as it is presently defined, is specific to schizophrenia. Squires-Wheeler and her colleagues (1988, 1989) have reported that the children of individuals with affective disorder have a significantly elevated likelihood of meeting SPD diagnostic criteria; the observation of elevated risk for latent schizophrenia in the biological relatives of adoptees with affective disorders has also been reported (Ingraham & Kety, 1988; Kety et al., 1994).

The studies of Silverman et al. (1993) and Yeung et al. (1993) have added to the evidence for limits in the specificity of DSM-III SPD to schizophrenia. Silverman et al. assessed the risk for schizophrenia-related and affective personality disorder traits in the first-degree relatives of 55 chronic schizophrenic and 67 personality disorder probands with either or both SPD or borderline personality disorder. Whereas SPD (where no comorbidity with borderline personality disorder was observed) was concentrated among the relatives of probands with schizophrenia (12.3% of relatives) or SPD alone (9.6% of relatives), SPD was also found among the relatives of individuals with borderline personality disorder (3.9%) or both schizotypal and borderline personality disorder (5.6%). In the study of Yeung et al., the prevalence of DSM-III personality disorders assessed through a self-report questionnaire were not found to differ among the relatives of 194 schizophrenic, bipolar, depressed, and atypical psychosis probands. In particular, the age-adjusted prevalence for SPD was 6.0% among the relatives of schizophrenic probands, and 9.1%, 8.3%, and 12.5% among the relatives of bipolar, depressed, and atypical psychosis probands respectively.

Confirmation of a familial–genetic link between schizophrenia and SPD

The Roscommon family study

Despite negative reports of the range and dimensionality of schizophrenia-like psychopathology observed in some of the family members of individuals with schizophrenia, the central observation of an increased risk for SPD in the families of individuals with schizophrenia is well supported.

The Roscommon family study of Kendler and colleagues (1993) used a case-controlled epidemiological family study design to investigate the familial relationship between schizotypal, paranoid, schizoid, avoidant, and borderline personality disorders and schizophrenia, other nonaffective psychoses, and affective illness. Personal interviews of 1,753 first-degree relatives of 303 schizophrenic probands, 99 affective disorder probands, and 150 controls were conducted blindly. Schizotypal personality disorder was observed five times more frequently among the relatives of schizophrenic probands than among the relatives of controls, with lifetime prevalences of 6.9% and 1.4%, respectively. The increased prevalence of SPD was specific to the relatives of probands with schizophrenia, SPD (prevalence 5.0%), and other nonaffective psychoses (prevalence 3.9%); no excess was observed among the relatives of probands with psychotic or nonpsychotic affective illness probands (prevalence 2.5%, 2.3%). Paranoid, schizoid, and avoidant personality disorder occurred at low rates among the relatives of schizophrenic probands (1.4%, 1.0%, 2.1% respective prevalences), but occurred at even lower rates among control relatives (0.4%, 0.2%, 0.2% respective prevalences), suggesting that these disorders may have a familial relationship with schizophrenia.

Kendler had previously predicted (Kendler, 1986) that if SPD represents a mild form of schizophrenia, then the rate of SPD might be expected to be higher in parents of schizophrenic probands than in siblings or offspring, since SPD in a parent might be associated with high familial liability to schizophrenia but less impairment of reproductive capacity. In the Roscommon family study (Kendler et al., 1993), SPD or paranoid personality disorder was observed in 13.9% of the parents of schizophrenic probands, but in only 6.8% of siblings, suggesting the operation of fitness effects in the transmission of schizophrenia and SPD.

The Provincial sample of the Danish–American adoption studies

Following the publication of results from the Copenhagen sample of the Danish–American adoption studies, Kety and his colleagues proceeded with a replication in order to test the generality of the original results. The replication was conducted in the provinces outside of Denmark following the procedures of the original study, and has become known as the Provincial sample.

Results from the Provincial sample are described in detail elsewhere (Kety et al., 1994); results relevant to SPD are presented here. Kety et al. retained the use of the diagnosis of latent schizophrenia rather than SPD, as the latent schizophrenia diagnosis had been more sensitive than DSM-III in the previous Copenhagen study, and in order to integrate the results of the Provincial sample with the Copenhagen sample. A diagnosis of latent schizophrenia was made where social withdrawal, affective flattening, changes in the form of thought and speech, or delusional (including paranoid) tendencies characteristic of chronic schizophrenia were present in the absence of frank delusions or other psychotic symptoms.

The results of the Provincial sample were similar to the findings of the Copenhagen sample. Latent schizophrenia was observed primarily among the biological relatives of the chronic schizophrenic index probands (8.2% of biological index relatives vs. 2.5% in biological control relatives), and occurred more frequently among these relatives than chronic schizophrenia (4.7%). As in the Copenhagen sample, schizoid personality did not discriminate between the biological relatives of schizophrenic probands and the biological relatives of controls. The replication of the original findings in a separate sample provides strong support for the association between latent and chronic schizophrenia; that these results were observed in a blind adoptees' relative design is evidence that the observed association is mediated through genetic means.

It is possible to pool the results of the two samples to give an overall picture of the risk for schizophrenia and related illnesses in the biological relatives of schizophrenic adoptees in Denmark. There is a highly significant concentration of schizophrenia (5.0% vs. 0.4% in controls) and latent schizophrenia (10.8% vs. 1.7% in controls) among the biological relatives of chronic schizophrenic adoptees. An excess of schizoid personality in the biological relatives of chronic schizophrenic adoptees was not observed.

In addition to the global diagnoses made by the original investigators (Kety et al., 1994), interviews from the Provincial sample were reviewed and given DSM-III diagnoses by Kendler and his colleagues (Kendler et al., 1994). When combined with the DSM-III diagnoses from the Copenhagen sample (Kendler et al., 1981b) to make a National sample, SPD was observed in 7.3% of the biological relatives of schizophrenic adoptees, and in 2.3% of the biological relatives of control adoptees ($p <.01$). Kendler's analysis of the risk of SPD in the relatives of adoptee probands diagnosed with either schizophrenia or SPD indicates a higher risk for SPD among the biological relatives of probands with SPD, suggesting that the genetic vulnerability to schizotypal traits may in part be transmitted independently of the risk to schizophrenia. Both the Kety et al. (1994) and the Kendler et al. (1994) reports provide further discussion of the results of the Danish–American adoption studies, and the interested reader is referred to them.

Investigation of the heritable components of SPD

Seeking the heritable components of SPD

Given substantial evidence of a heritable liability for a nonpsychotic schizophrenia-like disorder in the relatives of schizophrenic individuals, several investigators have applied family–genetic designs to attempt to define more precisely the manifestations of the transmitted liability.

Analysis of material from the interviews in the Copenhagen sample of the Danish–American Adoption Studies by Kendler et al. (1982b) provided empirical investigation of individual characteristics observed in the biological relatives of schizophrenic individuals using a design that avoided the effects of nongenetic familial influences. Relatives' descriptions of themselves as children indicated that the biological relatives of schizophrenic adoptees were more likely to characterize themselves as having been withdrawn or antisocial (but not more anxious) than were the relatives of controls, and that the biological relatives of schizophrenic adoptees who reported childhood social withdrawal were at high risk as adults to develop a schizophrenia spectrum disorder.

The Norwegian twin study

Analysis of individual symptoms of the Present State Examination (PSE; Wing, Cooper, & Sartorius, 1974) by Torgersen (1984) in a study of twins with SPD indicated that genetic factors were important in the transmission of SPD, and that the heritable aspects of SPD measured by the PSE consisted primarily of paranoid-like (ideas of reference) and schizoid (social anxiety) features, but not psychotic-like cognitive or perceptual distortions. Torgersen also noted that the risk of SPD was considerably higher than the risk of schizophrenia in the co-twins of twins with SPD, such that an increased risk for schizophrenia was not observed in his sample.

More recently, Torgersen and his colleagues have conducted a twin study investigating personality disorders among the co-twins and other first-degree biological relatives of twin probands with either schizophrenia or major depression (Torgersen et al., 1993). Schizotypal personality disorder was more common among the biological relatives of schizophrenic probands, and further analysis of the SPD criteria indicated that odd speech, inappropriate affect, odd behavior, and excessive social anxiety were significantly more common among the relatives of schizophrenic probands. The prevalences of these criteria were similar in monozygotic co-twins, dizygotic co-twins, and other first-degree relatives, supporting the role of both genetic and nongenetic factors in their development.

Continuing investigation of the specific liabilities observed in the families of schizophrenic individuals has been conducted by Pogue-Geile and his colleagues in a series of analyses of the siblings of schizophrenic patients and controls. As in Torgersen's study, the siblings of schizophrenic probands had little evidence of psychotic-like traits (Huxley et al., 1993), and showed impaired social functioning (Brunke et al., 1991). Additionally, Pogue-Geile et al. have reported observing increased thought disorder in response to proverbs (see Hall et al., 1991), but no differences in negative symptoms (Crown et al., in press) among the siblings of schizophrenic patients.

Support for the interpretation that the impaired social functioning observed by investigators in some of the relatives of schizophrenic individuals may be related to genetic factors rather than family environment is provided by the finding of increased self-reported social withdrawal in the biological relatives of schizophrenic adoptees when compared with the biological relatives of controls (Ingraham, 1993).

Prevalence of SPD criteria in the biological relatives of schizophrenic adoptees

In addition to approaches that survey a range of behaviors and symptoms to characterize the heritable components of SPD, it is possible to focus on the present set of diagnostic criteria and investigate to what extent individual criteria are more frequently observed in the biological relatives of schizophrenic probands in comparison with controls. This approach can suggest which of the criteria are most strongly associated with a familial liability to schizophrenia, and, in the case of twin and adoption designs, which criteria are associated with genetic material shared with a schizophrenic proband.

Methods

The present analysis was based on interviews conducted as part of the investigation of the Provincial sample of the Danish–American adoption studies; the basic methods have been briefly described earlier in this report. Blinded interviewers completed a rating form covering the interviewees' report of physical and mental health in childhood through adulthood, and the interviewers' rating of observed physical, cognitive, emotional, and social functioning. In all, over 500 individual items were rated and further supplemented by a narrative description of the interview.

These items were reviewed to select those which reflect each of the nine criteria for DSM-IV SPD. For most of the criteria, several items were closely related to one another and to the criterion, so that an initial set of 38 potentially useful items was identified.

For this and subsequent analyses, the group of control probands was screened to eliminate control probands with a psychotic illness or with latent schizophrenia. Relatives with chronic schizophrenia were also eliminated from the present analyses, as more cases of schizophrenia (and thus more schizophrenia-like symptoms) had been observed in the relatives of the index probands, and the present focus was on relatives with milder, if any, illness.

Items from the interviews of the biological relatives of index probands were compared with interviews of biological relatives of controls using the nonparametric Mann–Whitney U statistic (SPSS Inc., 1988). Probability was evaluated from a one-tailed perspective, since an excess of SPD criteria was expected only in the biological relatives of schizophrenic probands. As there might be considerable covariance among items attempting to measure the same SPD criteria, and as there is in addition potential covariance among the set of SPD criteria, a strict Bonferroni adjustment for multiple comparisons was not applied. Rather, a moderate approach of increasing alpha to .01 (.05/5) to reflect five (or fewer) potentially separate domains being assessed was followed; this may be overly conservative if there were considerable covariance among criteria, and overly liberal if the items chosen to measure each criteria were poorly correlated.

Results

Three items were observed with a significantly greater frequency among the relatives of schizophrenic probands (Tables 2.1–2.3): suspicion, flat or spotty affectivity, and seclusive/withdrawn behavior. These results are consistent with those of Torgersen (1984, Torgersen et al., 1993) and Pogue-Geile's group (Brunke et al., 1991; Huxley et al., 1993), and suggest that suspiciousness and social withdrawal may be more frequently observed among the non-schizophrenic relatives of individuals with schizophrenia, but that psychotic-like phenomena are not. The failure to find evidence of an increased prevalence of additional criteria for SPD suggests that the current criteria may not be optimal in defining a genetically transmitted schizophrenia-like syndrome observed in some relatives of schizophrenic individuals.

The present results are limited in that they rely on analysis of items not specifically designed to assess DSM-IV criteria for SPD. Nevertheless, the findings are consistent with and support the findings of other investigators, and they extend them to an adoptee design where nongenetic familial influence is unlikely to play a significant role. The lack of observed differences for some criteria in the present study may be due either to inadequate assessment or to a real absence of differences. A final concern is that the present analyses are based on the assumption that SPD and schizophrenia are not in some cases independent disorders with independent transmission; if so, it would be inappropriate to screen our controls for SPD but not our schizophrenic probands (Kendler, 1990).

Discussion

The body of family–genetic research in schizophrenia provides considerable empirical evidence for the presence of a nonpsychotic syndrome characterized by milder forms of the symptoms of chronic schizophrenia in some of the biological relatives of schizophrenic individuals, a syndrome described in DSM-IV as SPD.

Considerable work remains to be done in the validation of SPD as a diagnostic category. While the boundary between schizophrenia and SPD seems relatively firm (with psychotic features as the main determinant), the boundaries between SPD and schizoid or paranoid personality disorders are less clear. Whether boundaries are even appropriate is actively being investigated; perhaps a dimensional model may be more appropriate. If so, the number and name of the dimensions remain to be completely specified.

Is SPD a personality orientation rather than a disorder? Investigators more

Table 2.1. *Interviewer's rating of suspicion (observed among the non-schizophrenic relatives of adoptees with chronic schizophrenia and of control adoptees free of major mental illness)*

Relative groups	Not present at all	Slightly present	Definitely present	Total relatives
Biological rels. of 29 adoptees with chronic schizophrenia	94 83%	4 4%	15 13%	113
Biological rels. of 24 control adoptees	74 96%		3 4%	77
Adoptive rels. of 29 adoptees with chronic schizophrenia	30 97%		1 3%	31
Adoptive rels. of 24 control adoptees	19 95%	1 5%		20

Note: Mann–Whitney U 1-tailed p biological index vs. control = .0035.

Table 2.2. *Interviewer's rating of flat or spotty affectivity (observed among the nonschizophrenic relatives of adoptees with chronic schizophrenia and of control adoptees free of major mental illness)*

Relative groups	Absent	Slight or doubtful	Confident is present	Total relatives
Biological rels. of 29 adoptees with chronic schizophrenia	103 87%	3 2%	13 11%	119
Biological rels. of 24 control adoptees	81 98%		2 2%	83
Adoptive rels. of 29 adoptees with chronic schizophrenia	31 97%		1 3%	32
Adoptive rels. of 24 control adoptees	18 86%		3 14%	21

Note: Mann–Whitney U 1-tailed p biological index vs. control = .0036.

comfortable with categories than dimensions question how dimensions may have reliable age of onset and gender distribution without underlying categorical mechanisms. As dimensions multiply, a simple genetic model of schizophrenia and related illness becomes more difficult to hold to.

Table 2.3. *Interviewer's rating of seclusive/withdrawn behavior (observed among the nonschizophrenic relatives of adoptees with chronic schizophrenia and of control adoptees free of major mental illness)*

Relative groups	Absent	Slight or doubtful	Clearly present	Total relatives
Biological rels. of 29 adoptees with chronic schizophrenia	92 78%	20 17%	6 5%	118
Biological rels. of 24 control adoptees	76 91%	7 8%	1 1%	84
Adoptive rels. of 29 adoptees with chronic schizophrenia	31 97%	1 3%		32
Adoptive rels. of 24 control adoptees	17 81%	4 19%		21

Note: Mann–Whitney U 1-tailed *p* biological index vs. control = .0089.

The nature of the specificity of SPD to schizophrenia also remains under discussion. This raises the question of the independence of SPD from schizophrenia, such that SPD may be a risk factor for schizophrenia, but independently heritable. Is SPD necessary for schizophrenia?

Despite the remaining questions, some interim conclusions seem possible:

1. There is increased risk for more than chronic schizophrenia in some relatives of individuals with schizophrenia.
2. Although broader than chronic schizophrenia, that risk is more narrow than for psychopathology in general.
3. That risk is for something more common than chronic schizophrenia.
4. That risk has an empirically demonstrated genetic basis.
5. There is evidence for social withdrawal and suspiciousness as components of that increased risk, and less evidence for psychotic-like experiences.

In general, based on the results from ongoing family–genetic studies of schizophrenia, it appears that there is a genetically based syndrome characterized by social withdrawal, suspiciousness, and restricted affect in a fraction of the biological relatives of individuals with chronic schizophrenia that is more common than schizophrenia itself in these relatives. We still have much to learn about how schizotypy is the same as schizophrenia, and how it is different.

Acknowledgments

I would like to acknowledge Dr. Seymour Kety and the Institute of Preventive Medicine, Copenhagen, for help in providing access to the adoption study data analyzed here. I am grateful to Tina Chan and Thalene Mallus, M.A., for their help in carrying out this project, and to Chris Aiken for his comments on the manuscript.

References

American Psychiatric Association. (1952). *Diagnostic and statistical manual of mental disorders.* Washington, D.C.: Author. (Cited as DSM-I).

American Psychiatric Association. (1968). *Diagnostic and statistical manual of mental disorders* (2nd ed.). Washington, DC: Author. (Cited as DSM-II).

American Psychiatric Association. (1980). *Diagnostic and statistical manual of mental disorders* (3rd ed.). Washington DC: Author. (Cited as DSM-III).

American Psychiatric Association. (1987). *Diagnostic and statistical manual of mental disorders* (3rd ed., revised). Washington, D.C.: Author. (Cited as DSM-III-R).

American Psychiatric Association. (1993). *Diagnostic and statistical manual of mental disorders* (4th ed.). Washington DC: Author. (Cited as DSM-IV).

Baron, M., Gruen, R., Asnis, L., & Kane, J. (1983) Familial relatedness of schizophrenia and schizotypal states. *American Journal of Psychiatry, 140,* 1437–1442.

Baron, M., Gruen, R., Rainer, J. D., Kane, J., Asnis, L., & Lord, S. (1985). A family study of schizophrenic and normal control probands: Implications for the spectrum concept of schizophrenia. *American Journal of Psychiatry, 142,* 447–455.

Battaglia, M., Gasperini, M., Sciuto, G., Scherillo, P., Diaferia, G., & Bellodi, L. (1991). Psychiatric disorders in the families of schizotypal subjects. *Schizophrenia Bulletin, 17,* 659–668.

Bleuler, E. (1991). *Dementia praecox, oder Gruppe der Schizophrenien.* Leipzig: Deuticke.

Bleuler, E. (1911/1950). Dementia praecox or the group of schizophrenias (J. Zinkin, trans.). New York: International Universities Press. (Original work published 1911).

Bleuler, E. (1924). *Textbook of psychiatry.* Authorized English edition by A. Brill. New York: Macmillan.

Brunke, J. J., Pogue-Geile, M. F., Garrett, A. H., & Hall, J. K. (1991). Impaired social functioning and schizophrenia: A familial association? *Schizophrenia Research, 4,* 250–251.

Coryell, W. H., & Zimmerman, M. (1988). The heritability of schizophrenia and schizoaffective disorder. A family study. *Archives of General Psychiatry, 45,* 323–327.

Coryell, W. H., & Zimmerman, M. (1989). Personality disorder in the families of depressed, schizophrenic, and never-ill probands. *American Journal of Psychiatry, 146,* 496–502.

Crown, J., Pogue-Geile, M. F., et al. (in press). Liability to schizophrenia: A sibling study of negative symptoms.

Deutsch, H. (1942). Some forms of emotional disturbance and their relationship to schizophrenia. *Psychoanalytic Quarterly, 11,* 310–321.

Dorfman, A., Shields, G., & DeLisi, L E. (1993). DSM-III-R personality disorder in parents of schizophrenic patients. *American Journal of Medical Genetics (Neuropsychiatric Genetics), 48,* 60–62.

Frangos, E., Athanassenas, G., Tsitourides, S., S. Katsanou, N., & Alexandrakou, P. (1985). Prevalence of DSM III schizophrenia among the first-degree relatives of schizophrenic probands. *Acta Psychiatrica Scandinavica, 72,* 382–386.

Fulton, M., & Winokur, G. (1993). A comparative study of paranoid and schizoid personality disorders. *American Journal of Psychiatry, 150,* 1363–1367.

Gershon, E. S., DeLisi, L E., Hamovit, J., Nurnberger, J. I., Jr., Maxwell, M. E., Schreiber, J., Dauphinais, D., Dingman, C. W., 2nd, & Guroff, J. J. (1988). A controlled family study of chronic psychoses: Schizophrenia and schizoaffective disorder. *Archives of General Psychiatry, 45,* 328–336.

Gunderson, J. G., Siever, L. J., & Spaulding, E. (1983). The search for a schizotype. Crossing the border again. *Archives of General Psychiatry, 40,* 15–22.

Hall, J. K., Pogue-Geile, M. F., Garrett, A. H., & Brunke, J. J. (1991). Though disorder in the siblings of schizophrenic patients. *Schizophrenia Research, 4,* 277–278.

Hoch, P. H., & Polatin, P. (1949). Pseudoneurotic forms of schizophrenia. *Psychiatric Quarterly, 23,* 248–276.

Huxley, N. A., Pogue-Geile, M. F., Garrett, A. H., Brunke, J. J., Hall, J. K., & Crown, J. (1993). Is there a familial relationship between psychotic-like symptoms and schizophrenia? *Schizophrenia Research, 9,* 118.

Ingraham, L. J. (1993). Social withdrawal in nonschizophrenic biological relatives of chronic schizophrenic adoptees. *Schizophrenia Research, 9,* 101.

Ingraham, L. J., & Kety, S. S. (1988). Schizophrenia spectrum disorders. In M. T. Tsuang & J. C. Simpson (Eds.), *Handbook of schizophrenia* (Vol. 3, pp. 117–137). Amsterdam: Elsevier.

Kallman, F. J. (1938). *The genetics of schizophrenia.* New York: J. J. Augustin.

Kendler, K. S. (1985). Diagnostic approaches to schizotypal personality disorder: A historical perspective. *Schizophrenia Bulletin, 11,* 538–553.

Kendler, K. S. (1986). Fitness and the risk of illness and 'spectrum disorder' in offspring, parents, and siblings. *Behavior Genetics, 16,* 417–431.

Kendler, K. S. (1990). The super-normal control group in psychiatric genetics: Possible artifactual evidence for coaggregation. *Psychiatric Genetics, 1,* 45–53.

Kendler, K. S., & Gruenberg, A. M. (1984). An independent analysis of the Danish adoption study of schizophrenia. VI. The relationship between psychiatric disorders as defined by DSM-III in the relatives and adoptees. *Archives of General Psychiatry, 41,* 555–564.

Kendler, K. S., Gruenberg, A. M., Jacobsen, B., Kinney, D. K., Jansson, L., & Faber, B. (1994). An independent analysis of the Provincial and National samples of the Danish adoption study of schizophrenia: The pattern of illness, as defined by DSM-III, in adoptees and relatives. *Archives of General Psychiatry, 51,* 456–468.

Kendler, K. S., Gruenberg, A. M., & Strauss, J. S. (1981a). An independent analysis of the Copenhagen sample of the Danish adoption study of schizophrenia. I. The relationship between anxiety disorder and schizophrenia. *Archives of General Psychiatry, 38,* 973–977.

Kendler, K. S., Gruenberg, A. M., & Strauss, J. S. (1981b). An independent analysis of the Copenhagen sample of the Danish adoption study of schizophrenia. II. The relationship between schizotypal personality disorder and schizophrenia. *Archives of General Psychiatry, 38,* 982–984.

Kendler, K. S., Gruenberg, A. M., & Strauss, J. S. (1981c). An independent analysis of the Copenhagen sample of the Danish adoption study of schizophrenia. III. The relationship between paranoid psychosis (delusional disorder) and the schizophrenia spectrum disorders. *Archives of General Psychiatry, 38,* 985–987.

Kendler, K. S., Gruenberg, A. M., & Strauss, J. S. (1982a). An independent analysis of the Copenhagen sample of the Danish adoption study of schizophrenia. IV. The relationship between major depressive disorder and schizophrenia. *Archives of General Psychiatry, 39,* 639–642.

Kendler, K. S., Gruenberg, A. M., & Strauss, J. S. (1982b). An independent analysis of the Copenhagen sample of the Danish adoption study of schizophrenia. V. The relationship between childhood social withdrawal and adult schizophrenia. *Archives of General Psychiatry, 39,* 1257–1261.

Kendler, K. S., Masterson, C. C., Ungaro, R., & Davis, K. L. (1984). A family history study of schizophrenia-related personality disorders. *American Journal of Psychiatry, 141,* 424–427.

Kendler, K. S., McGuire, M., Gruenberg, A. M., O'Hare, A., Spellman, M., & Walsh, D. (1993). The Roscommon Family Study. III. Schizophrenia-related personality disorders in relatives. *Archives of General Psychiatry, 50,* 781–788.

Kety, S. S., Rosenthal, D., Wender, P. H., & Schulsinger, F. (1968). The types and prevalence of mental illness in the biological and adoptive families of adopted schizophrenics. In D. Rosenthal & S. S. Key (Eds.), *The transmission of schizophrenia* (pp. 345–362). Oxford: Pergamon Press. Also in *Journal of Psychiatric Research* 1968; *6*(Suppl.), 345–362.

Kety, S. S., Rosenthal, D., Wender, P. H., Schulsinger, F., & Jacobsen, B. (1975). Mental illness in the biological and adoptive families of adopted individuals who have become schizophrenic: A preliminary report based upon psychiatric interviews. In R. Fieve, D. Rosenthal, & H. Brill (Eds.), *Genetic research in psychiatry* (pp. 147–165). Baltimore & London: The Johns Hopkins University Press.

Kety, S. S., Wender, P. H., Jacobsen, B., Ingraham, L. J., Jansson, L., Faber, B., & Kinney, D. (1994). Mental illness in the biological and adoptive relatives of schizophrenic adoptees: Replication of the Copenhagen study in the rest of Denmark. *Archives of General Psychiatry, 51,* 442–455.

Kretschmer, E. (1925). *Physique and character: An investigation of the nature of constitution and of the theory of temperament,* 2nd ed. (English transl. by WJH Sprott). New York: Harcourt, Brace:

Lowing, P. A., Mirsky, A. F., & Pereira, R. (1983). The inheritance of schizophrenia spectrum disorders: A reanalysis of the Danish adoptee study data. *American Journal of Psychiatry, 140,* 1167–1171.

McGlashan, T. H. (1986). Schizotypal personality disorder; Chestnut Lodge follow-up study: VI. Long term follow-up perspectives. *Archives of General Psychiatry, 43,* 329–334.

Meehl, P. E. (1962). Schizotaxia, schizotypy, schizophrenia. *American Psychologist, 17,* 827–838.

Meehl, P. E. (1989). Schizotaxia revisited. *Archives of General Psychiatry, 46,* 935–944.

Onstad, S., Skre, I., Edvardsen, J., Torgersen, S., & Kringlen, E. (1991). Mental disorders in first-degree relatives of schizophrenics. *Acta Psychiatrica Scandinavica, 83,* 463–467.

Rado, S. (1953). Dynamics and classification of disordered behavior. *American Journal of Psychiatry, 110,* 406–416.

Rosanoff, A. J. (1911). A study of heredity in insanity in light of the Mendelian theory. *American Journal of Insanity, 68,* 211–261.

Rosenthal, D. (1975). The spectrum concept in schizophrenic and manic-depressive disorders. *Research Publications of the Association for Research in Nervous and Mental Disorders, 54,* 19–25.

Shields, J., Heston, L. L., & Gottesman, I. I. (1975). Schizophrenia and the schizoid:

The problem for genetic analysis. In R. Fieve, D. Rosenthal, & H. Brill (Eds.), *Genetic research in psychiatry* (pp. 167–197). Baltimore & London: The Johns Hopkins University Press.
Siever, L. J., Kalus, O. F., & Keefe, R. S. (1993). The boundaries of schizophrenia. *Psychiatric Clinics of North America, 16,* 217–244.
Siever, L. J., Silverman, J. M., Horvath, T. B., Klar, H., Coccaro, E., Keefe, R. S., Pinkham, L., Rinaldi, P., Mohs, R. C., & Davis, K. L. (1990). Increased morbid risk for schizophrenia-related disorders in relatives of schizotypal personality disordered patients. *Archives of General Psychiatry, 47,* 634–640.
Silverman, J. M., Siever, L. J., Horvath, T. B., Coccaro, E. F., Klar, H., Davidson, M., Pinkham, L., Apter, S. H., Mohs, R. C., & Davis, K. L. (1993). Schizophrenia-related and affective personality disorder traits in relatives of probands with schizophrenia and personality disorders. *American Journal of Psychiatry, 150,* 435–442.
Slater, E. (1953). *Psychotic and neurotic illnesses in twins.* London: Her Majesty's Stationery Office.
SPSS Inc. (1988). *SPSS-X User's guide,* 3rd ed. Chicago: Author.
Spitzer, R. L., Endicott, J., & Gibbon, M. (1979). Crossing the border into borderline personality and borderline schizophrenia. *Archives of General Psychiatry, 36,* 17–24.
Squires-Wheeler, E., Skodol, A. E., Bassett, A., & Erlenmeyer-Kimling, L. (1989). DSM-III-R schizotypal personality traits in offspring of schizophrenic disorder, affective disorder, and normal control parents. *Journal of Psychiatric Research, 23,* 229–239.
Squires-Wheeler, E., Skodol, A. E., Friedman, D., & Erlenmeyer-Kimling, L. (1988). The specificity of DSM-III schizotypal personality traits. *Psychological Medicine, 18,* 757–765.
Stangl, D., Pfohl, B., Zimmerman, M., Bowers, W., & Corenthal, C. (1985). A structured interview for the DSM-III personality disorders. A preliminary report. *Archives of General Psychiatry, 42,* 591–596.
Thaker, G., Adami, H., Moran, M., Lahti, A., & Cassady, S. (1993). Psychiatric illnesses in families of subjects with schizophrenia-spectrum personality disorders: High morbidity risks for unspecified functional psychoses and schizophrenia. *American Journal of Psychiatry, 150,* 66–71.
Torgersen, S. (1984). Genetic and nosological aspects of schizotypal and borderline personality disorders. A twin study. *Archives of General Psychiatry, 41,* 546–554.
Torgersen, A., Onstad, S., Skre, I., Edvardsen, J., & Kringlen, E. (1993). "True" schizotypal personality disorder: A study of co-twins and relatives of schizophrenic probands. *American Journal of Psychiatry, 150,* 1661–1667.
Tsuang, M. T., Kendler, K. K., & Gruenberg, A. M. (1985). DSM-III schizophrenia: Is there evidence for familial transmission? *Acta Psychiatrica Scandanavica* [*Suppl. 319*], *71,* 77–83.
Wender, P. (1963). Dementia praecox: The development of the concept. *American Journal of Psychiatry, 119,* 1143–1151.
Wing, J. K., Cooper, J. E., & Sartorius, N. (1974). *Measurement and classification of psychiatric symptoms: An instruction manual for the PSE and CATEGO Program.* Cambridge: Cambridge University Press.
World Health Organization (1957). *Manual of the International Statistical Classification of Diseases, Injuries, and Causes of Death,* 7th revision, Vols. 1 & 2. Geneva: World Health Organization. (Cited as ICD-7).
World Health Organization (1967–9). *Manual of the International Statistical Classifi-*

cation of Diseases, Injuries, and Causes of Death, 8th revision, Vols. 1 & 2. Geneva: World Health Organization. (Cited as ICD-8).

Yeung, A. S., Lyons, M. J., Waternaux, C. M., Faraone, S. V., & Tsuang, M. T. (1993). A family study of self-reported personality traits and DSM-III-R personality disorders. *Psychiatry Research, 48,* 243–255.

Zilboorg, G. (1941). Ambulatory schizophrenia. *Psychiatry, 4,* 149–155.

3

Schizotypal personality disorder characteristics associated with second-trimester disturbance of neural development

RICARDO A. MACHÓN, MATTI O. HUTTUNEN, SARNOFF A. MEDNICK, and JOSÉ LaFOSSE

In this chapter we examine the hypothesis that second-trimester neural developmental disturbance is associated with increased presence of schizotypal personality disorder characteristics, which in turn increases the risk for adult schizophrenia. First, we review the literature on schizophrenia and neurodevelopment and the literature on schizotypal personality disorder (SPD) and neurodevelopment. Second, we report on findings relevant to the abovementioned hypothesis emanating from the Helsinki Influenza Project, which has studied a cohort of individuals exposed in utero to the 1957 type A2/Singapore influenza epidemic (Mednick, Machón, Huttunen, & Bonett, 1988).

Literature review

Schizophrenia and neurodevelopment

Central nervous system deficits were posited to underlie the disorder of schizophrenia since Kraepelin (1919) first formulated the term "dementia praecox." Advances in technology have now provided empirical support of this earlier speculation. There now exists a solid body of evidence that schizophrenia may have as one of its bases an underlying neurodevelopmental etiology (Akbarian et al., 1993a,b; Mednick, Cannon, Barr, & LaFosse, 1991; Mednick, Machón, Huttunen, & Bonett, 1988; Waddington, Torrey, Crow, &

Hirsch, 1991; Weinberger, 1986). Cytoarchitectonic studies have implicated brain areas and processes important in the development of positive schizophrenic symptoms; anatomical disturbances have been reported in the hippocampus and entorhinal cortex (Altshuler, Conrad, Kovelman, & Scheibel, 1987; Arnold, Hyman, Van Hoesen, & Damasio, 1991). Positron emission tomography (PET) and postmortem studies have, on the other hand, implicated brain structures/processes important in the development of negative symptoms; dysfunction and anatomical disturbances have been reported in the dorsolateral prefrontal cortex (Akbarian et al., 1993a,b; Tamminga et al., 1992).

The findings from the above studies, as a whole, have been interpreted as supporting a neurodevelopmental origin of schizophrenia (Machón & Mednick, 1994). Specifically, it has been proposed that at least one form of schizophrenia is due to a disruption of normal brain development during a critical risk period, namely the second trimester. This, in turn, increases the probability that an individual will develop adult schizophrenia. Psychiatric epidemiological studies examining the association between prenatal exposure to influenza and adult schizophrenia have played a major role in defining this critical period of gestation (Mednick, Machón, Huttunen, & Bonett, 1988).

SPD and neurodevelopment

Meehl, in 1962, first proposed a diathesis–stress paradigm to understanding the etiology of schizophrenia. He hypothesized that the disorder has at its basis an inherited neural integrative deficit based on a single gene that caused a prenatal structural aberration. Meehl further suggested that persons with this genotype, which he termed "schizotypy," develop the core traits of "schizophrenia" (cognitive slippage, anhedonia, and interpersonal alienation), which he termed "schizotaxia," over time – triggered by social factors. This basic interactional model has been expanded by subsequent evidence implicating a polygenic model of schizophrenia (Gottesman & Shields, 1973) and the findings of nonsocial factors (such as perinatal complications) which might trigger the underlying schizotypy into schizophrenia (Mednick & Schulsinger, 1968).

In earlier papers we proposed that the basic genetic disorder of the schizophrenia spectrum is expressed as a disruption of neural development during a critical period in the second trimester of gestation. We have also stated that this genetically caused schizophrenogenic neurodevelopmental disruption may be mimicked by a teratogenic agent, such as an influenza infection, disturbing the development of the fetus during the second-trimester critical period (Mednick, Cannon, Barr, & LaFosse, 1991). The phenotypic manifestation of the basic genetic disorder of the "schizophrenia spectrum" consists of characteristics summarized by the diagnosis "schizotypal personality disorder" (SPD). [Schizophrenia is a complication of this basic genetic disorder which is produced by unfortunate environmental circumstances (e.g., perinatal complications and/or unstable early family conditions).]

Hypotheses

From the considerations above, it follows that second-trimester disruption of neural development following a teratogenic event, such as an influenza infection, may increase risk for SPD. In the context of an epidemiological study (the Helsinki Influenza Study) examining the psychiatric sequelae of prenatal influenza exposure in Helsinki, Finland, we have reported that Helsinki residents exposed to the 1957 type A2 influenza epidemic during their second trimester of gestation evidenced a significantly increased risk of adult schizophrenia (Mednick, Machón, Huttunen, & Bonett, 1988). It is conceivable that the influenza may have increased the rate of SPD among those infected during their second trimester of gestation. Our observation of a significant increase in the rate of schizophrenia may be attributable to the increased risk of schizophrenia among individuals with SPD.

In order to provide a test of the influenza–SPD–schizophrenia relationship, we undertook a study utilizing the schizophrenic subjects from the Helsinki Influenza Study. We coded the hospital records of the Index and Control schizophrenics for evidence of SPD symptomatology and hypothesized that those who were exposed to an influenza epidemic in their second trimester of fetal life would evidence an elevated level of SPD characteristics as compared to their controls.

Helsinki influenza study

Research design

The type A2 influenza epidemic lasted from October 8 to November 14, 1957. The index year cohort consisted of (1) all children born in Uusimaa County, which encompasses Greater Helsinki, Finland, (2) from November 15, 1957, to August 14, 1958, and (3) diagnosed schizophrenic (ICD-8 and ICD-9 code: 295) and admitted before the age of 29 years and 10 months as an inpatient to one or more of the eight psychiatric hospitals serving the county of Uusimaa. The controls for the present phase of the study comprised all children (1) born in Uusimaa County (2) from November 15, 1955, to August 14, 1956, and (3) diagnosed schizophrenic and admitted before the age of 29 years and 10 months as an inpatient to one or more of these same eight hospitals. For this study, only subjects with a hospital diagnosis of schizophrenia were included.

There were a total of 71 index schizophrenics born in the three trimesters; we were able to code clinical hospital data for 68 of these (19, 32, and 17 in each of the respective trimesters).

Controls were born November 15, 1955, to August 14, 1956. A review of epidemiological data had revealed that this year was a relatively low influenza period. Since the type A2/Singapore virus appeared for the first time in Europe in the summer and fall of 1957, it is impossible for the controls to have suffered a type A2/Singapore viral infection during their fetal development. There was a total of 90 control schizophrenics born 1955–6; we were able to code clinical hospital data for 80 of these (28, 26, and 26 in each of the respective trimesters).

Control or index hospital records were usually not available because either the patient was currently in the hospital or someone else was examining the patient.

We employed for these analyses information pertaining to psychiatric admissions before the age of 29 years and 10 months. Additional details about the study's design may be found in Mednick, Machón, Huttunen, and Bonett (1988).

Diagnosis

Subjects born in the index or control years were first identified as having a WHO International Classification of Disease (ICD-8 and -9) hospital diagnosis of schizophrenia. The hospital records for those with an ICD diagnosis of schizophrenia were reviewed, and a DSM-III-R (American Psychiatric Association, 1987) diagnosis was made (by coauthor M.O.H.). Information from the hospital records was used to complete the Present State Examination, ninth edition (Wing, Cooper, & Sartorius, 1974) and a modified version of the Personality Disorder Examination (PDE) (Loranger et al., 1984) interview forms, including Andreasen's Scales for the Assessment of Negative and Positive Symptoms (Andreasen, 1982; Andreasen & Olsen, 1982); the coded information from the hospital records forms the data of this paper.

SPD scale score

Items that represent each of the nine DSM-III-R criteria for SPD were selected from the PDE. If any one of the items representing each of the nine criteria for SPD was scored positively, that criterion was given a score of "1." Therefore, SPD scale scores could range from 0 through 9.

Raine et al. (1994) have factor-analyzed the SPD criteria and found three factors – Interpersonal Deficit, Cognitive–Perceptual Deficit, and Disorganized. This same factor structure has been also found by Gruzelier et al. (in press). The nine DSM-III-R criteria for SPD and the items chosen to represent them are presented in Table 3.1. Scores were obtained for each of these factors by summing the scores for the constituent items as follows: Cognitive Perceptual Deficit: SPD items 1, 3, 4, and 9; Interpersonal Deficit: SPD items 2, 6, 8, and 9; and Disorganized: SPD items 5 and 7. The total SPD score was computed by adding SPD items 1–9.

Results

T-tests were performed comparing index and control schizophrenic subjects separately for each of the three trimesters on the total SPD score and the three Raine factor scores. Schizophrenics exposed in trimester 1 or 3 did not differ from their controls on any of the *t*-test comparisons for the total SPD score, or three SPD factor scores. Index trimester-2 schizophrenics were rated as having significantly higher mean scores on the SPD Total Scale [$t(54) = 2.5$, $p < .016$] and Cognitive Perceptual Deficit factor [$t(54) = 2.8$, $p < .008$] as compared to controls. The Interpersonal Deficit factor score differences almost reached significance [$t(54) = 1.93$, $p < .058$]. The effect sizes (*d*) were .66, .77, and .53, respectively. The magnitude of the difference between index trimester-2 schizophrenics and their controls on the Disorganized factor was small ($d = .30$), and the difference was not statistically significant. These results, presented in Figure 3.1, support the research hypothesis.

Post hoc analyses were then performed on the nine individual SPD items in order to ascertain the possible source of the above-mentioned significant results. Trimester-1 and -3 exposed schizophrenics did not differ from their controls on any of the *t*-test comparisons for the nine SPD criteria scores. Index trimester-2 schizophrenics were rated as having significantly higher mean scores on SPD item 7 (Odd speech) [$t(54) = 2.4$, $p < .02$] and SPD item 9 (Suspiciousness or Paranoid ideation) [$t(53) = 3.3$, $p < .002$], as compared to their controls. The effect size for SPD item 7 was .74. The effect size for SPD item 9 was .90, which is greater than the criterion for a large effect size (.80) as defined by Cohen (1988). These results are presented in Figure 3.2. The second-trimester index and control schizophrenics did not significantly differ from each other on individual SPD items 1 through 6, and 8.

Since SPD item 9 (Suspiciousness or Paranoid ideation) loaded on both

Table 3.1. *Composition of DSM-III-R schizotypal personality disorder (SPD) criteria*

SPD 1: Ideas of reference (excluding delusions of reference)
"Reads hidden threatening meanings into benign remarks."

SPD 2: Excessive social anxiety, e.g., extreme discomfort in social situations involving unfamiliar people
"Guarded and secretive."
"Hypervigilant."

SPD 3: Odd beliefs or magical thinking, influencing behavior and inconsistent with subcultural norms e.g., superstitiousness, belief in clairvoyance, telepathy or "sixth sense," "others can feel my feelings"
"Bizarre apparently nondelusional thought content: seems preoccupied with very strange or esoteric subjects, or expresses extremely unusual ideas or opinions about a subject."

SPD 4: Unusual perceptual experiences, e.g., illusions, sensing the presence of a force or person not actually present
"Have you had the feeling recently that things around you were unreal?" (derealization)
"Have you felt yourself unreal, that you were not a person, not in the living world?" (depersonalization)

SPD 5: Odd or eccentric behavior or appearance, e.g., unkempt, usual mannerisms, talks to self
"Dress inappropriate or unusual."
"Unkempt."

SPD 6: No close friends or confidants (or only one) other than first-degree relatives
"Relationships with friends and peers – the patient may have few or no friends and may prefer to spend all of his time isolated."

SPD 7: Odd speech (without loosening of associations or incoherence), e.g., speech that is impoverished, digressive, vague, or inappropriately abstract
"Word approximations (metonyms) – meaning is evident but word usage is unusual or bizarre, because words are used in idiosyncratic or unconventional ways or as approximations of more exact ones."

SPD 8: Inappropriate or constricted affect, e.g., silly, aloof, rarely reciprocates gestures or facial expressions, such as smiles or nods
"Little or no variation in vocal pitch, volume or inflection."
"Unchanging facial expression – the patient's face appears wooden, changes less than expected as emotional content of discourse changes."
"Affective nonresponsivity – the patient fails to smile or laugh when prompted."

SPD 9: Suspiciousness or paranoid ideation
"Suspicious."

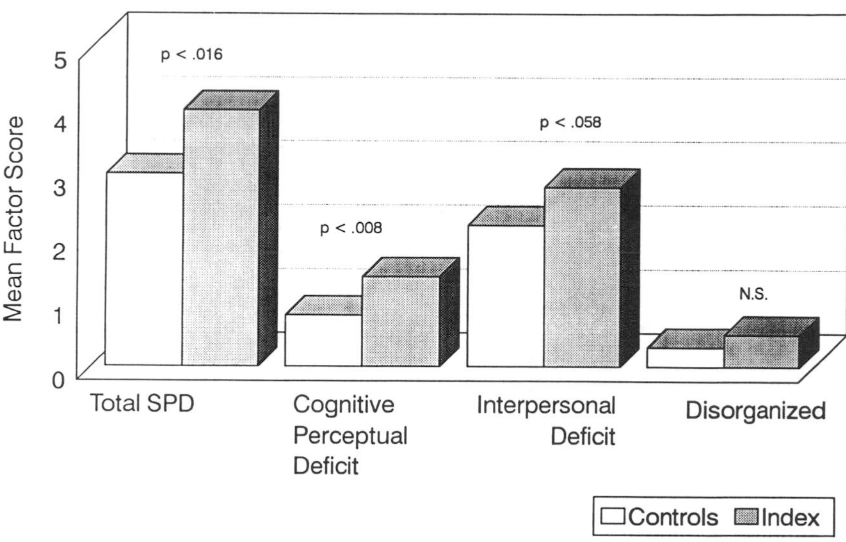

Fig. 3.1. Mean scores on Raine's SPD factors for trimester 2 exposed.

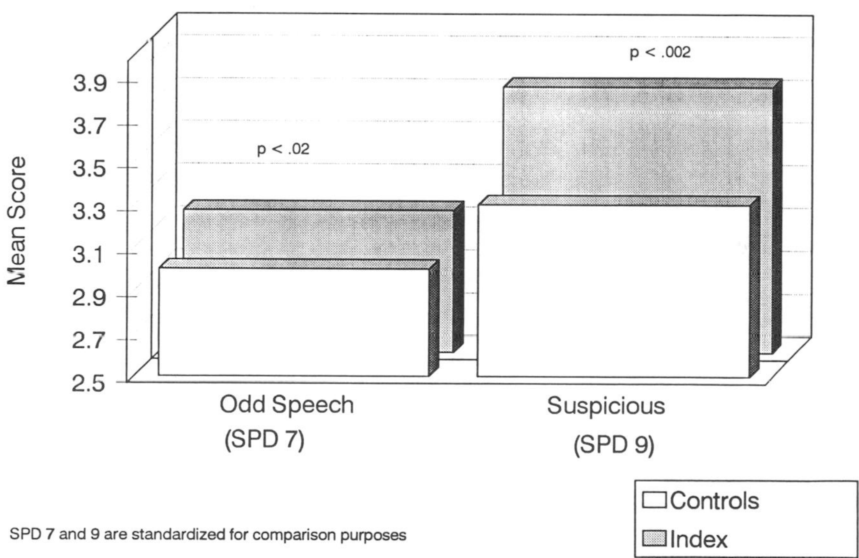

Fig. 3.2. Mean scores on SPD criteria for trimester 2 exposed.

Perceptual Deficit and Interpersonal Deficit factor scores, we explored the possibility that the observed differences between index and controls on these factor scores were due to the impact of this single item. We recomputed the composite scores for both of these factor scores leaving out SPD item 9. The differences between the second-trimester index and control schizophrenics on both factor scores disappeared, suggesting that the observed differences on these two factors are, to a large extent, attributable to the significant elevation of Suspiciousness and Paranoid ideation for the index trimester-2 subjects.

Since no significant differences were observed between trimester-1 and -3 exposed schizophrenics, we decided to group them together and compare this combined group with index second-trimester-exposed schizophrenics. As compared to the index 1 plus 3 combined group, index second-trimester-exposed schizophrenics were not significantly rated higher on Total SPD scale, Cognitive Perceptual Deficit factor, and Disorganized factor, though the means were in the expected direction. The index second-trimester-exposed schizophrenics did have a nonsignificant trend toward higher scores on Interpersonal Deficit factor score [$t(65) = 1.7$, $p < .09$] as compared to index 1 plus 3 combined group. Post-hoc analyses were also performed on the nine individual SPD items. The index second-trimester-exposed schizophrenics had a significantly higher score on SPD item 9 (Suspicious and Paranoid ideation) [$t(64) = 2.4$, $p < .02$] as compared to the index first- and third-trimester group; both groups did not significantly differ from each other on SPD items 1 through 8.

The pattern of the above results supports the hypothesis that second-trimester exposure to influenza increases the risk for SPD symptoms, with a concomitant increase in the risk for later, adult schizophrenia. However, since this study is based on clinical ratings of subjects who were already schizophrenic, it is possible that schizophrenic symptomatology may somehow account for the increased SPD symptom picture that we observe. To control for this possibility, we undertook a series of analyses comparing the index and control second-trimester schizophrenics on the various SPD scales while holding "acute schizophrenic symptomatology" constant. As measures of acute, schizophrenic symptoms, we used the Delusions subscale score from Andreasen's Scale for the Assessment of Positive Symptoms (SAPS) and the SAPS total score (Andreasen & Olsen, 1982). Analyses of covariance were performed using the Delusions subscale score and total SAPS score separately as covariates to test for differences between index and control second-trimester schizophrenics on Total SPD score, Cognitive Perceptual Deficit, Interpersonal Deficit, and SPD items 7 and 9. The results of the ANCOVAs we performed revealed that the differences we had observed between the second-trimester index and controls on the SPD scales remained significant, even when controlling for the effects of schizophrenic positive symptoms. After controlling for the SAPS Delusions subscale score, index second-trimester schizophrenics still had a significantly higher score on SPD total score ($F[1,53] = 11.1$, $p < .002$); Cognitive Perceptual Deficit factor ($F[1,53] = 7.8$, $p < .007$); Interpersonal Deficit factor ($F[1,53] = 5.1$, $p < .03$); Disorganized factor ($F[1,53] = 4.8$, $p < .03$); SPD item 7 (Odd Speech) ($F[1,53] = 5.5$, $p < .02$); and SPD item 9 (Suspiciousness and Paranoid ideation) ($F[1,52] = 9.7$, $p < .003$). Identical results were obtained from the set of ANCOVAs that controlled for total SAPS score.

We then examined the population rates of schizophrenia (per 1,000 live-born) for those index schizophrenics rated as "suspicious" and "not suspicious" by trimester of exposure. These results are presented in Figure 3.3. The reader will note that the population rates of schizophrenia for those rated as "not suspicious" are quite similar across the three trimesters. For those rated as "suspicious," the rate of schizophrenia for those exposed in their second trimester is about 2.5 times as high as those rated suspicious but exposed in trimester 1 or 3. These results suggest that the increase in the rates of schizophrenia among those exposed in the second trimester is accounted for by those rated as "suspicious."

Figure 3.4 presents the number of index schizophrenics rated as "suspicious" distributed by month of exposure. As can be seen, there is a steady increase in the number of schizophrenics rated as "suspicious" who were exposed in months 4, 5, and 6 relative to those exposed in months 1 through 3. The reader will also note that the number of schizophrenics rated as suspicious drops off dramatically after month 6.

Conclusions and synthesis

We have presented evidence that supports the initial, hypothesis-driven set of analyses, suggesting that exposure to the influenza epidemic in the second trimester of gestation produces a disorganization in the brain that is expressed behaviorally as SPD symptoms, especially suspiciousness and paranoid ideation. The neurodevelopmental disruption underlying these SPD symptoms, in turn, increases the risk for later, adult schizophrenic breakdown. The increased risk of schizophrenia for those exposed to the epidemic during their second trimester of neural development is found only among those schizophrenics described as exhibiting "suspiciousness and paranoid ideation" in their psychiatric hospital records.

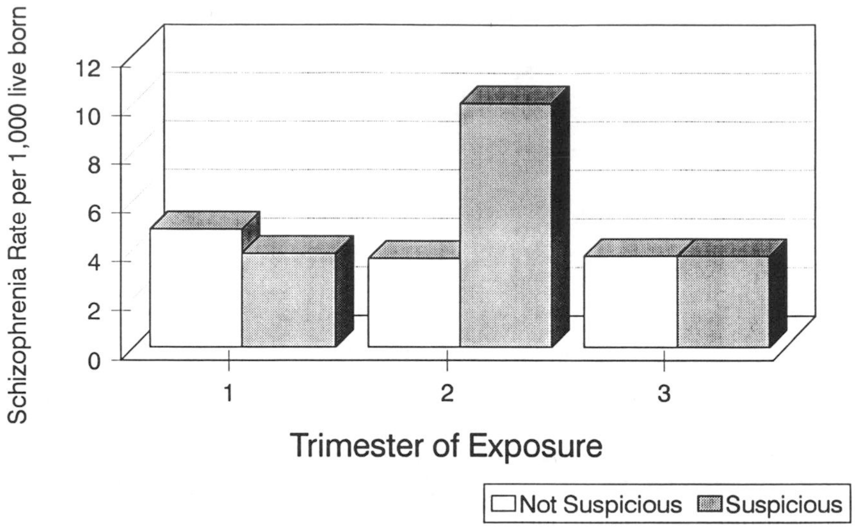

Fig. 3.3. Population-based rates of schizophrenia for index subjects rated as "suspicious" and "not suspicious."

Conceptual issues

While it can be suggested that our significant findings are attributable to the schizophrenic positive symptom profile of our subjects, two important points argue against this possibility. First, the finding that index subjects had significantly more schizotypal symptoms than control subjects – selectively in the second trimester – cannot be solely accounted for by schizophrenic symptoms since *all* the subjects in this study are schizophrenic. Second, the results remained significant even when controlling for positive schizophrenic symptomatology. This finding is not very surprising, given that SPD symptoms reflect more enduring personality characteristics than their parallel schizophrenic symptoms. These results suggest that the pattern of increased SPD symptoms among the second-trimester-exposed schizophrenics remains significant after the effects of the patients' positive symptom picture are statistically removed.

The more specific importance of "suspicious and paranoid ideation" is attested to by the measures of effect size. The effect size for the difference on SPD total score between index trimester-2 schizophrenics and their controls was .66. Suspiciousness or paranoid ideation (SPD item 9) was one of nine items on this scale. The effect size for Raine's Cognitive Perceptual Deficit factor was .76, of which item 9 was one of four constituent items. When item

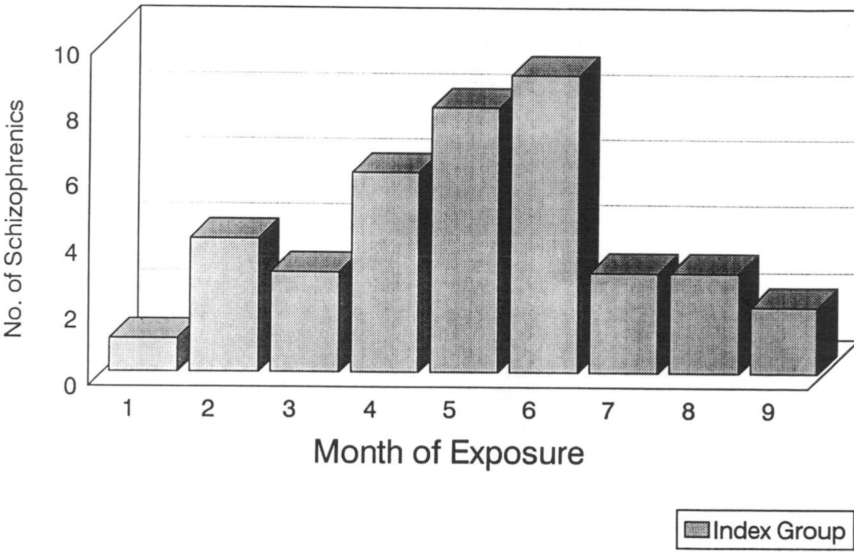

Fig. 3.4. Number of index schizophrenics rated as "suspicious" (by month of exposure).

9 was analyzed by itself, the effect size was .90, greater than Cohen's (1988) criteria for a large effect (.80). Effect size conveys the magnitude of the phenomenon of interest as a standardized mean difference between groups (Cohen, 1988). Ultimately, effect size is more important than statistical significance, and it protects against the inferential invalidity of type I and type II errors.

Directions for future research

These findings of increased SPD symptoms, especially suspiciousness and paranoid ideation, must be interpreted with caution, however. We rated the psychiatric hospital records of adult schizophrenic patients and ascertained their status as to SPD symptoms. Our hypothesis-driven theory of the influenza–SPD–schizophrenia relationship assumes that SPD symptoms *preceded* the onset of schizophrenic symptoms; unfortunately, we are unable to test this assumption. We await independent attempts to replicate these findings in a population that prospectively measures SPD symptomatology before the onset of schizophrenia symptomatology.

As noted above, one limitation of the present study is that we examined SPD characteristics in subjects all of whom were schizophrenic. Another effective way to assess whether influenza infection during the second trimester of fetal life is associated with an elevated level of SPD characteristics would be to study nonschizophrenic subjects that had been exposed to the same influenza epidemic. We are preparing to do this soon.

References

Akbarian, S., Bunney, W. E., Jr., Potkin, S. G., Wigal, S. B., Hagman, J. O., Sandman, C. A., & Jones, E. G. (1993a). Altered distribution of nicotinamide-adenine dinucleotide phosphate-diaphorase cells in frontal lobe of schizophrenics implies disturbances of cortical development. *Archives of General Psychiatry, 50,* 169–177.

Akbarian, S., Vinuela, A., Kim, J. J., Potkin, S. G., Bunney, W. E., Jr., & Jones, E. D. (1993b). Distorted distribution of nicotinamide-adenine dinucleotide phosphate-diaphorase neurons in temporal lobe of schizophrenics implies anomalous cortical development. *Archives of General Psychiatry, 50,* 178–187.

Altshuler, L. L., Conrad, A., Kovelman, J. A., & Scheibel, A. (1987). Hippocampal pyramidal cell orientation in schizophrenia. *Archives of General Psychiatry, 44,* 1094–1098.

American Psychiatric Association. (1987). *Diagnostic and statistical manual of mental disorders* (3rd ed., rev.). Washington, DC: Author.

Andreasen, N. C. (1982). Negative symptoms in schizophrenia: Definition and reliability. *Archives of General Psychiatry, 39,* 784–788.

Andreasen, N. C., & Olsen, S. (1982). Negative vs. positive schizophrenia: Definition and validation. *Archives of General Psychiatry, 39,* 789–794.

Arnold, S. E., Hyman, B. T., Van Hoesen, G. W., & Damasio, A. R. (1991). Some cytoarchitectural abnormalities of the entorhinal cortex in schizophrenia. *Archives of General Psychiatry, 48,* 625–632.

Cohen, J. (1988). *Statistical power analysis for behavioral sciences.* New York: Academic Press.

Gottesman, I. I., & Shields, J. (1973). Genetic theorizing and schizophrenia. *British Journal of Psychiatry, 22,* 15–30.

Gruzelier, J. H., Burgess, A., Stygall, J., Irving, G., & Raine, A. (in press). Hemisphere imbalance and syndromes of schizotypal personality. *Psychiatry Research.*

Kraepelin, E. (1919). *Dementia praecox and paraphrenia.* New York: Robert E. Krieger.

Loranger, A. W., Oldham, J. M., Russakoft, L. M., & Susman, V. L. (1984). *Personality disorder examination: A structured interview for making DSM III axis II diagnoses (PDE).* White Plains, N.Y.: The New York Hospital–Cornell Medical Center.

Machón, R. A., & Mednick, S. A. (1994). Adult schizophrenia and early neurodevelopmental disturbances. *Confrontations Psychiatriques* Paris: Specia Rhône-Poulenc Rorer.

Mednick, S. A., Cannon, T. D., Barr, C. E., & LaFosse, J. M. (Eds.). (1991). *Developmental neuropathology of schizophrenia.* New York: Plenum Press.

Mednick, S. A., Machón, R. A., Huttunen, M. O., & Bonett, D. (1988). Adult schizophrenia following prenatal exposure to an influenza epidemic. *Archives of General Psychiatry, 45,* 189–192.

Mednick, S. A., & Schulsinger, F. (1968). Some premorbid characteristics related to breakdown in children with schizophrenic mothers. In D. Rosenthal & S. Kety (Eds.), *The transmission of schizophrenia.* Oxford: Pergamon Press.

Meehl, P. E. (1962). Schizotaxia, schizotypy, schizophrenia. *American Psychologist, 17,* 827–838.

Raine, A., Reynolds, C., Scerbo, A., & Lencz, T. (1994). Cognitive/perceptual, interpersonal, and disorganized features of schizotypal personality. *Schizophrenia Bulletin, 20,* 191–201.

Tamminga, C. A., Thaker, G. K., Buchanan, R., Kirkpatrick, B., Alphs, L. D., Chase, T. N., & Carpenter, W. T. (1992). Limbic system abnormalities identified in schizophrenia using positron emission tomography with fluorodeoxyglucose and neocortical alterations with deficit syndrome. *Archives of General Psychiatry, 49,* 522–530.

Waddington, J. L., Torry, E. F., Crow, T. J., & Hirsch, S. R. (1991). Schizophrenia, neurodevelopment, and disease: The Fifth Biannual Winter Workshop on Schizophrenia. Badgastein, Austria, January 28 to February 3, 1990. *Archives of General Psychiatry, 48,* 271–273.

Weinberger, D. R. (1986). The pathogenesis of schizophrenia: A neurodevelopmental theory. In H. A. Nasrallah & D. R. Weinberger (Eds.), *The handbook of schizophrenia: The neurology of schizophrenia.* Amsterdam: Elsevier Science.

Wing, J. R., Cooper, J. E., & Sartorius, N. (1974). *The measurement and classification of psychiatric symptoms.* Cambridge: Cambridge University Press.

4

Neurodevelopmental processes in schizophrenia and schizotypal personality disorder

ELAINE F. WALKER and SUSAN GALE

As defined by contemporary diagnostic criteria (DSM-III-R), schizotypal personality disorder (SPD) does not necessarily involve either subjective distress or impairment in occupational/academic functioning. Thus, in contrast to most other psychiatric disorders, the significance of SPD does not primarily lie in its negative consequences for the patient or society. Instead, its importance is due to its presumed association with more severe psychopathology – specifically, schizophrenia.

One prevalent notion, which receives tentative support from the research literature, is that some cases of SPD reflect a partially expressed genotype for schizophrenia (Clementz, Grove, Katsanis, & Iacono, 1991; Kendler, Ochs, Gorman, Hewitt, Ross, & Mirsky, 1991; Meehl, 1989, 1990; Schultz et al., 1986). This assumption raises the questions that are the primary focus of this chapter; namely, what neuropathological process might SPD and schizophrenia share in common, and what triggering mechanism(s) might be responsible for determining whether this constitutional vulnerability is behaviorally expressed in the clinical syndrome of schizophrenia versus SPD? We generate some hypothetical answers to these questions by drawing upon research findings on the developmental course of schizophrenia, as well as on theoretical models of the neuropathology underlying the disorder. Specifically, we explore the manner in which neurodevelopmental processes might interact with exogenous stressors in determining the extent of the behavioral expression of the diathesis.

The link between SPD and schizophrenia

As defined by contemporary diagnostic criteria, the "negative" symptoms of social withdrawal and constricted affect are a prominent feature of the SPD syndrome, and the boundaries are broad for these symptoms, in that they can vary in severity from mild to severe. In contrast, by definition, the ideational and perceptual abnormalities of SPD must not cross the clinical threshold into delusions and hallucinations. Thus, compared with the schizophrenic syndrome, SPD involves more subtle florid or positive symptoms, whereas the negative symptoms of withdrawal and blunting may be as pronounced as those observed in many schizophrenic patients. Consequently, the severity of the positive signs is the primary factor distinguishing between SPD and schizophrenia.

In addition to the overlap between SPD and schizophrenia at the level of phenomenology (Siever, 1985; Siever et al., 1990), there is substantial evidence that SPD is linked with schizophrenia both genetically and developmentally. It has been shown that biological relatives of schizophrenic patients manifest an elevated rate of SPD and related symptoms (Clementz et al., 1991; Kendler et al., 1991; Silverman et al., 1993), even in the absence of shared environmental experiences (Kendler, 1988a; Kety, 1987, 1988). With respect to developmental trajectories, research findings suggest that individuals who meet diagnostic criteria for SPD in young adulthood, or who show some of its symptoms, are at heightened risk for developing schizophrenia (Angst & Clayton, 1986; Fenton & McGlashan, 1989; Kendler, 1985; Mehlum et al., 1991; Peralta, Cuesta, & deLeon, 1991; Wolff, Townshend, McGuire, & Weeks, 1991). Thus, SPD represents the prodromal phase of schizophrenia in some patients. The genetic and developmental links between SPD and schizophrenia strongly suggest that the two disorders share some underlying neuropathological determinants.

However, despite these links, SPD and schizophrenia are clearly separate syndromes, and their partial independence suggests that some features of their underlying neuropathology are not shared in common. Although the evidence is sparse, it appears that many, perhaps most, individuals who manifest SPD are not subsequently diagnosed with schizophrenia (Fenton & McGlashan, 1989). Thus the schizophrenic syndrome is not an inevitable *outcome* of SPD. The question of whether SPD is an inevitable *precursor* of schizophrenia is more difficult to answer. There is certainly evidence that a substantial proportion of schizophrenic patients manifest premorbid behavioral abnormalities, and they appear to worsen as the onset of the illness approaches. Included among these abnormalities are some of the defining symptoms of SPD – social withdrawal and ideational abnormalities (Angst & Clayton, 1986;

Fenton & McGlashan, 1989; Kendler, 1985; Peralta et al., 1991). However, because most studies of premorbid functioning are based on retrospective accounts of behavior that may not be highly reliable, it is impossible to estimate the proportion of schizophrenic patients who would have met diagnostic criteria for SPD in the past. If highly reliable data on the premorbid period were available, we might find that virtually all schizophrenic patients showed SPD prior to meeting diagnostic criteria for schizophrenia. In sum, the available data clearly indicate that SPD is not "sufficient" to predict schizophrenia, although we cannot rule out the possibility that it is a "necessary" or inevitable precursor.

The theoretical significance of the relation between SPD and schizophrenia

Many researchers in the field of psychopathology have viewed SPD as part of the spectrum of schizophrenic disorders, with the implicit assumption that the two represent different points on the continuum of severity and phenotypic expression (Baron & Risch, 1987; Clementz, Cerri, Medus, & Iacono, 1991; Kendler et al., 1991; Kety, 1988; Meehl, 1989). Thus, some have assumed that individuals with SPD possess an unexpressed, or partially expressed, genotype for schizophrenia. Further, some assume that the genotype is not expressed owing to the absence of sufficient environmental stressors; only when such stressors exceed a critical threshold do they serve to trigger a first episode of schizophrenia.

Support for the assumption of unexpressed genetic liabilities for schizophrenia comes from two primary sources: studies of monozygotic (MZ) twins and studies of the biological offspring of MZ twins. Averaging across studies, the concordance rate for schizophrenia in MZ twins is about 50% (Gottesman, 1991), and some recent reports suggest that the most accurate MZ concordance rate may be under 30% (Torrey, 1992; Walker, Downey, & Caspi, 1991). Given that members of MZ twin pairs are presumed to be genetically identical, these data suggest that there is a high rate of unexpressed genotypes. Of course, this conclusion rests on the assumption that hereditary factors are primary in the etiology of schizophrenia. Further, it leads to the prediction that the biological offspring of both affected and unaffected members of the discordant MZ pairs will show elevated, and comparable, rates of schizophrenia. Although the findings of two studies are consistent with this prediction (Fischer, 1971; Gottesman & Bertelsen, 1989), one research group found no elevation in the rate of schizophrenia for offspring of unaffected co-twins of schizophrenics (Kringlen & Cramer, 1989).

The notion of unexpressed genetic liabilities for schizophrenia is an appealing one; however, it should be kept in mind that at the present time there is no overwhelming evidence to support its validity. For example, it is possible that the affected twin in discordant MZ pairs acquired, rather than inherited, a constitutional vulnerability for schizophrenia. Obstetrical complications are a likely candidate in such an etiologic process (Cannon, Barr, & Mednick, 1991; Schulsinger et al., 1984). In this case, the unaffected co-twin would not possess a genotype for schizophrenia. Alternatively, there is evidence that abnormalities in the differentiation of the two zygotes, or mutations that occur in only one zygote, can result in MZ pairs in which the two members are *not* genetically identical (Porreco, 1990; MacGillivray, Nylander, & Corney, 1975). Thus, vulnerability to schizophrenia could be genetically determined, yet not hereditary, in the affected co-twin.

If we follow this line of thinking, we might assume that environmental stressors are irrelevant to the expression of the genotype for schizophrenia. Patients who manifest SPD that does not lead to schizophrenia may possess a different genotype or acquired constitution, compared to SPD patients who develop schizophrenia. In other words, the neurodevelopmental process(es) that lead to both SPD and schizophrenia may be relatively fixed, such that the ultimate phenotypic outcome is preordained to unfold in a specific manner by nature of the individual's constitution. For some patients, SPD may be a transitional period in the constitutionally determined developmental trajectory leading to schizophrenia. For others, SPD may be the clinical endpoint of the trajectory.

However, the demonstrated familial and developmental links between SPD and schizophrenia suggest that the two share at least some determinants in common. For purposes of the present discussion, therefore, we make the assumption that at least some cases of SPD reflect a nonexpressed liability for schizophrenia. More specifically, we assume that vulnerability to schizophrenia will be expressed as SPD when biopsychosocial stressors do not exceed a critical threshold. In the next section, we briefly explore the developmental aspects of dysfunction in schizophrenia and SPD.

The developmental course of schizophrenia and SPD

As previously mentioned, the primary goal of this chapter is to offer some speculations on the neuropathological substrate that gives rise to both SPD and schizophrenia, and the process by which the transition from SPD to schizophrenia might be triggered. In addressing the first issue, we begin by examining the developmental phenomenology of schizophrenia and SPD. Although our knowledge of the developmental precursors of SPD is relatively limited, the available data suggest that SPD and schizophrenia share some precursors in the domains of neuromotor and interpersonal functions.

Schizophrenia

Recent findings from our research (Walker & Lewine, 1990; Walker, Savoie, & Davis, 1993) confirm earlier reports (Fish, Marcus, Hans, Auerbach & Perdue, 1992) of neuromotor abnormalities in preschizophrenic children that are especially pronounced during the first two years of life. Extending beyond this, the results of our investigation suggest that a substantial proportion of preschizophrenic infants show subclinical involuntary movements and posturing (i.e., dyskinesias) of the limbs.

It is of interest to note that studies of unmedicated adult schizophrenic patients also reveal involuntary movements (Casey & Hansen, 1984; Khot & Wyatt, 1991). Further, the rate of spontaneous dyskinesias increases with advanced age, and elderly schizophrenics show a much higher rate of dyskinesias than age-matched normal comparison subjects. Thus, although motor dysfunction is apparent across the life-span in schizophrenic patients, movement abnormalities appear to be most pronounced early and late in the life course. This suggests that schizophrenic patients show an exaggerated version of the U-shaped relation between age and movement abnormalities that has been observed in nonschizophrenic subjects.

In the domain of social behavior, the manifestation of abnormalities shows a very different relation with age. As with motor functions, there is evidence of social and cognitive dysfunction, ranging from subtle to severe, across the life-span of schizophrenic patients (Aylward, Walker, & Bettes, 1984; Walker, 1991; Watt, 1978; Watt, Anthony, Wynne, & Rolf, 1984). But the severity of premorbid social dysfunction increases with age. Studies of high-risk children have shown that those who eventually manifest schizophrenia were characterized by increased social withdrawal and disruptive behavior in adolescence (John, Mednick, & Schulsinger, 1982). Similarly, follow-back studies have revealed that preschizophrenic children tend to show a gradually escalating rate of behavior problems with age (Watt, 1978). Recent findings from our research indicate that preschizophrenic children are distinguishable from their healthy siblings by the early elementary school years, and the diagnostic group differences become more pronounced over time (Walker, Weinstein, & Baum, in press). Like previous investigators, we find that preschizophrenic males show more disruptive behavior, whereas females show a more "internalized" syndrome. Both sexes, however, manifest interpersonal deficits. Using a more microlevel approach, our analyses of childhood home movies indicate that preschizophrenic children show abnormalities in facial expression of emotion that are apparent as early as infancy (Walker, Grimes, Davis, & Smith, 1993).

Of course, the most severe impairments in interpersonal behavior and thought processes typically occur in conjunction with the onset of the florid symptoms of psychosis in late adolescence/early adulthood. The period prior to the first episode is often marked by a significant deterioration of functional capacities. Then, after the first episode, there may be further deterioration. However, this eventually plateaus, and a large proportion of patients show substantial improvement with advanced age (Harding & Strauss, 1985; Ram, Bromet, Eaton, Pato, & Schwartz, 1992). The most marked improvement is in the positive or florid symptoms, which appear to show a significant age-related decline (Bridge, Cannon, & Wyatt, 1978). Thus, an inverted "U" best describes the relation between age and the disturbances in interpersonal behavior and thought that are associated with psychosis.

With respect to their longitudinal course, there appears to be an important distinction between the positive and negative symptoms of psychosis. Several studies have shown that ratings of negative symptoms are more highly correlated with premorbid behavioral function than are ratings of positive symptoms (Peralta et al., 1991; for a review, see Walker & Lewine, 1990). There is also evidence that negative symptoms are more stable and persistent over time. Thus, negative symptoms may, in part, reflect a more longstanding aspect of the neuropathological process underlying schizophrenia. It is important to emphasize, however, that positive and negative symptoms do not appear to be wholly independent symptom dimensions; ratings of positive and negative symptoms in schizophrenic patients tend to be moderately, positively correlated. Obviously, the correlation obtained would be much larger if the two types of symptoms were rated in samples representing a broader range of psychiatric status.

SPD

As indicated, relatively little is known about the developmental course of SPD. However, the available data suggest that it, like schizophrenia, is preceded by subclinical motor and behavioral dysfunction in childhood. Research on the biological offspring of schizophrenic patients indicates that those who are diagnosed with SPD in adulthood showed neuromotor abnormalities in infancy (Fish et al., 1992). Subjects who manifest SPD in adulthood are also characterized by greater behavior problems in childhood, including deficits in interpersonal behavior (John et al., 1982). However, SPD and schizophrenia differ in the nature of their childhood behavioral precursors. Both SPD and schizophrenia are preceded by childhood social withdrawal; however, it appears that only schizophrenia is preceded by behavioral disinhibition (Goldstein & Jones, 1977; John et al., 1982).

A neurodevelopmental model of neurocircuitry malfunction in schizophrenia

A comprehensive neurodevelopmental model of any disorder must account for its changing manifestations of dysfunction across the life course. In the case of schizophrenia, we must account for the evidence of neuromotor dysfunction – in particular, dyskinesia – that is most pronounced early and late in the life course, and florid psychotic symptoms that are most pronounced in early adulthood. In pursuit of this goal, we have recently proposed a neurodevelopmental model of schizophrenia which assumes that maturational events in the CNS modulate the expression of a congenital abnormality in subcortical regions of the brain (Walker, 1994; Walker et al., in press). More specifically, we propose that schizophrenia involves an overactivation of dopamine (DA) transmission in the striatum – a brain region that is one component of multiple, functionally segregated circuits that involve various regions of the cortex. We briefly describe this model here, then turn to a discussion of how it might be modified to account for SPD as both a clinical outcome and transitional state.

Because neuromotor abnormalities are so consistently found in schizophrenia, their underlying pathophysiology is pertinent to our model. Dyskinesias, such as those observed in preschizophrenic infants and adult schizophrenic patients, are known to be associated with abnormalities in the basal ganglia (Penney & Young, 1983, 1986). Further, dyskinesias can be induced or exacerbated by DA agonists, particularly in individuals with known or suspected CNS damage (Klawans, 1988; Klawans & Weiner, 1975). Of course, it is well known that DA agonists, such as amphetamine, can also induce psychotic symptoms in human subjects (Davis, Kahn, Ko, & Davidson, 1991). Similarly, DA agonists produce movement abnormalities, stereotypies, and disruptions in the social behavior of nonhuman primates and rats (for an overview, see Walker, 1994; Walker, Davis, & Baum, 1993a).

Recent theorizing on the specific neural mechanisms underlying dyskinesias focuses on the motor circuit that links the basal ganglia with the motor cortex (Alexander, Crutcher, & DeLong, 1990). A model of this hypothetical circuit is illustrated in Figure 4.1. Ascending DA neurons from the substantia

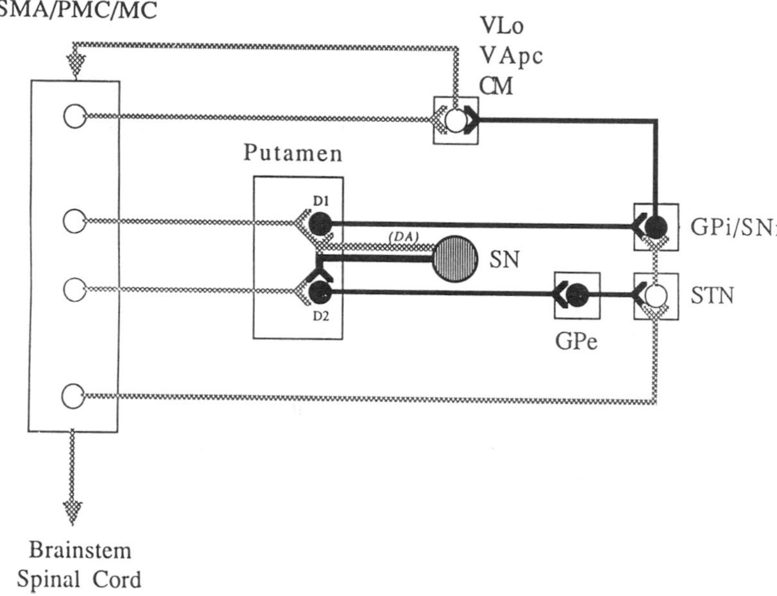

Fig. 4.1. Hypothesized motor circuit. Solid lines represent inhibitory effects, and broken lines represent excitation. CM, centrum medianum; DA, dopamine; GABA, gamma-aminobutyric acid; Glu, glutamate; Gpe, globus pallidus, external segment; Gpi, globus pallidus, internal segment; MC, primary motor cortex; PMC, premotor cortex; SMA, supplementary motor area; SN, substantia nigra; SNr, substantia nigra, pars reticulata; STN, subthalamic nucleus; VApc, ventralis anterior, pars parvocellularis; VLo, ventralis lateralis, pars oralis. (Modified from Alexander et al., 1990.)

nigra pars compacta (SNc) provide excitatory or inhibitory input to neurons in the putamen. These neurons, in turn, either (1) project directly to the globus pallidus\substantia nigra pars reticulata (GPi\SNr), or (2) project indirectly via the globus pallidus (external segment (GPe) and subthalamic nucleus (STN). For both the direct and indirect pathway, the circuit continues with projections to the thalamic nuclei (VLo, VApc, and CM) which provide excitatory input to the motor cortex (SMA, PMC, and MC). The loop is completed by excitatory descending projections from the motor cortex to the putamen. It has been suggested that dyskinesias are produced by relative overactivation of the DA-mediated, indirect pathway linking the striatum with its output nuclei, while tonic activity in the direct pathway is preserved (Alexander et al., 1990). As shown in Figure 4.1, recent data indicate that the indirect pathway is specifically mediated by inhibitory D_2 DA receptors on striatal neurons (Gerfen, 1992).

Although a review of the literature linking schizophrenia with DA overactivation is beyond the scope of this paper (for a review, see Davis et al., 1991), two recent findings are relevant to our model. First, enlargement of the striatum (i.e., caudate and putamen) and abnormalities in the metabolic activity of the striatum have been found in schizophrenic patients (Bogerts et al., 1990a,b; Buchsbaum, 1990; Buchsbaum et al., 1987, 1992a,b; Heckers, Heinsen, Heinsen, & Beckmann, 1991; Resnick, Gur, Alavi, Gur, & Reivich, 1988; Szechtman et al., 1988). Second, an increase in D_2 DA striatal receptors, or the ratio of D_2 to D_1 receptors, in schizophrenic patients has been reported by several groups of investigators (Cross, Crow, & Owen, 1981; Farde et al., 1990; Joyce, Lexow, Bird, & Winokur, 1988; Wong et al., 1986). Thus, there is evidence to support the notion that striatal abnormalities – in particular, excess D_2 DA striatal receptor activity – is involved in the neuropathology of schizophrenia. Given the neural circuit model of dyskinesia described above, we would, therefore, expect to see an increased rate of spontaneous dyskinesias in schizophrenia.

The "motor" circuit linking the basal ganglia with the cortex is assumed to be just one of several circuits linking various regions of the cortex with the basal ganglia. Alexander et al. (1990) have proposed that there are, minimally, three other parallel and functionally segregated circuits: oculomotor, limbic, and frontal. The limbic and frontal circuits are illustrated in Figures 4.2 and 4.3, respectively. Like the motor circuit shown in Figure 4.1, the limbic and frontal circuits are presumed to involve both direct and indirect pathways from the striatum that are mediated by D_1 and D_2 DA receptors, respectively. The circuits differ, however, in the striatal, pallidal, and thalamic regions they transverse, and they project to functionally distinct regions of the cortex.

Several writers have suggested that the limbic circuitry is involved in the manifestation of florid or positive psychotic symptoms (e.g., Swerdlow & Koob, 1987; Weinberger, 1987). Specifically, they have proposed that DA overactivation in this circuitry is responsible for these symptoms. Swerdlow and Koob (1987) suggested that overactivation of DA pathways in the striatum resulted in a "phasic" interruption of the thalamocortical feedback loop, specifically the thalamus-to-limbic cortex circuit. Thus, the same DA overactivation that is expressed as dyskinesia through the motor circuit may be expressed as psychotic symptoms through the limbic circuit.

Drawing on the notion of multiple, functionally segregated circuits, we turn to the question of how brain maturation might alter circuitry function and dysfunction. Findings from research on human CNS maturational changes indicate that during infancy the motor cortex is maximally, metabolically activated relative to other cortical regions, including the frontal and limbic

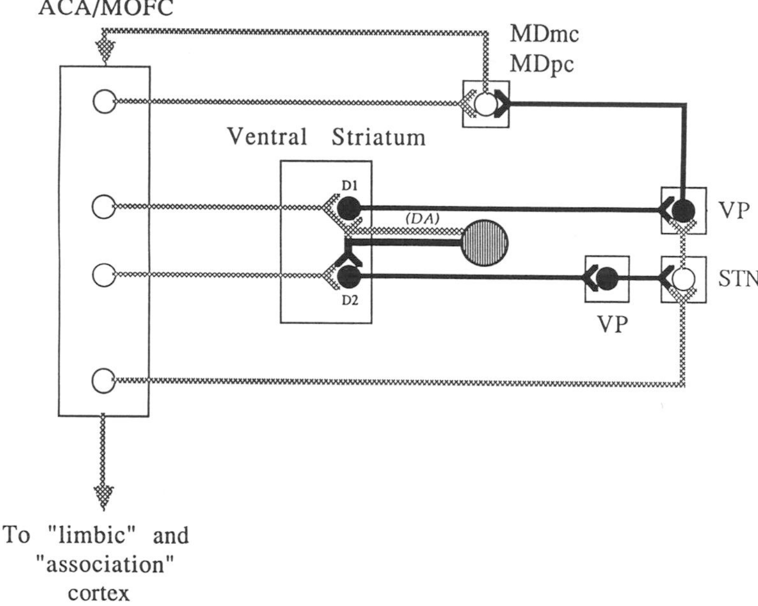

Fig. 4.2. Hypothesized limbic circuit. Solid lines represent inhibitory effects, and broken lines represent excitation. ACA, anterior cingulate area; DA, dopamine; MDmc, medialis dorsalis pars multiformis; MDpc, medialis dorsalis pars parvicellularis; MOFC, medial orbitofrontal cortex; STN, subthalamic nucleus; VP, ventral pallidum. (Modified from Alexander et al., 1990.)

regions (Chugani, 1992; Chugani & Phelps, 1986). With respect to myelination, it is also the most mature cortical region in infancy (Gibson, 1991; Konner, 1991). It would, therefore, be predicted that abnormalities in the striatum would be predominantly expressed in functions subserved by the motor circuit during infancy. This is consistent with the observations of more pronounced neuromotor signs during the first two years of life in preschizophrenic children, as well as in children suspected of having experienced CNS insult (Knobloch & Pasamanick, 1974; Saint-Anne Dargassies, 1982).

Late adolescence/early adulthood is marked by several CNS maturational processes that may deem it the critical period for the manifestation of psychotic symptoms. Relative to other cortical regions, the frontal and limbic areas show greater metabolic activation at this time (Chugani, 1992). Paralleling this, these regions show the most protracted process of myelination, which appears to be completed in adolescence (Konner, 1991). Most notable, myelination of certain critical limbic pathways occurs in adolescence (Benes, 1991). This period is also characterized by a peak in synaptic pruning,

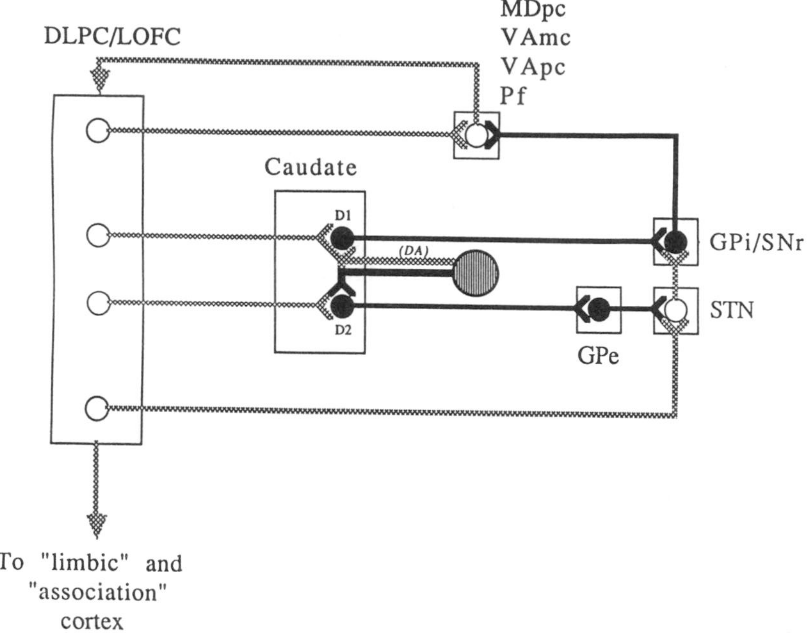

Fig. 4.3. Hypothesized frontal circuit. Solid lines represent inhibitory effects, and broken lines represent excitation. DA, dopamine; DLPC, dorsolateral prefrontal cortex; GPe, globus pallidus, external segment; GPe, globus pallidus, internal segment; LOFC, lateral orbitofrontal cortex; MDpc, medialis dorsalis pars paravicellularis; Pf, parafascicularis; SNr, substantia nigra, pars reticulata; STN, subthalamic nucleus; VAmc, ventralis anterior, pars magnocellularis; VApc, ventralis anterior, pars parvocellularis. (Modified from Alexander et al., 1990.)

which is believed to refine cortical interconnections (Huttenlocher, 1979, 1990), and heightened DA activation that appears to be linked with hormonal changes (McGeer & McGeer, 1981; Morgan, May, & Finch, 1987). Taken together, these changes, especially the maturation of limbic circuitry and heightened DA activity, may explain the dramatic increase in the risk rate for first-episode psychosis in late adolescence/early adulthood.

With advanced age, there is a decline in neuronal and synaptic density (Huttenlocher, 1979, 1990) and metabolic activity (Obrist, 1980) in the cortex. However, the motor regions of the brain undergo less deterioration (Rapaport, 1991). Thus, as in infancy, the motor circuit may be relatively more dominant with advanced age. This may account for the apparent exacerbation of movement abnormalities in elderly schizophrenic patients (Jeste & Wyatt, 1987). In addition, there is a reduction in DA receptors, especially the

D_2 subtype, with age (Farde, Wiesel, Nordstrom, & Sedvall, 1988; Rinne, Lonnberg, & Marjamaki, 1990; Wong et al., 1984). In combination with the reduction in limbic circuitry activation, this may account for the decrease in florid symptoms in elderly patients.

In summary, we propose that schizophrenia involves a congenital abnormality that entails a functional excess of DA activity in the striatum. This subcortical region is one component of multiple neural circuits that involve various regions of the cortex which are differentially activated by brain maturational processes. Thus, the behavioral expression of the abnormality changes as a function of maturational stage.

It is important to emphasize that the empirical data indicate that developmental changes in neural circuitry are gradual, perhaps with the exception of those associated with the onset of puberty. Thus, developmental changes in the relative activation of neural circuits will be gradual, so that an abnormality in DA transmission in the striatum might impact on the motor, limbic, and frontal circuits to varying degrees across the life-span. This is consistent with the evidence that schizophrenic subjects manifest deficits in both motor and social behavior throughout life.

The transition from SPD to schizophrenia

We now turn to the question of how the proposed neurodevelopmental process might either culminate in SPD or evolve into schizophrenia. In order to address this question, we extend the neural circuitry model, described above, and assume that both SPD and schizophrenia are subserved by DA overactivation in the striatum. Further, we suggest that malfunction of the prefrontal circuit (Figure 4.3) is primarily responsible for the syndrome labeled SPD, as well as for the social withdrawal and affective flattening (i.e., negative symptoms) observed in schizophrenia. Malfunction of the limbic circuit, in contrast, is the neural substrate for the expression of the subclinical perceptual abnormalities of SPD and the positive symptoms that are the defining features of schizophrenia.

As previously mentioned, several writers have suggested that the limbic circuit plays a role in the expression of positive symptoms. It has also been proposed that the circuitry linking the frontal cortex with subcortical regions is involved in the manifestation of negative symptoms (Carpenter, Buchanan, Kirkpatrick, Tamminga, Thaker, & Breier, 1992; Tamminga et al., 1992; Weinberger, 1987). This notion is partially based on evidence that schizophrenic patients display a reduction in brain metabolic activity in the frontal regions (Andreasen et al., 1992; Weinberger & Berman, 1988), and that the level of metabolic activity is inversely correlated with ratings of negative or deficit symptoms (Tamminga et al., 1992; Wolkin, Sanfilipo, Wolf, Angrist, Brodie, & Rotrosen, 1992). Research on both animal and human subjects has shown a reciprocal relation between subcortical and frontal dopamine activity, as well as subcortical and frontal metabolic activity (for an overview, see Weinberger, 1987). The neural mechanisms responsible for this are not known. However, it is known that frontal lobe dysfunction is associated with a behavioral syndrome that includes "negative" features, such as asociality and affective blunting (Wolkin et al., 1992). This association has led to the suggestion that negative symptoms in schizophrenia may originate in subcortical DA hyperactivation which leads to frontal hypoactivation (Weinberger, 1987).

As indicated earlier, research on the longitudinal course of symptoms suggests that negative symptoms are more persistent than positive symptoms, and that negative symptoms are more strongly associated with premorbid social deficits (Walker & Lewine, 1988). When individual negative symptoms are separately examined, significant longitudinal stability is found for social withdrawal. Peralta et al. (1991) presented data on the pre- and postmorbid course of schizophrenia which led them to conclude that negative symptoms are persistent schizoid traits that predate the onset of psychotic symptoms. These findings suggest that the frontal circuitry responsible for SPD and negative symptoms comes "on-line" earlier than the limbic circuitry that subserves the expression of positive or florid symptoms.

What this suggests, then, is that malfunction of the limbic circuitry may be the primary substrate distinguishing schizophrenia from SPD. The obvious question this raises is, What factor(s) are responsible for triggering limbic circuit malfunction at a level of severity necessary to produce florid psychotic symptoms? Two classes of variables may be relevant to this process: (1) the CNS maturational changes mentioned above, and (2) stage-related psychosocial stressors that serve to increase DA activation.

If it is true, as we and other authors (Benes, 1989, 1991; Feinberg, 1982; Weinberger, 1987) have suggested, that CNS changes occurring in adolescence can serve to trigger psychotic symptoms in vulnerable individuals, then individual differences in maturation may partially determine whether a schizophrenic episode is triggered (Saugstad, 1989). For example, if the pubertal rise in DA activation or the changes in limbic neuronal interconnections are less pronounced, the vulnerable individual may manifest the interpersonal and subtle ideational abnormalities of SPD, but not the positive symptoms necessary for the diagnosis of a schizophrenic syndrome.

It is also possible that psychosocial stressors play a role in triggering malfunction of limbic circuitry. Environmental stress increases DA transmission (Antelman & Chiodo, 1984). Human adolescence may be associated with a unique increase in psychosocial stressors that deem this developmental period a very critical one with respect to perturbations of circuitry involving DA transmission. Psychosocial stressors may, therefore, play a role in determining whether SPD is a transitional state or the final psychiatric outcome.

The literature on the effects of DA agonists on individuals with known or suspected CNS damage provides a framework for understanding how neurohormonal events might interact with preexisting abnormalities to produce clinical symptoms. It has been shown that amphetamine and other DA agonists can induce dyskinesias (Tolosa & Alom, 1988), and this effect may be most pronounced, or occur exclusively, in individuals with damage to subcortical brain regions (Klawans, 1988). Thus, DA activity that exceeds a threshold might serve to trigger the expression of subcortical abnormality.

Up to this point, we have paid little attention to the origins of the neuropathology underlying SPD and schizophrenia. Genetic factors are one well-established source of constitutional vulnerability (Gottesman, 1991). Within the past decade, evidence supporting a role for obstetric complications has accumulated. It is of particular interest that prenatal viral infection in the second trimester is one complication that has been reported with some consistency (Machon, Huttunen, Mednick, & LaFasse, Chapter 3, this volume). The second trimester is a critical period for the development of subcortical regions, especially the basal ganglia (Towbin, 1986). Thus, prenatal complications are a potential source of damage to the striatum, and may lead to abnormalities in the cytoarchitecture of this region (Gerfen, 1992).

Conclusions and directions for further research

In summary, then, both SPD and schizophrenia are hypothesized to involve overactivation of D_2 DA-mediated pathways in the striatum. This abnormality will be manifested in behavioral dysfunction that changes in nature with development. Early in life, functions subserved by the motor circuit encompassing the striatum will be most affected. Gradually, as the frontal circuit matures, social and affective dysfunction will become more apparent. These two "stages" of the neuropathological process will be shared by SPD and schizophrenia. Ultimately, the extent to which the limbic circuitry is disrupted will determine whether the transition is made from SPD to schizophrenia.

The ideas presented here are admittedly highly speculative. However, they generate some testable hypotheses about differences between patients with SPD and schizophrenia. Specifically, they predict that SPD and schizophrenia will involve similar abnormalities in frontal and motor circuits, but significant differences in limbic circuitry structure and/or function. To date, there is evidence that both SPD and schizophrenia are associated with deficits in frontal structure and function (Raine, Sheard, Reynolds, & Lenez, 1992; Tien, Costa, & Eaton, 1992); however, limbic circuit structure and function have not been examined in SPD.

Differences between SPD and schizophrenia may be revealed by positron emission tomography (PET) in studies of receptor activity in the limbic striatum. Postmortem investigations will be needed to identify differences between SPD and schizophrenia in myelination and cytoarchitectonics of the limbic circuitry. Finally, studies of psychosocial stressors and indices of pubertal maturation may shed light on "triggering" mechanisms that differentiate SPD and schizophrenia (Walker, Downey, & Bergman, 1989).

References

Alexander, G. E., Crutcher, M. D., & DeLong, M. R. (1990). Basal ganglia-thalamocortical circuits: Parallel substrates for motor, oculomotor, "prefrontal" and "limbic" functions. *Progress in Brain Research, 85,* 119–145.

American Psychiatric Association. (1987). *Diagnostic and statistical manual of mental disorders* (3rd ed., rev.). Washington, D.C.: Author. (Cited as DSM-III-R).

Andreasen, N. C., Rezai, K., Alliger, R., Swayze, V. W., II, Flaum, M., Kirchner, P., Cohen, G., & O'Leary, D. S. (1992). Hypofrontality in neuroleptic-naive patients and in patients with chronic schizophrenia: Assessment with xenon-133 single-photon emission computed tomography and the tower of London. *Archives of General Psychiatry, 49,* 943–956.

Angst, J., & Clayton, P. (1986). Premorbid personality of depressive, bipolar, and schizophrenic patients with special reference to suicidal issues. *Comprehensive Psychiatry, 27,* 511–532.

Antelman, S. M., & Chiodo, L. A. (1984). Stress: Its effect on interactions among biogenic amines and role in the induction and treatment of disease. In L. L. Iversen, S. D. Iversen, & S. H. Snyder (Eds.), *Handbook of psychopharmacology* (Vol. 18, pp. 279–341). New York: Plenum Press.

Aylward, E., Walker, E., & Bettes, B. (1984). Intelligence in schizophrenia: Meta-analysis of the research. *Schizophrenia Bulletin, 10,* 430–459.

Baron, M., & Risch, N. (1987). The spectrum concept of schizophrenia: Evidence for a genetic–environmental continuum. *Journal of Psychiatric Research, 21,* 257–267.

Benes, F. M. (1989). Myelination of cortical hippocampal relays during late adolescence. *Schizophrenia Bulletin, 15,* 585–593.

Benes, F. M. (1991). Toward a neurodevelopmental understanding of schizophrenia and other psychiatric disorders. In D. Cicchetti & S. L. Toth (Eds.), *Rochester Symposium on Developmental Psychopathology, 3,* 161–184.

Bogerts, B., Ashtari, M., Degreef, G., Alvir, J. M., Bilder, R. M., & Lieberman, J. A. (1990a). Reduced temporal limbic structure volumes on magnetic resonance images in first episode schizophrenia. *Psychiatry Research, 35,* 1–13.

Bogerts, B., Falkai, P., Haupts, M., Greve, B., Ernst, S., Tapernon, F. U., & Heinzmann, U. (1990b). Post-mortem volume measurements of the limbic system and basal ganglia structures in chronic schizophrenics. *Schizophrenia Research, 3,* 295–301.

Bridge, T. P., Cannon, H. E., & Wyatt, R. J. (1978). Burned-out schizophrenia: Evidence for age effects on schizophrenic symptomatology. *Journal of Gerontology, 33,* 835–839.

Buchsbaum, M. S. (1990). The frontal lobes, basal ganglia, and temporal lobes as sites for schizophrenia. *Schizophrenia Bulletin, 16,* 379–389.

Buchsbaum, M. S., Haier, R. J., Potkin, S. G., Nuechterlein, K., Bracha, H. S., Katz, M., Lohr, J., Wu, J. C., Lottenberg, S., Jerabek, P. A., Trenary, M., Tafalla, R., Reynolds, C., & Bunney, W. E., Jr. (1992a). Frontostriatal disorder of cerebral metabolism in never-medicated schizophrenics. *Archives of General Psychiatry, 49,* 935–942.

Buchsbaum, M. S., Potkin, S. G., Marshall, J. F., Lottenberg, S., Teng, C., Heh, C. W., Tafalla, R., Reynolds, C., Abel, L., Plon, L., & Bunney, W. E., Jr. (1992b). Effects of clozapine and thiothixene on glucose metabolic rate in schizophrenia. *Neuropsychopharmacology, 6,* 155–163.

Buchsbaum, M. S., Wu, J. C., DeLisi, L. E., Holcomb, H. H., Hazlett, E., Cooper-Langston, K., & Kessler, R. (1987). Positron emission tomography studies of basal ganglia and somatosensory cortex neuroleptic drug effects: Differences between normal controls and schizophrenic patients. *Biological Psychiatry, 22,* 479–494.

Cannon, T. D., Barr, C. E., & Mednick, S. A. (1991). Genetic and perinatal factors in the etiology of schizophrenia. In E. F. Walker (Ed.), *Schizophrenia: A life-course developmental perspective* (pp. 9–31). San Diego: Academic Press.

Carpenter, W. T., Buchanan, R. W., Kirkpatrick, B., Tamminga, C., Thaker, G., & Breier, A. (1992). The neuroanatomy of the deficit syndrome. *Schizophrenia Research, 6,* 166 (abstract).

Casey, D. E., & Hansen, T. E. (1984). Spontaneous dyskinesias. In D. V. Jeste & R. J. Wyatt (Eds.), *Neuropsychiatric movement disorders* (pp. 68–95). Washington, D.C.: American Psychiatric Press.

Chugani, H. T. (1992). Development of regional brain glucose metabolism in relation to behavior and plasticity. In G. Dawson & K. Fischer (Eds.), *Human behavior and the developing brain.* New York: Guilford Press.

Chugani, H. T., & Phelps, M. E. (1986). Maturational changes in cerebral function in infants determined by ^{1}8FDG positron emission tomography. *Science, 231,* 840–843.

Clementz, B. A., Cerri, A., Medus, C., & Iacono, W. G. (1991). Familial prevalence and coaggregation of schizotypy indicators: A multitrait family study. *Journal of Abnormal Psychology, 100,* 115–121.

Clementz, B. A., Grove, W. M., Katsanis, J., & Iacono, W. G. (1991). Psychometric detection of schizotypy: Perceptual aberration and physical anhedonia in relatives of schizophrenics. *Journal of Abnormal Psychology, 100,* 607–612.

Cross, A. J., Crow, T. J., & Owen, F. (1981). ^{3}H-Flupenthixol binding in post-mortem brains of schizophrenics: Evidence for a selective increase in dopamine D_2 receptors. *Psychopharmacology, 74,* 122–124.

Davis, K. L., Kahn, R. S., Ko, G., & Davidson, M. (1991). Dopamine in schizophrenia: A review and reconceptualization. *American Journal of Psychiatry, 148,* 1474–1486.

Dworkin, R., Cornblatt, B. A., Friedmann, R., Kaplansky, L. M., Lewis, J. A., Rinaldi, A., Shilliday, C., & Erlenmeyer-Kimling, L. (1993). Childhood neuromotor and attentional precursors of affective versus social deficits in adolescents at risk for schizophrenia. *Schizophrenia Bulletin, 19,* 563–577.

Farde, L., Wiesel, F. A., Nordstrom, A. L., & Sedvall, G. (1988). PET examination of human D-1 and D-2 characteristics. *Psychopharmacology, 96* (Suppl.), 79.

Farde, L., Wiesel, F. A., Stone-Elander, S., Halldin, C., Nordstrom, A. L., Hall, H., & Sedvall, G. (1990). D_2 dopamine receptors in neuroleptic-naive schizophrenic patients: A positron emission tomography study with [^{11}C]raclopride. *Archives of General Psychiatry, 47,* 213–219.

Feinberg, I. (1982). Schizophrenia: Caused by a fault in programmed synaptic elimination during adolescence? *Journal of Psychiatric Research, 17,* 319–334.

Fenton, W. S., & McGlashan, T. H. (1989). Risk of schizophrenia in character disorder patients. *American Journal of Psychiatry, 146,* 1280–1284.

Fischer, M. (1971). Psychosis in the offspring of schizophrenic monozygotic twins and their normal co-twins. *British Journal of Psychiatry, 118,* 43–52.

Fish, B., Marcus, J., Hans, S. L., Auerbach, J. G., & Perdue, S. (1992). Infants at risk for schizophrenia: Sequelae of a genetic neurointegrative defect. *Archives of General Psychiatry, 49,* 221–235.

Gerfen, C. R. (1992). The neostriatal mosaic: Multiple levels of compartmental organization in the basal ganglia. *Annual Review of Neurosciences, 15,* 285–320.

Gibson, K. (1991). Myelination and behavioral development. In K. Gibson & A. Peterson (Eds.), *Brain maturation and cognitive development* (pp. 29–64). New York: Aldine De Gruyter.

Goldstein, M. J., & Jones, J. E. (1977). Adolescent and familial precursors of borderline and schizophrenic conditions. In P. Hartocollis (Ed.), *Borderline personality disorder*. New York: International University Press.

Gottesman, I. I. (1991). *Schizophrenia genesis.* New York: W. H. Freeman.

Gottesman, I. I., & Bertelsen, A. (1989). Confirming unexpressed genotypes for schizophrenia. *Archives of General Psychiatry, 46,* 867–872.

Harding, C., & Strauss, J. (1985). The course of schizophrenia: An evolving concept. In M. Alpert (Ed.), *Controversies in schizophrenia.* New York: Guilford.

Heckers, S., Heinsen, H., Heinsen, Y., & Beckmann, H. (1991). Cortex, white matter, and basal ganglia in schizophrenia: A volumetric postmortem study. *Biological Psychiatry, 29,* 556–566.

Huttenlocher, P. R. (1979). Synaptic density in human frontal cortex – developmental changes and effects of aging. *Brain Research, 163,* 195–205.

Huttenlocher, P. R. (1990). Morphometric study of human cerebral cortex development. *Neuropsychologia, 28,* 517–527.

Jeste, D., & Wyatt, R. J. (1987). Aging and tardive dyskinesia. In N. Miller & G. Cohen (Eds), *Schizophrenia and aging* (pp. 275–283). New York: Guilford Press.

John, R. S., Mednick, S. A., & Schulsinger, F. (1982). Teacher reports as predictor of schizophrenia and borderline schizophrenia. *Journal of Abnormal Psychology, 91,* 399–413.

Joyce, J. N., Lexow, N., Bird, E., & Winokur, A. (1988). Organization of dopamine D_1 and D_2 receptors in human striatum: Receptor autoradiographic studies in Huntington's disease and schizophrenia. *Synapse, 2,* 546–557.

Kendler, K. S. (1985). Diagnostic approaches to schizotypal personality disorder: A historical perspective. *Schizophrenia Bulletin, 11,* 538–553.

Kendler, K. S. (1988a). Familial aggregation of schizophrenia and schizophrenia spectrum disorders. *Archives of General Psychiatry, 45,* 377–386.

Kendler, K. S., Ochs, A. L., Gorman, A. M., Hewitt, J. K., Ross, D. E., & Mirsky, A. F. (1991). The structure of schizotypy: A pilot multitrait twin study. *Psychiatry Research, 36,* 19–36.

Kety, S. (1987). The significance of genetic factors in the etiology of schizophrenia:

Results from the national study of adoptees in Denmark. *Journal of Psychiatric Research, 21,* 423–429.

Kety, S. (1988). Schizophrenic illness in the families of schizophrenic adoptees: Findings from the Danish national sample. *Schizophrenia Bulletin, 14,* 217–222.

Khot, V., & Wyatt, R. J. (1991). Not all that moves is tardive dyskinesia. *American Journal of Psychiatry, 148,* 661–666.

Klawans, H. L. (1988). The pathophysiology of drug-induced movement disorders. In J. Jankovic & E. Tolosa (Eds.), *Parkinson's disease and movement disorder* (pp. 315–324). Baltimore: Urban & Schwarzenberg.

Knobloch, H., & Pasamanick, B. (1974). *Developmental diagnosis.* New York: Harper & Row Publishers.

Konner, M. (1991). Universals of behavioral development in relation to brain myelination. In K. Gibson & A. Peterson (Eds.), *Brain maturation and cognitive development* (pp. 181–224). New York: Aldine De Gruyter.

Kringlen, E., & Cramer, G. (1989). Offspring of monozygotic twins discordant for schizophrenia. *Archives of General Psychiatry, 46,* 873–877.

MacGillivray, L., Nylander, P. S., & Corney, G. (1975). *Human multiple reproduction.* London: Saunders.

McGeer, P. L., & McGeer, E. G. (1981). Neurotransmitters in the aging brain, In A. M. Darrison & R. H. Thompson (Eds.), *The molecular basis of neuropathology* (pp. 631–648). London: Edward Arnold.

Meehl, P. E. (1989). Schizotaxia revisited. *Archives of General Psychiatry, 46,* 935–944.

Meehl, P. E. (1990). Toward an integrated theory of schizotaxia, schizotypy, and schizophrenia. *Journal of Personality Disorders, 4,* 1–99.

Mehlum, L., Friis, S., Irion, T., Johns, S., Karterud, S., Vaglum, P., & Vaglum, S. (1991). Personality disorders 2–5 years after treatment: A prospective follow-up study. *Acta Psychiatrica Scandinavica, 84,* 72–77.

Morgan, D. G., May, P. C., & Finch, C. E. (1987). Dopamine and serotonin systems in human and rodent brain: Effects of age and neurodegenerative disease. *Journal of the American Geriatrics Society, 35,* 334–345.

Obrist, W. D. (1980). Cerebral blood flow and EEG changes associated with aging and dementia. In E. W. Busse & D. G. Blazer (Eds.), *Handbook of geriatric psychiatry* (pp. 83–101). New York: Van Nostrand Reinhold.

Penney, J. B., & Young, A. B. (1983). Speculations on the functional anatomy of basal ganglia disorders. *Annual Review of Neuroscience, 6,* 73–94.

Penney, J. B., & Young, A. B. (1986). Striatal inhomogeneities and basal ganglia function. *Movement Disorders, 1,* 3–15.

Peralta, B., Cuesta, M. J., & deLeon, J. (1991). Premorbid personality and positive and negative symptoms in schizophrenia. *Acta Psychiatrica Scandinavica, 84,* 336–339.

Porreco, R. P. (1990). Twin gestation. *Clinical Obstetrics and Gynecology, 33,* 1–54.

Raine, A., Sheard, C., Reynolds, G. P., & Lencz, T. (1992). Prefrontal structural and functional deficits associated with individual differences in schizotypal personality. *Schizophrenia Research, 7,* 237–247.

Ram, R., Bromet, E. J., Eaton, W. W., Pato, C., & Schwartz, J. E. (1992). The natural course of schizophrenia: A review of first-admission studies. *Schizophrenia Bulletin, 18,* 185–207.

Rapaport, S. I. (1991). Positron emission tomography in Alzheimer's disease in relation to disease pathogenesis: A critical review. *Cerebrovascular and Brain Metabolism Reviews, 3,* 297–335.

Resnick, S. M., Gur, R. E., Alavi, A., Gur, R. C., & Reivich, M. (1988). Positron emission tomography and subcortical glucose metabolism in schizophrenia. *Psychiatry Research, 24,* 1–11.

Rinne, J. O., Lonnberg, P., & Marjamaki, P. (1990). Age-dependent decline in human brain dopamine D_1 and D_2 receptors. *Brain Research, 508,* 349–352.

Saint-Anne Dargassies, S. (1982). *The neuromotor and psychoaffective development of the infant.* Amsterdam: Elsevier.

Saugstad, L. (1989). Social class, marriage and fertility in schizophrenia. *Schizophrenia Bulletin, 15,* 9–43.

Schulsinger, F., Parnas, J., Petersen, E. T., Schulsinger, H., Teasdale, T. W., Mednick, S. A., Moller, L., & Silverton, L. (1984). Cerebral ventricular size in the offspring of schizophrenic mothers: A preliminary study. *Archives of General Psychiatry, 41,* 602–606.

Schultz, P. M., Schultz, S. C., Solomon, C., Goldberg, C., Ettigi, P., Resnick, R. J., & Friedel, R. O. (1986). Diagnoses of the relatives of schizotypal outpatients. *Journal of Nervous and Mental Disease, 174,* 457–463.

Siever, L. J. (1985). Biological markers in schizotypal personality disorder. *Schizophrenia Bulletin, 11,* 564–575.

Siever, L. J., Keefe, R., Bernstein, D. P., Coccaro, E. F., Klar, H. M., Zemishlany, Z., Peterson, A. E., Davidson, M., Mahon, T., Horvath, T., & Mohs, R. (1990). Eye tracking impairment in clinically identified patients with schizotypal personality disorder. *American Journal of Psychiatry, 147,* 740–745.

Silverman, J. M., Siever, L. J., Horvath, T. B., Coccaro, E. F., Klar, H., Davidson, M., Pinkham, L., Apter, S. H., Mohs, R. C., & Davis, K. L. (1993). Schizophrenia-related and affective personality disorder traits in relatives of probands with schizophrenia and personality disorders. *American Journal of Psychiatry, 150,* 435–442.

Swerdlow, N. R., & Koob, G. F. (1987). Dopamine, schizophrenia, mania, and depression: Toward a unified hypothesis of cortico-striato-pallido-thalamic function. *Behavioral and Brain Sciences, 10,* 197–245.

Szechtman, H., Nahmias, C., Garnett, E. S., Firnau, G., Brown, G. M., Kaplan, R. D., & Cleghorn, J. M. (1988). Effect of neuroleptics on altered cerebral glucose metabolism in schizophrenia. *Archives of General Psychiatry, 45,* 523–532.

Tamminga, C. A., Thaker, G. K., Buchanan, R., Kirkpatrick, B., Alphs, L. D., Chase, T. N., & Carpenter, W. T. (1992). Limbic system abnormalities identified in schizophrenia using positron emission tomography with fluorodeoxyglucose and neocortical alterations with deficit syndrome. *Archives of General Psychiatry, 49,* 522–530.

Tien, A. Y., Costa, P. T., & Eaton, W. W. (1992). Covariance of personality, neurocognition, and schizophrenia spectrum traits in the community. *Schizophrenia Research, 7,* 149–158.

Tolosa, E., & Alom, J. (1988). Drug-induced dyskinesias. In J. Jankovic & E. Tolosa (Eds.), *Parkinson's disease and movement disorders* (pp. 327–347). Baltimore: Urban & Schwarzenberg.

Torrey, E. F. (1992). Are we overestimating the genetic contributions to schizophrenia? *Schizophrenia Bulletin, 18,* 159–170.

Towbin, A. (1986). Obstetric malpractice litigation: The pathologist's view. *American Journal of Obstetrics and Gynecology, 155,* 927–935.

Walker, E. (Ed.). (1991). *Schizophrenia: A life-course developmental perspective.* New York: Academic Press.

Walker, E. (1994). Developmentally moderated expression of the neuropathology underlying schizophrenia. *Schizophrenia Bulletin, 20,* 453–480.

Walker, E., Davis, D., & Baum, B. (1993a). Social withdrawal. In C. Costella (Ed.), *Symptoms of schizophrenia* (pp. 227–260). New York: Wiley.

Walker, E., Downey, G., & Bergman, A. (1989). The effects of parental psychopathology and maltreatment on child behavior: A test of the diathesis–stress model. *Child Development, 60,* 15–24.

Walker, E., Downey, G., & Caspi, A. (1991). Twin studies of psychopathology: Why do the concordance rates vary? *Schizophrenia Research, 4,* 1–12.

Walker, E., Grimes, K., Davis, D., & Smith, A. (1993b). Childhood precursors of schizophrenia: Facial expressions of emotion. *American Journal of Psychiatry, 150,* 1654–1660.

Walker, E., & Lewine, R. (1988). The positive/negative symptom distinction in schizophrenia: Validity and etiological relevance. *Schizophrenia Research, 1,* 315–328.

Walker, E. F., & Lewine, R. J. (1990). The prediction of adult-onset schizophrenia from childhood home-movies of patients. *American Journal of Psychiatry, 147,* 1052–1056.

Walker, E., Savoie, T., & Davis, D. (1994). Neuromotor precursors of schizophrenia. *Schizophrenia Bulletin, 20,* 441–451.

Walker, E., Weinstein, J., & Baum, K. (in press). Antecedents of schizophrenia: Moderating influences of age and biological sex. In H. Hafner & W. Gottey (Eds.), *Search for the causes of schizophrenia.* New York: Springer-Verlag.

Watt, N. F. (1978). Patterns of childhood social development in adult schizophrenics. *Archives of General Psychiatry, 36,* 160–165.

Watt, N. F., Anthony, E. J., Wynne, L., & Rolf, T. E. (1984). *Children at risk for schizophrenia.* Cambridge: Cambridge University Press.

Weinberger, D. (1987). Implications of normal brain development for the pathogenesis of schizophrenia. *Archives of General Psychiatry, 44,* 660–669.

Weinberger, D. R., & Berman, K. F. (1988). Speculation on the meaning of cerebral metabolic hypofrontality in schizophrenia. *Schizophrenia Bulletin, 14,* 157–168.

Wolff, S., Townshend, R., McGuire, R. J., & Weeks, D. J. (1991). 'Schizoid' personality in childhood and adult life. II: Adult adjustment and the continuity with schizotypal personality disorder. *British Journal of Psychiatry, 159,* 620–629, 634–635.

Wolkin, A., Sanfilipo, M., Wolf, A. P., Angrist, B., Brodie, J. D., & Rotrosen, J. (1992). Negative symptoms and hypofrontality in chronic schizophrenia. *Archives of General Psychiatry, 49,* 959–965.

Wong, D. F., Wagner, H. N., Jr., Dannals, R. F., Links, J. M., Frost, J. J., Ravert, H. T., Wilson, A. A., Rosenbaum, A. E., Gjedde, A., Douglass, K. H., Petroms, K. A., Folstein, J. D., Toung, J. K. T., Burns, H. D., & Kuhar, M. J. (1984). Effects of age on dopamine and serotonin receptors measured by positron emission tomography in the living human brain. *Science, 226,* 1393–1396.

Wong, D. F., Wagner, H. N., Jr., Tune, L. E., Dannals, R. F., Pearlson, G. D., Links, J. M., Tamminga, C. A., Broussolle, E. P., Ravert, H. T., Wilson, A. A., Toung, J. K. T., Malat, J., Williams, J. A., O'Tuama, L. A., Snyder, S. H., Kuhar, M. J., & Gjedde, A. (1986). Positron emission tomography reveals elevated D2 dopamine receptors in neuroleptic-naive schizophrenics. *Science, 234,* 1558–1563; correction, *235,* 623 (1987).

PART III
Assessment

5

Scales for the measurement of schizotypy

JEAN P. CHAPMAN, LOREN J. CHAPMAN, and THOMAS R. KWAPIL

More than a dozen pencil-and-paper questionnaires or scales have been developed in an attempt to measure the interrelated constructs of schizotypy, the predisposition to schizophrenia or to psychosis, and schizotypal personality disorder. The attraction of this research is its potential for major payoff should it be completely successful. If researchers could use measures of traits and symptoms to identify schizophrenia-prone persons in advance of clinical decompensation, they would have a powerful tool for studying many of the important questions about schizophrenia. They could better seek the events that precipitate the disorder in predisposed persons or, conversely, identify protective factors that help prevent decompensation. They could study the biological substrate of the predisposition before the disruptive intrusion of the psychotic episode and the side effects of treatment. Geneticists could determine the mode of genetic transmission of the predisposition to schizophrenia and determine whether some schizophrenia-prone persons carry a genetic predisposition whereas others do not. Clinicians could attempt prophylactic intervention in advance of the disaster of the schizophrenic episode.

We review these scales together with some evidence for the validity of each, giving most detailed attention to five scales developed in our own laboratory. Our review is, of necessity, a very selective one. The majority of the numerous publications on these scales are not covered. In particular, our discussion of the validity of the scales focuses on the evidence provided by interviews for schizotypal and psychotic-like symptoms in high-scoring persons on the scales. We do not examine the large literature of laboratory studies of deviant scorers. The laboratory studies mainly test hypotheses about poor performance on tasks on which schizophrenics perform badly. Edell (in press) and Miller and Yee (1994) provided reviews of laboratory studies of such subjects. In our review of the validity of the five scales from our own laboratory, we focus on a 10-year follow-up study in which psychotic decompensation was observed.

We do not review every published scale for schizotypy. Less widely used scales to be omitted for lack of space include the Hallucination Scale (Launay & Slade, 1981), the Social Fear Scale (Raulin & Wee, 1984), and the Ambivalence Scale (Raulin, 1984).

The Psychoticism Scale

Eysenck and Eysenck (1975, 1976) were impressed with the abundance of reports that sociopathic personality and criminality are elevated in the families of schizophrenic probands. Several studies have found that the relatives of schizophrenics include an excess of criminals, alcoholics, and/or psychopaths (Heston, 1966; Kallmann, 1938; review by Planansky, 1972). The Eysencks conjectured that schizophrenia is the endpoint of a dimension of psychoticism, which, like the traits of neuroticism and extroversion, they describe as dimensions of normal personality. The Eysencks suggested that sociopaths and criminals are high on psychoticism and that schizophrenics are the highest of all. Accordingly, the Eysencks built their Psychoticism Scale primarily around aspects of personality often found in sociopaths and criminals.

Eysenck and Eysenck (1976) wrote a formal trait specification to guide the writing and selection of items. They described the high psychoticism subject as "cold, impersonal, hostile, lacking in sympathy, unfriendly, untrustful, odd, unemotional, unhelpful, antisocial, lacking in human feelings, inhumane, generally bloody-minded, lacking in insight, strange, with paranoid ideas that other people were against him" (p. 47). They sought items that would not be rejected by subjects as overly odd.

The Eysencks have published a series of versions of the Psychoticism Scale. The most widely used is a 25-item version from the Eysenck Personality Questionnaire, or EPQ (Eysenck & Eysenck, 1975). Illustrative items, together with the response that contributes to a high score, are:

Do you stop to think things over before doing anything? (No)
Would being in debt worry you? (No)
Do you enjoy hurting people you love? (Yes)
Do good manners and cleanliness matter to you? (No)

The investigators intermixed candidate items with established measures of extroversion and neuroticism and administered them to groups of normal subjects. Items that correlated positively with other psychoticism items but not with extroversion or neuroticism were retained.

Reliability

Eysenck and Eysenck (1976) reported coefficient-alpha reliability values ranging from .68 to .74. In contrast, Chapman, Chapman, and Miller (1982) reported values of .52 for male college students and .58 for females. The Eysencks (1976) reported retest reliabilities for various groups averaging .71, with one month intervening between testings.

Validity

The evidence, as a whole, strongly supports the hypothesis that criminals, psychopaths, alcoholics, and drug addicts score high on the scale, substantially higher than psychotics. Several scholars have criticized the scale on the grounds that psychotics do not score especially high on it, pointing out, in effect, that the Psychoticism Scale is a doubtful measure of the trait for which it is named (Bishop, 1977; Block, 1977; Davis, 1974; Zuckerman, 1991). Eysenck has responded vigorously to such criticisms, most recently providing a lengthy scholarly recapitulation of his argument (Eysenck, 1992). He suggests that schizophrenics dissemble on the scale, and he points to their high scores on the Minnesota Multiphasic Personality Inventory (MMPI) Lie Scale. He believes that nonpsychotics dissemble less and that the scale is a valid measure of their psychoticism, although it is not for schizophrenics.

Perhaps the most direct validity data are provided by Raine's (1987) study. Raine administered the Psychoticism Scale, together with other scales, to 37 male prisoners who were rated on each symptom of DSM-III schizotypal personality disorder (SPD). Raine found no significant relationship between these ratings and Psychoticism Scale scores, despite finding significant relationships between the ratings and scores on six other widely used scales of schizotypal disorder.

It should also be pointed out that the meaning of the heightened criminality and antisociality in the families of schizophrenics is unclear. Rosenthal (1975) has argued that criminals and psychopaths are found in the families of schizophrenics not necessarily because antisociality leads to psychosis, but rather, because female schizophrenics tend to mate with psychopaths. Additional supportive data for such selective mating are found in Fowler and Tsuang (1975). On the other hand, Silverton (1988) found heightened criminality in the families of schizophrenics without selective mating of schizophrenics with psychopaths.

We would also suggest that finding antisociality and criminality in the relatives of schizophrenics is not strong evidence that antisocial persons are at risk for psychosis. Of greater relevance to Eysenck's conjecture is the converse, that is, whether the relatives of antisocial individuals and criminals include an excess of schizophrenics. The results of such studies have been largely negative (Cadoret, 1978; Crowe, 1972, 1974; Hutchings & Mednick, 1975; Schulsinger, 1974). This is not surprising when one considers the heterogeneity of criminality. Even if some antisocial persons are schizophrenia prone, one might expect great difficulty confirming an excess of schizophrenics among the relatives of criminals. A few criminals may carry a predisposition to psychosis, but most appear to have other sources of their criminality. This being the case, high scores on a scale of antisocial attitudes, like the Eysencks' scale, would be expected to identify more false positives for psychosis proneness than valid positives. This suggestion is consistent with the data which, on the whole, show that the Eysencks' Psychoticism Scale does not identify people for whom psychosis proneness can be readily confirmed by other criteria, such as schizotypal symptoms.

The Schizotypal Personality Scale

Claridge and his collaborators began their development of the Schizotypal Personality Scale in response to their experience with the Eysencks' Psychoticism Scale. Claridge was favorably impressed with the Eysencks' conjecture that psychosis is the extreme point of a normal personality dimension and was somewhat favorably disposed toward the Eysencks' Psychoticism Scale. He suggested, however, that the personality dimension relevant to psychoticism might, in addition, be measured by items derived from the clinical symptoms of schizophrenia. Claridge and his collaborators used the DSM-III diagnostic criteria for SPD and for borderline personality disorder to guide the construction of two new sets of items. These are the 37-item Schizotypal Personality Scale (usually referred to as the STA Scale) and the 18-item Borderline Personality Scale (usually referred to as the STB Scale). We focus here on the STA Scale. Illustrative items include:

Do you often feel that people have it in for you? (Yes)
Are you easily distracted from work by daydreams? (Yes)
Do you ever feel that your thoughts don't belong to you? (Yes)
Have you ever felt that you were communicating with someone else telepathically? (Yes)

Reliability

Claridge and Broks (1984) published their items but did not report the psychometric features of the scales or psychometric procedures, if any, that they used for the selection and screening of candidate items. However, Claridge and Hewitt (1987) remedied this by reporting psychometric information for the scale, using data from 403 subjects. The distribution of scores was approximately normal, and the coefficient-alpha estimate of reliability was .86. The average item endorsement was 39%, which indicates that the investigators were successful in their attempt to cast the DSM-III schizotypal symptoms in terms of common experiences of normal people. On the other hand, all of the items are worded so that an affirmative answer contributes to a high schizotypy score. As a result, the scale is expected to be subject to acquiescence response bias more than it would be otherwise.

Validity

Unlike the Psychoticism Scale, the STA Scale yields markedly higher scores for partially recovered schizophrenics and other psychotics than for control subjects (Jackson & Claridge, 1991). The scores of relatives of schizophrenics were not found, however, to exceed those of either normal subjects or the relatives of neurotic subjects, but instead were significantly lower than both groups (Claridge, Robinson, & Birchall, 1983). The investigators very reasonably attributed this unexpected finding to the extreme defensiveness of relatives who know that they are being tested because they are relatives of schizophrenics and who recognize that many items of the scale represent schizophrenic symptoms.

Claridge and Hewitt (1987) did an interesting study of the heritability of schizotypy using these scales. They gave the STA and STB scales to a large sample of monozygotic and dizygotic twin pairs. They obtained a heritability estimate of 53% for the STA Scale and 55% for the STB Scale.

The Schizophrenism Scale

Nielsen and Petersen (1976) developed a scale of schizophrenism, which they defined as a subschizophrenic trait indexed by withdrawal and cognitive peculiarities. They wrote a pool of items based on published reports of experiences of premorbid or early schizophrenics, taking care to avoid items that subjects might recognize as associated with mental illness. They used interitem correlations to select the final 14-item scale. Illustrative items are:

I am easily distracted when I read or talk to someone. (True)
I do not like to mix with other people. (True)
I often daydream. (True)
I often change between positive and negative feelings toward the same person. (True)

All of the items were worded so that an affirmative response contributes toward a high score, a feature that would be expected to make the scale vulnerable to acquiescence response bias.

Reliability and validity

The authors reported item–scale correlations that were extraordinarily high – all of them falling between .53 and .78. The closest thing to validation of Nielsen and Petersen's Schizophrenism Scale is provided by studies of Venables et al.'s Schizophrenism Scale, which borrowed many of Nielsen and Petersen's items. Those studies will be reviewed below.

The Rust Inventory of Schizotypal Cognitions

The Rust Inventory of Schizotypal Cognitions or RISC (Rust, 1987, 1988, 1989) consists of 26 items. Rust started with a pool of items tapping a broad range of content, but used factor analysis to restrict the content to paranoid items and items that tap general schizophrenic symptoms. Items were also chosen on the basis of item–scale correlations and with special attention to obtaining a normal distribution in the general population. Half of the items are worded so that agreement contributes to a high schizotypy score and half are worded in the opposite direction, a precaution that prevents acquiescence response set from artifactually producing extreme scores. Examples of RISC items are:

Sometimes my thoughts seem so loud, I can almost hear them. (True)
Sometimes I feel I am ugly and at other times that I am attractive. (True)
Secret organizations have no real power or influence on our lives. (False)
It has never occurred to me that the world may be a figment of my imagination. (False)

Rust claimed that a special virtue of the scale is that true or false responses to the items are not obviously good or bad. As evidence he pointed out that no item on the RISC is accepted or rejected by less than 20% of the normal population. Frequency of endorsement, however, is a separate issue from the extent to which social desirability determines responses. One can readily construct items on which answers are determined primarily by the social desirability of the response at any given level of endorsement frequency.

Reliability and validity

The RISC manual reports that coefficient-alpha values for various groups have been found to range from .68 to .81. Split-half reliability for a much larger group was .71 and test–retest reliability was .87 for 131 subjects with an interval between testings of 2 weeks to 3 months.

The manual reports that RISC scores of schizophrenics are substantially higher than those of normal control subjects. Moreover, the manual briefly mentions a validity study in which 36 chronic schizophrenic patients who responded to the RISC were rated by a psychiatrist on the extent of schizotypal symptoms. The two measures correlated .52 ($p < .001$), thus sharing 27% of their variance. No data have been published on the relation of inventory scores to schizotypal symptoms in less disturbed samples.

Comment

Rust has published his scale commercially, apparently viewing its validity as sufficiently well established that it can be recommended for general clinical use. However, he has not reported much data relevant to such a recommendation. More standardization information is needed for a clinical instrument that is used for making judgments about individuals than for a research instrument used for comparisons of groups. Rust states that the RISC was designed to tap the "cognitive schizotypal dimension" in the normal population. The usual reason for inquiring about schizotypal cognitions in clinical practice is to diagnose SPD. Before adopting a clinical instrument for making diagnostic decisions, one would need data on the percentage of persons of any given score who would be expected to be valid positives and the percentage who would be expected to be false positives. There does not appear, however, to be any evidence that this scale detects SPD in a nonpsychotic population, much less any data on its diagnostic specificity.

Venables et al.'s Schizotypy Scale

Venables et al. (1990) needed a schizotypy scale for a research project in Mauritius and found that none of the previously published scales quite met their needs. They wanted a scale to measure both positive and negative symptoms of schizotypy, types of symptoms that they believed might correspond to positive and negative schizophrenia. They also wanted the scale to be short, and they were especially concerned that the items not be recognizable to the subjects as probing abnormal behavior. Accordingly, they developed a new scale largely consisting of items borrowed from previous scales.

The investigators pointed out that both positive symptoms (perceptual, cognitive, and attentional dysfunction), and negative symptoms (anhedonia and withdrawal) have been described as aspects of schizotypy but have been found not to be significantly correlated. For positive-symptom schizotypy, which they call schizophrenism, the investigators used items from Nielsen and Petersen's (1976) Schizophrenism Scale, plus selected items from several other scales. For negative symptom schizotypy, they relied largely on items borrowed from Chapman, Chapman and Raulin's (1976) Physical Anhedonia and Social Anhedonia scales, which we review later in this chapter. Venables et al.'s final scale is the result of a series of factor analyses that confirmed their expectation of a two-factor solution – one factor for schizophrenism and one for anhedonia.

Reliability and validity

Venables et al.'s final 30-item scale has coefficient-alpha values of .82 for the schizophrenism factor and .76 for the anhedonia factor.

Raine's (1987) data provided striking evidence for the validity of the Venables et al. Schizophrenism subscale. Using his group of 37 male prisoners, Raine found that scores on the subscale correlated .66 with the sum of symptom ratings for SPD. Anhedonia, however, had no such relationship.

Venables (1990) used the scale with the Mauritius sample. They rated subjects on Quay and Peterson's (1987) Psychotic Behavior Scale and found that rated psychotic behavior was positively correlated with the Schizophrenism Scale score but not the Anhedonia Scale score.

Studies using the MMPI

A number of researchers have investigated the usefulness of various MMPI scales and indicators for the detection of schizotypy. Grove (1982) and Walters (1983) reviewed several such studies. Both of these reviewers concluded that the MMPI has not proved very sensitive in the detection of schizotypy.

A recent series of studies by Moldin and his collaborators have combined many of the MMPI scales and indicators derived from the MMPI to yield a single conjoint marker of schizotypy. The guiding principle of this work was that indicators of schizotypy should also be indicators of schizophrenia. The subjects were all participants in the New York High Risk Project, which is a study of the developmental outcomes for the children of schizophrenics.

Moldin, Gottesman, and Erlenmeyer-Kimling (1987a,b) began by testing the power of each of a large number of MMPI indicators to discriminate 31 patients, who included 14 schizophrenic and 17 schizoaffective patients who were mainly schizophrenic, from affectively disordered patients and normal control subjects. Using a variety of statistical procedures, the investigators selected 13 MMPI candidate indicators of schizophrenia that were prominent in the literature and had proved most successful in distinguishing schizophrenics from nonschizophrenics in their own studies. These indicators were scales L, F, K, and 4; a linear combination of scales 2, 7, 8, and 0; the Paranoid Schizophrenia Scale (Pz, Rosen, 1962); the 8-6 scale pattern; and six Wiggins (1966) Content Scales – namely, Social Maladjustment, Religious Fundamentalism, Psychoticism, Phobias, Manifest Hostility, and Hypomania.

Moldin et al. (1990a) administered these scales to 35 offspring of schizophrenic parents, 43 offspring of affectively disordered parents, and 93 control offspring of normal parents. Presumably many, or all, of the parents were the same subjects whose performance had aided in the selection of the 13 indicators. The investigators performed a series of sophisticated analyses to distinguish the groups. They computed for each subject a deviancy score on each variable (with the effects of age, gender, and social class regressed out) and assigned the subject a score of "1" if the score fell in the deviant upper 5% for normal subjects, or a zero if it did not. Summing across the 13 indicators, this procedure yielded, for each subject, a total deviancy score that ranged from 0 to 13. The investigators found that a cutoff score of "3" on total deviancy identified 23% of the offspring of schizophrenics, 7% of the offspring of affectively disordered patients, and 2% of the offspring of normal control subjects. Thus, the combined score appears to be a valid indicator of schizophrenia proneness.

In a second publication, Moldin et al. (1990b), using the same subjects, performed an elegant admixture analysis. They used the sum of the residual scores on the 13 indicators to plot the distribution of a combined score of the 13 indicators for 171 subjects from the three groups: the offspring of schizophrenics, of affectively disordered subjects, and of normal control subjects. The distribution appeared bimodal. Use of the admixture analysis allowed the scores to be separated into two classes and yielded a nonarbitrary cutoff between deviant and nondeviant subjects. Seventeen percent of the offspring of schizophrenics, 7% of the offspring of affectively disordered patients, and 2% of the normal control group were identified as deviant. Six of the 11 deviant subjects were offspring of schizophrenics. Moreover, three of the deviant subjects who were offspring of schizophrenics already showed, in their early twenties, either schizophrenia or schizophrenia-spectrum illness.

Comment

The finding that the children were identified as deviant using the indicators derived from study of their parents may lack generality for the relation of the indicators to schizotypy. After all, patterns of performance on these scales would be expected to be similar in parents and children as a result of both genetic and environmental factors. If, instead, the original selection had been based on indices discovered using patients not related to the children, then one could have ruled out the possibility that the results were due to the correlation between the parents' and children's performance. Also, the number of schizophrenic parents was small and the number of candidate measures was large, so that the investigators may have capitalized on chance in the selection of some indicators and may have overlooked other indicators. Despite these limitations, the methodology is appealing in its elegance and its sophistication, and the 13 scales do enjoy some face validity. It is important to test these indicators on samples other than the children of the patients on whom the indicators were derived. Regardless of the outcome, the innovative methodological approach of these studies should be a valuable addition to the tools of investigators of schizotypal signs.

Schizoidia Scale

Schizoidia, in Meehl's usage, is the underlying syndrome that gives rise to schizotypal symptoms. In response to the apparent insensitivity of the various traditional MMPI indicators of schizotypy, Golden and Meehl (1979) proposed a radically different approach. Using elegant taxometric theory and methods, they derived a seven-item scale from the MMPI item pool. The authors based their selection of the seven items in part on the statistical power of the items to discriminate between schizophrenics and nonschizophrenics. Their theory required them to seek items that are independent of one another – that is, that have low interitem correlations in a sample in which schizotypal and nonschizotypal subjects are not intermixed. They pointed out that a small number of items that are not correlated with one another, but yet are correlated with the criterion, can together have a high validity. In addition, the investigators required that each item not be correlated with decompensation variables such as severity of illness, and that the items not discriminate highly among diagnosed subtypes of schizophrenia or among other psychoses. The seven items are:

I have not lived the right kind of life. (True)
I have been disappointed in love. (True)
My sex life is satisfactory. (False)
I am more sensitive than most other people. (True)
I am sure I am being talked about. (True)
I usually work things out for myself rather than get someone to show me how. (False)
I enjoy many different kinds of play and recreation. (False)

In their discussion of the schizoid taxon, Golden and Meehl also advocated the use of the sum of the scores on the MMPI scales 2, 7, 8, and 0 as an index of schizoidia. The investigators computed a factor analysis of the MMPI scales for 211 psychiatric male inpatients with nonpsychotic diagnoses and found that these four scales loaded on a single factor. They suggested that a successful scale of schizoidia should correlate highly with these four scales. They found that the schizoidia scale correlated .81 with a combined score based on these four MMPI scales.

Reliability

Chapman et al. (1982) reported coefficient-alpha values of .16 for male and .27 for female college students on the Schizoidia Scale. These reliability values are very low, but Golden and Meehl, unlike most test developers, deliberately sought low internal consistency. Miller, Streiner, and Kahgee (1982) reported a retest correlation on psychiatric patients of .54 with a mean retest interval of 141 days.

Validity

The Schizoidia Scale has been used in a few studies with mixed results. Miller et al. (1982) investigated whether or not the Schizoidia Scale would differentiate schizophrenics from acutely depressed control patients. The scale failed to do so, as might be expected from its modest retest reliability. Fifty-three percent of the schizophrenics were identified as members of the schizoid taxon, whereas 71% of the nonschizophrenics were so identified. This is not an encouraging finding. Similarly, Nichols and Jones (1985) found that this scale did not discriminate among patients with schizophrenia, affective disorders, and nonpsychotic illnesses. Grove et al. (1991) found that the

Schizoidia Scale failed to discriminate either schizophrenic probands or their relatives from control subjects.

A more positive finding was reported by Raine (1987), from his study of the relation of measures of schizotypy to rated SPD in prisoners. Raine found a significant correlation of .54 for the Schizoidia Scale.

A possible problem with the use of the Schizoidia Scale is that, in its derivation, the final seven items had been presented in the context of the rest of the MMPI items. In subsequent use of the Schizoidia Scale by other investigators, these seven items were apparently usually given in isolation. A context effect might account for some of the inconsistency of findings.

The Schizotypal Personality Questionnaire

Raine (1991) developed the Schizotypal Personality Questionnaire, or SPQ, specifically to measure DSM-III-R (American Psychiatric Association, 1987) schizotypal personality disorder. The questionnaire consists of nine subscales, each of which is designed to correspond to one of the nine symptoms of schizotypal personality disorder that the DSM-III-R manual recommends for use in diagnosis.

Raine obtained most of his items from published questionnaires and interview schedules for schizotypal features but also wrote new items modeled on examples of schizotypal traits in the DSM-III-R manual. After administering a pool of candidate items to 302 undergraduate students, he selected items on the basis of percentage endorsements and item–scale correlations. The final version of the scale consists of 74 items that yield a score on each of 9 subscales – namely, ideas of reference, excessive social anxiety, odd belief or magical thinking, unusual perceptual experiences, odd or eccentric behavior, lack of close friends, odd speech, constricted affect, and suspiciousness. Examples of items are:

I am aware that people notice me when I go out for a meal or to see a film. (True)
I get anxious when meeting people for the first time. (True)
Do you believe in telepathy (mind-reading)? (Yes)
Do everyday things seem unusually large or small? (Yes)

Unfortunately, all of the items are worded so that a "True" or "Yes" response contributes to a high score on the trait measured. As a result, differences in acquiescent response tendencies are expected to be one source of high or low scores on the scale.

Reliability and validity

The available reliability and validity data are on an earlier 66-item version of the scale, rather than on the 74-item scale discussed above. Coefficient-alpha for the entire 66-item SPQ scale was .91, and the alpha values for the 9 subscales ranged from .71 to .78. These are high values for scales of this length.

Using the earlier 66-item version of the scale, the author selected for interview 11 subjects who scored in the top decile of total score and 14 subjects who scored in the bottom decile. Six of the 11 subjects from the top decile were found to qualify for a diagnosis of SPD, whereas none of the 14 low-scoring subjects did so. These findings are strong evidence for the validity of the scale.

Comment

Raine's SPQ should prove to be a valuable tool for research on DSM-III-R SPD. If Raine's finding has generality that about 55% of subjects in the top decile on the SPQ qualify for a clinical diagnosis of DSM-III-R SPD, then any investigator with large samples of college students can easily obtain a sample of subjects with that diagnosis. Also, as Raine (1991) pointed out, the scale should be useful for screening samples of control subjects who are to be compared with patients. Since subjects who volunteer for research are frequently more deviant than the general population, eliminating those volunteers who are schizotypal should improve the sensitivity of comparisons of schizophrenic and normal control subjects.

Scales developed in our own laboratory

We developed scales to measure five traits or symptoms of schizophrenia proneness. The scales were based on Meehl's (1964) description of schizotypy and Hoch and Cattell's (1959) description of pseudoneurotic schizophrenia. We started this research in the late 1960s as a study of schizophrenia proneness but switched to focus more broadly on psychosis proneness both because of our findings and because of the narrowing of the diagnostic category of schizophrenia in DSM-III.

Descriptions of the five scales

The Physical Anhedonia Scale

The Revised Physical Anhedonia Scale (PhyAnh), described in Chapman et al. (1976), consists of 61 true–false items that inquire about the sensory and aesthetic pleasures of taste, touch, sex, temperature, movement, smell, sight, and sound. Examples of items are:

I have always loved having my back massaged. (False)
I have never found a thunderstorm exhilarating. (True)
The beauty of sunsets is greatly overrated. (True)
Sex is okay, but not as much fun as most people claim it is. (True)

The Perceptual Aberration Scale

The 35-item Perceptual Aberration Scale (PerAb), described in Chapman, Chapman, and Raulin (1978), consists of 28 items designed to tap grossly schizophrenic-like distortions in the perception of one's own body and 7 items for other perceptual distortions. Representative items are:

Parts of my body occasionally seem dead or unreal. (True)
Sometimes I have had the feeling that I'm united with an object near me. (True)
My hands or feet have never seemed far away. (False)

The Magical Ideation Scale

The 30-item Magical Ideation Scale (MagicId), described by Eckblad and Chapman (1983), measures belief in forms of causation that by conventional standards of our dominant culture are regarded as invalid and magical. Most of the items inquire about the subject's interpretation of his or her personal experiences rather than mere belief in magical forms of causation. The experiences include common superstitions, thought transmission, precognition, spirit influences, ideas of reference, the transfer of psychic energies between people, and other schizophrenic-like deviant beliefs. Several, but not all, of these experiences receive some subcultural support.

Representative items are:

I almost never dream about things before they happen. (False)
I have sometimes felt that strangers were reading my mind. (True)
It is not possible to harm others merely by thinking bad thoughts about them. (False)
I have sometimes had the momentary feeling that someone's place has been taken by a look-alike. (True)

MagicId and PerAb were found to correlate .68 for males ($N = 2{,}500$) and .70 for females ($N = 3{,}067$) (Chapman et al., 1982). Therefore, high-scoring subjects on the two scales were combined into a single group which we refer to as the Perceptual Aberration–Magical Ideation (Per-Mag) group.

The Impulsive Nonconformity Scale

The 51-item Impulsive Nonconformity Scale (NonCon), described by Chapman et al. (1984), was designed to reveal a failure of incorporation of societal norms, a lack of empathy for the pain of others, and an unrestrained yielding to impulse and self-gratification. We initially relied on Eysenck and Eysenck's (1975) Psychoticism Scale. However, preliminary work (Chapman et al., 1984) suggested that psychotic-like symptoms were related to the impulsive and nonconforming items, but not the sadistic and paranoid items. Further, the reliability of the Psychoticism Scale was quite low. Therefore, Chapman et al. (1984) devised the NonCon Scale with the goal of including the kinds of items in the Eysencks' scale that relate best to psychotic-like symptoms. Representative items are:

When I want something, delays are unbearable. (True)
I would probably purchase stolen merchandise if I knew it was safe. (True)
I always stop at red lights. (False)

The Revised Social Anhedonia Scale

The 40-item Revised Social Anhedonia Scale (SocAnh) measures schizoid indifference to other people. Our project's original Social Anhedonia Scale (Chapman et al., 1976) included items that reflected social anxiety and hypersensitivity as well as schizoid withdrawal. Because the original version of this scale was not predictive of psychotic-like and schizotypal symptoms, Eckblad et al. (1982) revised the scale to eliminate items reflecting social anxiety and to add new items tapping schizoid asociality. The resulting Revised Social Anhedonia Scale was found to relate substantially to psychotic-like experiences and schizotypal symptoms (Mishlove & Chapman, 1985). Representative items are:

Having close friends is not as important as many people say. (True)
Just being with friends can make me feel really good. (False)
In many ways, I prefer the company of pets to the company of people. (True)

Scale development

The development of these questionnaires followed, for the most part, the sequential steps that D. N. Jackson (1970) recommended for general use in personality scale development. We prepared a formal trait specification for each symptom to help ensure that each scale bears a high congruence with the trait as specified by various clinical writers. This was an essay describing the characteristics of people who have this symptom or trait. The trait specification was given to item writers, together with a statement of characteristics of good items.

Groups of several hundred subjects each were used to screen items for gender bias, discriminant validity, social desirability, acquiescence, and for frequency of endorsement. Items were altered or dropped if answered by more than 95% of the subjects in the normal direction or by more than 80% in the direction of a high score on the trait. Most of the retained items have less than 50% response in the direction of a high score on the trait. We preferred items with a low trait-endorsement frequency because they maximize discriminations at the high end of the traits scales, where schizotypes are expected to score. Different investigators have based their scale construction on different theories of schizotypy. Many of the investigators whose scales we have reviewed, like Eysenck, consider schizophrenia, schizotypy, and normality to lie on a continuum. Others, following the lead of Meehl, consider schizotypy and normality to be discontinuous, with schizotypy arising genetically. These different theories yield different psychometric approaches to the measurement of schizotypy.

Those investigators who follow a continuity model usually seek a questionnaire that yields a normal distribution of scores, with the average item endorsement centered near 50%. Test theory indicates that scales such as these have their point of maximal discrimination among subjects in the middle of the range of the dimension studied and have poorer discrimination among subjects who are very high or very low on the dimension. Scales of this type yield a metric that is useful for investigating correlates of the dimension in a normal sample. The scores are amenable to correlational analysis and factor analysis but are not optimally discriminating of extremely deviant subjects.

The alternative view, which considers schizotypy to be a discrete category discontinuous with normality, encourages a different approach to scale construction. When the purpose of the scale is to select subjects who are extremely deviant on the dimension, the desired point of maximal discrimination is toward the deviant end of the scale. If, for example, one wishes to identify the top 10% of the population on a dimension, items with median item endorsement of around 10%, rather than 50%, should be used. A scale constructed in this fashion yields a very skewed distribution that is less suitable for correlational analysis and factor analysis. In our research, we have been concerned with the identification of subjects who are at risk for psychosis, and thus we have constructed scales designed to discriminate at the upper end of the dimensions studied.

Screening for discriminant validity

Ever since Campbell and Fiske's (1959) classic article on discriminant validity, one criterion for validity of a test has been a higher correlation of a scale with other measures of the same trait than with measures of different traits. Jackson (1970) has pointed out that this criterion is most reasonably invoked at the item selection stage rather than after the scale is completed. Accordingly, the correlation of each item on a given scale was computed with scores on scales measuring other traits, with the requirement that the item correlate more highly with its own scale than with any other scale. Items were also dropped that lacked a substantial correlation with the whole scale. The correlation was also computed between each item and an independent measure of the need to represent oneself in a socially desirable light, such as the Crowne–Marlowe (1964) Social Desirability Scale. Items that did not correlate higher with their own scale than with the Social Desirability Scale were dropped. Items were also dropped when gender markedly influenced either frequency of endorsement or susceptibility to social desirability bias.

Screening items for acquiescence bias

We omitted items that correlated highly with an independent measure of acquiescence, such as Jackson and Messick's (1962) DY-3 scale of acquiescence. We found that such items tended to be vaguely worded and that the correlation could be reduced by making the wording more specific.

Reliabilities of the five scales

The coefficient-alpha measures of reliability for the NonCon, MagicId, PerAb, PhyAnh, and SocAnh scales, for very large groups of college students, ranged from .79 to .89, whereas test–retest reliabilities ranged from .75 to .84 (Chapman et al., 1982; Mishlove & Chapman, 1985).

Validity of the five scales

We do not review here our earlier published findings concerning scale validity because that evidence is superseded by the recent 10-year follow-up study of Chapman et al. (1994). This follow-up study, described below, includes data on psychotic decompensation which is the best available evidence on psychosis proneness.

The 10-year follow-up study

Subjects

The psychosis-proneness screening questionnaires were administered to approximately 7,800 undergraduate students enrolled in introductory psychology courses at the University of Wisconsin–Madison during the late 1970s and early 1980s. Subjects who scored deviantly high on the PhyAnh, PerAb, MagicId, or NonCon were invited to participate in the study. We also included an additional group of 33 subjects who did not qualify for deviancy on any one scale but earned a high combined sum of the z scores of the four scales. We chose as control subjects persons whose scores were lower than one-half of a standard deviation above the mean on each of the four scales. SocAnh was not used to select subjects, although scores were obtained for all subjects on the scale.

Subjects were interviewed shortly after identification, again two years later, and finally at a 10-year follow-up. We reinterviewed 95% of our original 534 subjects at the 10-year assessment.

Materials

The follow-up evaluation consisted of a diagnostic interview which included assessment of overall functioning, psychosis, and psychotic-like experiences, schizophrenia-spectrum personality disorders, mood disorders, mental health treatment, and family psychopathology.

The Interview measure of psychotic-like experiences

We expected that psychosis-prone subjects would demonstrate transient and milder forms of the symptoms of psychotic patients. In order to measure such psychotic-like experiences, Chapman and Chapman (1980) developed a scoring manual that provides for ratings of experiences on an 11-point continuum of deviancy covering the range from normal to severely psychotic. The manual provides scoring criteria for six broad classes of psychotic and psychotic-like experiences. These include (1) transmission of thoughts, (2) passivity experiences, (3) voice experiences and other auditory hallucinations, (4) thought withdrawal, (5) other personally relevant aberrant beliefs, and (6) aberrant visual experiences. Scoring an experience as psychotic in this system does not necessarily mean that the person is clinically psychotic in the DSM-III-R sense but, rather, that the person has had the kind of experience that characterizes clinical psychosis. Although this rating scale gives scores for both psychotic-like experiences and full-blown psychotic experiences, we refer to it, for convenience of exposition, as a scale for psychotic-like experiences. We assessed deviancy of each subject's psychotic-like experiences by his or her single highest (most deviant) psychotic-like experience score.

We hypothesized in advance of data collection that subjects who reported at the initial interview at least one experience that was rated at least moderately psychotic-like (score of "4" or above) would show an elevated incidence at follow-up of both psychosis and other indications of psychosis proneness.

Results

The full findings of this longitudinal study are reported by Chapman et al. (1994). We report here a summary of those findings.

Prediction of psychosis at 10-year follow-up

Fourteen subjects reported a history of DSM-III-R psychosis at the follow-up interview. Thirteen of these experienced their first clinical psychosis during the follow-up period, and one Per-Mag subject had developed a psychosis during adolescence but did not reveal it until the follow-up interview. Table 5.1 displays the group membership and diagnosis of the psychotic subjects. Only the Per-Mag group significantly exceeded the control group on the frequency of clinical psychosis.

The three Per-Mag subjects listed in Table 5.1 as suffering from DSM-III-R Psychosis Not Otherwise Specified (NOS) all had developed full-fledged schizophrenic syndromes of several years' duration except for deterioration of functioning. All three subjects reported bizarre delusions, hallucinations, and other schizophrenic symptoms as pervasive features of everyday life. Two of them reported passivity experiences. Nevertheless, all three maintained responsible employment and none had been hospitalized for psychosis. Three other subjects (all Per-Mags) were labeled as possibly psychotic.

Prediction of psychosis in relatives

The percentage of subjects in each group who reported clinical psychosis in one or more relatives of either first or second degree were Per-Mag, 15%; NonCon, 6%; PhyAnh, 9%; Combined Score, 6%; and Control, 7%. Only the Per-Mag group differed significantly from the control group ($p < .05$).

Table 5.1. *DSM-III-R psychoses found at 10-year follow-up in each of five groups*

	Per-Mag (n = 182)	NonCon (n = 71)	PhyAnh (n = 70)	Combined score (n = 32)	Control (n = 153)
Schizophrenia	3	0	1	0	1
Psychosis NOS	3	0	0	0	0
Delusional dis.	1	0	0	0	0
Bipolar	3	0	0	0	0
Major depression	0	0	1	0	1
Total	10	0	2	0	2

Mood disorder

The five groups were compared on rates of DSM-III-R major depression. The percentage of each group who reported major depression at follow-up was Per-Mag, 35%; NonCon, 32%; PhyAnh, 16%; Combined Score, 16%; and Control, 20%. Only the Per-Mag group differed significantly from the control group. Similarly, the Per-Mag group exceeded the control group on the proportion of subjects who developed DSM-III-R mania or hypomania.

Improvement of prediction of psychosis by use of initial psychotic-like experiences

Psychosis was found at the follow-up in 9 of the 66 Per-Mag subjects with moderately psychotic-like experiences (rating of "4" or more) at the first interview, as compared to only 1 of the 125 Per-Mag subjects with low psychotic-like experiences (rating of 1 to 3). (For this analysis, we included in the Per-Mag group 9 subjects whose primary group was NonCon but who also qualified for the Per-Mag group.) The difference was significant. Those individuals with initial moderately high psychotic-like experiences were also more deviant at the follow-up on both psychotic-like experiences, and schizotypal dimensional score.

Psychotic-like experiences at follow-up

The above results support the validity of our measure of psychotic-like experiences at the first interview as an indicator of psychosis proneness and supports the use of psychotic-like experiences at the 10-year interview as an additional outcome measure of psychosis proneness. At both interviews, the Per-Mag group and the NonCon group significantly exceeded the control group on ratings of most deviant psychotic-like experience.

Prediction of schizophrenia spectrum personality disorders at follow-up

The Personality Disorder Examination (PDE) interview (Loranger, 1988) was used to assess schizotypal, schizoid, and paranoid personality disorders at follow-up. None of the experimental groups differed from the control group on rate of such diagnoses. However, the PDE dimensional scores did yield differences between groups. The Per-Mag group was found to exceed the control group on both schizotypal and paranoid dimensional score, whereas the NonCon group exceeded the Control group on paranoid dimensional score.

Studying only the Per-Mag subjects, we performed a hierarchical regression analysis using the independent variables of psychotic-like experiences at first interview, PerAb, MagicId, NonCon, SocAnh, and report of psychotic relatives, and using the PDE schizotypal dimensional score as the dependent variable. The significant predictors were the subject's psychotic-like experiences from the first interview, MagicId, SocAnh, and psychotic relatives.

A second regression analysis was computed with the same seven independent variables but using psychotic-like experiences at follow-up as the dependent variable. The same significant predictors were found as for schizotypal dimensional score. The subjects who were most deviant on either of these dependent variables at follow-up were those who were high at the initial interview on all three psychotic-like experiences, MagicId, and SocAnh.

A search for deviant subgroups within the Per-Mag group

We examined the scores of the Per-Mag subjects to see if there might be a pattern that distinguishes those who became psychotic. Eight of the 10 Per-Mag subjects who were found clinically psychotic at follow-up initially had high scores (standard score of 1.96 or greater) on MagicId. Four had high scores on PerAb, but all 4 of these also had high scores on MagicId. Thus, MagicId appears to predict better than PerAb, although the groups were too small to test this statistically.

Seven of the 8 psychotic subjects who had high scores on MagicId also had SocAnh scores above the mean of the total group tested (score of 7). There were, altogether, 33 subjects who scored that high on both MagicId and SocAnh (MagicId–SocAnh group). This group's 21% psychosis rate compares with 5% for the total Per-Mag group, 14% for those who both were high on Per-Mag and reported moderately psychotic-like experiences at the first interview, and 1.3% for the control group.

The combination of MagicId and SocAnh is not, however, a predictor of general psychopathology. A regression analysis was computed using depression at the follow-up as the dependent variable and with independent variables of PerAb, MagicId, NonCon, PhyAnh, SocAnh, and initial interview scores for rated depression, number of schizotypal signs, and psychotic-like symptoms. The only significant predictors were initial rated depression, NonCon, and number of schizotypal signs, all of which had a positive relationship.

Discussion

The findings strongly support the validity of the Perceptual Aberration, Magical Ideation, and Social Anhedonia Scales as indicators of psychosis proneness. At 10-year follow-up, the Per-Mag subjects exceeded control subjects on measures of psychosis proneness, including DSM-III-R psychosis, reports of psychotic relatives, schizotypal dimensional score, and psychotic-like experiences. The high scores at follow-up on these latter two measures indicate that psychosis proneness is an enduring characteristic even in many subjects who have not become psychotic. Psychotic-like experiences of at least moderate deviancy at initial interview are also an excellent indicator of psychosis proneness.

Despite our encouraging findings, we do not know what portion of any of our groups are genuinely psychosis prone; that is, we do not know the valid positive and false positive rates. These rates cannot be determined by the portion who actually became psychotic by the time of the 10-year follow-up. The genetic literature shows clearly that many genetically psychosis-prone subjects never became psychotic (Gottesman, 1991; Gottesman & Bertelsen, 1989). Moreover, our subjects have not yet passed through their entire age of risk. Exactly what portion of risk remains at their mean age of 30.0 is difficult to estimate. Presumably, the number of psychotics in our sample will eventually be much higher than found thus far.

Our finding that subjects whom we originally identified as hypothetically schizophrenia prone developed mood psychoses as well as schizophrenia was unexpected from the formulations of both Meehl (1964, 1973, 1990, 1993) and of Hoch and Cattell (1959). The finding is not inconsistent, however, with recent research evidence on the correlates of schizotypal symptoms. Schizotypal symptoms have been found to be as elevated in the first-degree relatives of mood-disordered patients as in those of schizophrenics (Squires-Wheeler, Skodol, Bassett, & Erlenmeyer-Kimling, 1989; Squires-Wheeler, Skodol, Friedman, & Erlenmeyer-Kimling, 1988). Conversely, mood disorder has been reported to be elevated in the first-degree relatives of schizotypal patients (Bornstein, Klein, Mallon, & Slater, 1988; Schulz, Schulz, Goldberg, Ettigi, Resnick, & Friedel, 1986). The results can also be seen as consistent with Crow's (1990) unitary psychosis theory as well as with Taylor's (1992) contention that schizophrenia and mood psychoses are not genetically distinguishable. On the other hand, it is possible that these two major psychoses are indeed distinct but that we have failed to measure the difference between their predispositions.

The PhyAnh Scale does not appear useful for predicting either psychosis or psychosis proneness. Neither did the NonCon scale predict psychosis at the 10-year follow-up nor did it relate to psychotic relatives. Thus, the NonCon scale appears to have only a modest relationship to psychosis proneness even though NonCon subjects differed from control subjects on psychotic-like symptoms.

Subjects who were deviant on MagicId and also above the mean on SocAnh had a high rate (21%) of clinical psychosis and exceeded the remaining Per-Mag subjects on psychotic-like experiences and on schizotypal dimensional score but not on reports of psychotic relatives. However, the extreme deviancy of this subgroup must be regarded as tentative because of the possibility that these findings capitalized on chance. Their special deviancy was not hypothesized. Scores on MagicId and SocAnh were, instead, chosen on the basis of their observed relationship to clinical psychosis, and their power to predict psychosis and psychosis proneness was tested on the same data that yielded the pairing of the two scores.

Cross-sectional research should be conducted to attempt to cross-validate the greater psychosis proneness of the MagicId–SocAnh subgroup than of other Per-Mag subjects. Substantial supporting data are possible without awaiting the results of an additional longitudinal study.

Directions for future research

Attempts to use questionnaires to measure proneness to schizophrenia or to psychosis have achieved a measure of success that encourages vigorous pursuit of the best possible measure or set of measures. Factor-analytic studies show that many of the instruments measure the same trait, and so most likely have some relationship to psychosis proneness. Although follow-up data are available only for our own scales, we would speculate that all of the scales that measure "positive trait schizotypy" may predict psychosis, rather than schizophrenia in particular. Factor analysis does not, however, indicate which questionnaire is most effective for identifying psychosis-prone persons. More studies are needed of multiple measures used with the same group of subjects. Although the best evidence for psychosis proneness is follow-up data on decompensation into psychosis, other strongly suggestive data are interviews for schizotypal symptoms, performance on some laboratory tasks, and biological correlates of schizotypy, such as smooth-pursuit eye tracking or brain structure anomalies.

The finding of a 21% psychosis rate in the MagicId–SocAnh group, and the fact that other researchers (Venables, Chapter 6, this volume) find that the two scales load on different factors, indicate that a syndromal approach to the identification of the psychosis prone may be superior to measurement of a factorially pure single trait. Traits that may have little relation to one another in the normal population may combine to produce an especially great susceptibility to psychosis.

In seeking traits for a potential syndrome of psychosis proneness, we prefer to test diverse traits, one at a time, rather than relying solely on the syndrome described in a diagnostic manual. The preferred criteria for schizotypal personality disorder are controversial and the list of criteria in the DSM-III-R manual represents the impressions of an expert committee rather than solid research evidence. For example, the list of criteria in the DSM-III-R manual includes social anxiety but not social anhedonia. Mishlove and Chapman (1985) found that social anhedonia predicts psychotic-like symptoms much better than does social anxiety. The findings of our follow-up study indicate that social anhedonia is very useful for predicting psychosis. Social anhedonia and social anxiety are easily confused because they both lead to the avoidance of other people. While we would not doubt that schizotypal persons are anxious, social anxiety is such a widespread symptom accompanying so many clinical syndromes that it is not at all specific to SPD.

Raine's (1991) SPQ is a powerful and useful research tool. If the scale's high hit rate holds up in a cross-validation study using a larger sample, it offers a means of rapid identification of persons who qualify for the diagnosis of DSM-III-R SPD. However, the DSM-III-R formal specification of this diagnostic category should not become the sole focus of research on the topic. It is not yet known how schizophrenia prone or how psychosis prone are persons who meet the DSM-III-R criteria for this diagnosis. It is also likely that future diagnostic manuals will be influenced by any new research findings concerning the traits of the psychosis prone.

Acknowledgments

This research was supported by Research Grant MH-31067 and by a Research Scientist Award to the second author, both from the National Institute of Mental Health.

References

American Psychiatric Association (1987). *DSM-III-R: Diagnostic and statistical manual of mental disorders* (3rd ed., rev.). Washington, DC: Author.

Bishop, D. V. M. (1977). The P scale and psychosis. *Journal of Abnormal Psychology, 86,* 127–134.

Block, J. (1977). P scale and psychosis: Continued concerns. *Journal of Abnormal Psychology, 86,* 431–434.

Bornstein, R. F., Klein, D. N., Mallon, J. C., & Slater, J. F. (1988). Schizotypal personality disorder in an outpatient population: Incidence and clinical characteristics. *Journal of Clinical Psychology, 44,* 322–325.

Cadoret, R. J. (1978). Psychopathology in adopted-away offspring of biologic parents with antisocial behavior. *Archives of General Psychiatry, 35,* 176–184.

Campbell, D. T., & Fiske, D. W. (1959). Convergent and discriminant validation by the multi trait–multi method matrix. *Psychological Bulletin, 56,* 81–105.

Chapman, L. J., & Chapman, J. P. (1980). Scales for rating psychotic and psychotic-like experiences as continua. *Schizophrenia Bulletin, 6,* 476–489.

Chapman, L. J., Chapman, J. P., Kwapil, T. R., Eckblad, M., & Zinser, M. C. (1994). Putatively psychosis prone subjects ten years later. *Journal of Abnormal Psychology, 103,* 171–183.

Chapman, L. J., Chapman, J. P., & Miller, E. N. (1982). Reliabilities and intercorrelations of eight measures of proneness to psychosis. *Journal of Consulting and Clinical Psychology, 50,* 187–195.

Chapman, L. J., Chapman, J. P., Numbers, J. S., Edell, W. S., Carpenter, B. N., & Beckfield, D. (1984). Impulsive nonconformity as a trait contributing to the prediction of psychoticlike and schizotypal symptoms. *Journal of Nervous and Mental Disease, 172,* 681–691.

Chapman, L. J., Chapman, J. P., & Raulin, M. L. (1976). Scales for physical and social anhedonia. *Journal of Abnormal Psychology, 85,* 374–382.

Chapman, L. J., Chapman, J. P., & Raulin, M. L. (1978). Body image aberration in schizophrenia. *Journal of Abnormal Psychology, 87,* 399–407.

Claridge, G., & Broks, P. (1984). Schizotypy and hemisphere function – I: Theoretical considerations and the measurement of schizotypy. *Personality and Individual Differences, 5,* 633–648.

Claridge, G., & Hewitt, J. K. (1987). A biometrical study of schizotypy in a normal population. *Personality and Individual Differences, 8,* 303–312.

Claridge, G., Robinson, D. L., & Birchall, P. (1983). Characteristics of schizophrenics' and neurotics' relatives. *Personality and Individual Differences, 4,* 651–664.

Crow, T. J. (1990). Nature of the genetic contribution to psychotic illness – a continuum viewpoint. *Acta Psychiatrica Scandinavica, 81,* 401–408.

Crowe, R. R. (1972). The adopted offspring of women criminal offenders: A study of their arrest records. *Archives of General Psychiatry, 27,* 600–603.

Crowe, R. R. (1974). An adoption study of antisocial personality. *Archives of General Psychiatry, 31,* 785–791.

Crowne, D. P., & Marlowe, D. (1964). *The approval motive.* New York: Wiley.

Davis, H. (1974). What does the P scale measure? *British Journal of Psychiatry, 125,* 161–167.

Eckblad, M., & Chapman, L. J. (1983). Magical ideation as an indicator of schizotypy. *Journal of Consulting and Clinical Psychology, 51,* 215–225.

Eckblad, M., Chapman, L. J., Chapman, J. P., & Mishlove, M. (1982). The Revised Social Anhedonia Scale. Unpublished test (copies available from authors), University of Wisconsin, Madison, Wis.

Edell, W. S. (in press). The psychometric measurement of schizotypy using the Wisconsin Scales of Psychosis Proneness. In G. A. Miller (Ed.), *The behavioral high-risk paradigm in psychopathology.* New York: Springer-Verlag.

Eysenck, H. J. (1992). The definition and measurement of psychoticism. *Personality and Individual Differences, 13,* 757–785.

Eysenck, H. J., & Eysenck, S. B. G. (1976). *Psychoticism as a dimension of personality.* London: Hodder and Stoughton.

Eysenck, S. B. G., & Eysenck, H. J. (1975). *Manual of the Eysenck Personality Questionnaire.* London: Hodder and Stoughton.

Fowler, R. C., & Tsuang, M. T. (1975). Spouses of schizophrenics: A blind comparative study. *Comprehensive Psychiatry, 16,* 339–342.

Golden, R. R., & Meehl, P. E. (1979). Detection of the schizoid taxon with MMPI indicators. *Journal of Abnormal Psychology, 88,* 217–233.

Gottesman, I. I. (1991). *Schizophrenia genesis: The origins of madness.* New York: Freeman.

Gottesman, I. I., & Bertelsen, A. (1989). Confirming unexpressed genotypes for schizophrenia: Risks in the offspring of Fischer's Danish identical and fraternal twins. *Archives of General Psychiatry, 46,* 867–872.

Grove, W. M. (1982). Psychometric detection of schizotypy. *Psychological Bulletin, 92,* 27–38.

Grove, W. M., Lebow, B. S., Clementz, B. A., Cerri, A., Medus, C., & Iacono, W. G. (1991). Familial prevalence and coaggregation of schizotypy indicators: A multitrait family study. *Journal of Abnormal Psychology, 100,* 115–121.

Heston, L. L. (1966). Psychiatric disorders in foster home reared children of schizophrenic mothers. *British Journal of Psychiatry, 112,* 819–825.

Hoch, P. H., & Cattell, J. P. (1959). The diagnosis of pseudoneurotic schizophrenia. *Psychiatric Quarterly, 33,* 17–43.

Hutchings, B., & Mednick, S. A. (1975). Registered criminality in the adoptive and biological parents of registered male criminal adoptees. In R. R. Fieve, D. Rosenthal, & H. Brill (Eds.), *Genetic research in psychiatry.* Baltimore: Johns Hopkins University Press.

Jackson, D. N. (1970). A sequential system for personality scale development. In C. D. Spielberger (Ed.), *Current topics in clinical and community psychology,* (Vol. 2, pp. 61–96). New York: Academic Press.

Jackson, D. N., & Messick, S. (1962). Response styles on the MMPI: Comparison of clinical and normal samples. *Journal of Abnormal and Social Psychology, 65,* 285–299.

Jackson, M., & Claridge, G. (1991). Reliability and validity of a psychotic traits questionnaire (STQ). *British Journal of Clinical Psychology, 30,* 311–323.

Kallmann, F. J. (1938). *The genetics of schizophrenia.* New York: Augustin.

Launay, G., & Slade, P. (1981). The measurement of hallucinatory predisposition in male and female prisoners. *Personality and Individual Differences, 2,* 221–234.

Loranger, A. W. (1988). *Personality Disorder Examination (PDE) manual.* Yonkers, N.Y.: DV Communications.

Meehl, P. E. (1964). *Manual for use with checklist of schizotypic signs.* Unpublished manuscript, University of Minnesota.

Meehl, P. E. (1973). *Psychodiagnosis: Selected papers.* Minneapolis: University of Minnesota Press.

Meehl, P. E. (1990). Toward an integrated theory of schizotaxia, schizotypy, and schizophrenia. *Journal of Personality Disorders, 4,* 1–99.

Meehl, P. E. (1993). The origins of some of my conjectures concerning schizophrenia. In L. J. Chapman, J. P. Chapman, & D. C. Fowles (Eds.), *Progress in experimental personality & psychopathology research* (Vol. 16, pp. 1–10). New York: Springer Publishing.

Miller, G. A., & Yee, C. M. (1994). Risk for severe psychopathology: Psychometric screening and psychophysiological assessment. In P. K. Ackles, J. R. Jennings, & M. G. H. Coles (Eds.), *Advances in Psychophysiology* (Vol. 5, pp. 1–54). London: Jessica Kingsley.

Miller, H. R., Streiner, D. L., & Kahgee, S. L. (1982). Use of the Golden–Meehl Indicators in the detection of schizoid-taxon membership. *Journal of Abnormal Psychology, 91,* 55–60.

Mishlove, M., & Chapman, L. J. (1985). Social anhedonia in the prediction of psychosis proneness. *Journal of Abnormal Psychology, 94,* 384–396.

Moldin, S. O., Gottesman, I. I., & Erlenmeyer-Kimling, L. (1987a). Psychometric validation of psychiatric diagnoses in the New York High-Risk Study. *Psychiatry Research, 22,* 159–177.

Moldin, S. O., Gottesman, I. I., & Erlenmeyer-Kimling, L. (1987b). Searching for the psychometric boundaries of schizophrenia: Evidence from the New York High-Risk Study. *Journal of Abnormal Psychology, 96,* 354–363.

Moldin, S. O., Gottesman, I. I., Erlenmeyer-Kimling, L., & Cornblatt, B. A. (1990a). Psychometric deviance in offspring at risk for schizophrenia: I. Initial delineation of a distinct subgroup. *Psychiatry Research, 32,* 297–310.

Moldin, S. O., Rice, J. P., Gottesman, I. I., & Erlenmeyer-Kimling, L. (1990b). Psychometric deviance in offspring at risk for schizophrenia: II. Resolving heterogeneity through admixture analysis. *Psychiatry Research, 32,* 311–322.

Nichols, D. S., & Jones, R. E. (1985). Identifying schizoid-taxon membership with the Golden–Meehl MMPI items. *Journal of Abnormal Psychology, 94,* 191–194.

Nielsen, T. C., & Petersen, K. E. (1976). Electrodermal correlates of extraversion, trait anxiety and schizophrenism. *Scandinavian Journal of Psychology, 17,* 73–80.

Planansky, K. (1972). Phenotypic boundaries and genetic specificity in schizophrenia. In A. R. Kaplan (Ed.), *Genetic factors in "schizophrenia"* (pp. 141–172). Springfield, Ill.: Charles C Thomas.

Quay, H. C., & Peterson, D. R. (1987). *Manual of the Revised Behavior Problem Checklist.*

Raine, A. (1987). Validation of schizoid personality scales using indices of schizotypal and borderline personality disorder in a criminal population. *British Journal of Clinical Psychology, 26,* 305–309.

Raine, A. (1991). The SPQ: A scale for the assessment of schizotypal personality based on DSM-III-R criteria. *Schizophrenia Bulletin, 17,* 555–564.

Raulin, M. L. (1984). Development of a scale to measure intense ambivalence. *Journal of Consulting and Clinical Psychology, 52,* 63–72.

Raulin, M. L., & Wee, J. L. (1984). The development and initial validation of a scale to measure Social Fear. *Journal of Clinical Psychology, 40,* 780–784.

Rosen, A. (1962). Development of the MMPI scales based on a reference group of psychiatric patients. *Psychological Monographs, 76,* 1.

Rosenthal, D. (1975). Discussion: The concept of subschizophrenic disorders. In R. R. Fieve, D. Rosenthal, & H. Brill (Eds.), *Genetic research in psychiatry* (pp. 199–208). Baltimore: Johns Hopkins University Press.

Rust, J. (1987). The Rust Inventory of Schizoid Cognitions (RISC): A psychometric measure of psychoticism in the normal population. *British Journal of Clinical Psychology, 26,* 151–152.

Rust, J. (1988). The Rust Inventory of Schizotypal Cognitions (RISC). *Schizophrenia Bulletin, 14,* 317–322.

Rust, J. (1989). *Handbook of the Rust Inventory of Schizotypal Cognitions.* London: The Psychological Corporation.

Schulsinger, F. (1974). Psychopathy: Heredity and environment. In S. A. Mednick, F. Schulsinger, J. Higgins, & B. Bell (Eds.), *Genetics, environment, and psychopathology* (pp. 177–195). New York: North-Holland, Elsevier.

Schulz, P. M., Schulz, S. C., Goldberg, S. C., Ettigi, P., Resnick, R. J., & Friedel, R. O. (1986). Diagnoses of the relatives of schizotypal outpatients. *Journal of Nervous and Mental Disease, 174,* 457–463.

Silverton, L. (1988). Crime and the schizophrenia spectrum: A diathesis stress model. *Acta Psychiatrica Scandinavica, 78,* 72–81.

Squires-Wheeler, E., Skodol, A. E., Bassett, A., & Erlenmeyer-Kimling, L. (1989). DSM-III-R schizotypal personality traits in offspring of schizophrenic disorder, affective disorder, and normal control parents. *Journal of Psychiatric Research, 23,* 229–239.

Squires-Wheeler, E., Skodol, A. E., Friedman, D., & Erlenmeyer-Kimling, L. (1988). The specificity of DSM-III schizotypal personality traits. *Psychological Medicine, 18,* 757–765.

Taylor, M. A. (1992). Are schizophrenia and affective disorder related? A selective literature review. *American Journal of Psychiatry, 149,* 22–32.

Venables, P. H., Wilkins, S., Mitchell, D. A., Raine, A., & Bailes, K. (1990). A scale for the measurement of schizotypy. *Personality and Individual Differences, 11,* 481–495.

Venables, P. H. (1990). The measurement of schizotypy in Mauritius. *Personality and Individual Differences, 11,* 965–971.

Walters, G. D. (1983). The MMPI and schizophrenia: A review. *Schizophrenia Bulletin, 9,* 226–246.

Wiggins, J. S. (1966). Substantive dimensions of self-report in the MMPI item pool. *Psychological Monographs, 80,* 1–42.

Zuckerman, M. (1991). *Psychobiology of personality.* Cambridge: Cambridge University Press.

6

Schizotypal status as a developmental stage in studies of risk for schizophrenia

PETER H. VENABLES

This chapter is concerned with the extent to which schizotypal status, which can be considered as productive of risk for later schizophrenia, may be more or less directly related to the type of schizophrenic status that the patient may eventually reach.

This problem may be approached in the first instance by examining the extent to which the divisions of schizophrenic symptomatology have parallels in dimensions of schizotypy. One of the origins of work on schizotypy is the seminal paper of Meehl (1962), who suggested that the common predisposition "schizotaxia" – an "integrative neural defect" (p. 829), "all that can properly be spoken of as inherited" (p. 830) – underlies both schizotypy and schizophrenia. Thus there is in this a clear suggestion that there is a commonality between schizotypy and schizophrenia in that their etiology is similar and, given the appropriate malign circumstances, schizotypy can develop into schizophrenia. It may thus be appropriate to think that the characteristics shown by schizotypics will have some relationship to those shown by schizophrenics, and that where schizotypic status is used as an indicator of increased risk for schizophrenia, the patient may develop the type of schizophrenia that is akin to those schizotypic characteristics shown in the premorbid state.

However, it is permissible to question this proposition, insofar as the characteristics shown by schizophrenics may be the result of growing up with a schizotypal personality which makes the "patient-to-be" less acceptable to his fellows; hence, for instance, the withdrawal shown by the schizophrenic patient may therefore be a secondary reaction to the "oddness" shown in the premorbid state. Another example would be that put forward by Mednick (1958), who suggested in his early theoretical model that it was the positive symptoms that arose secondarily, as a means of lowering the increasing disturbance which the patient felt due to the process of "reciprocal augmentation of anxiety."

It is also likely that the condition in the schizotypic state is not a direct parallel of that shown in the schizophrenic condition, but rather the precursor of that condition. For instance, it is less easy to envisage the possibility that the positive symptoms, hallucinations, and delusions may have parallels in the schizotypic state than it is to consider that negative symptoms, such as poverty of speech, may have direct counterparts in normal behavior. It may thus be that prodromal forms of positive schizophrenic symptoms may be reported as disorders of attention and perception. As the behaviors that result in a person being labeled as a patient are those that the public, or the person him- or herself, finds unacceptable (and these are most often the positive symptoms), it is unlikely that the schizotypic would report fully blown positive symptoms; otherwise by definition he or she would be a patient.

Another viewpoint on this problem is that of Zubin (1985), who, putting forward his "vulnerability theory" (e.g., Zubin & Steinhauer, 1981), makes the following statement: "For the vulnerability theorist, premorbid handicaps are independent (i.e., non–illness related) personality variables that interact with the patient's liability to episodes of schizophrenia" (p. 466). Thus from this standpoint there may be no necessary relation between what is measured premorbidly and the type of schizophrenia eventually shown by the patient.

Both the viewpoint of Meehl and that starting from the data reviewed by Ingraham (Chapter 2, this volume), suggesting that there is a genetic link between schizophrenia and schizotypy, imply a biological predisposition for both concepts, and both have tended, if not explicitly, originally to suggest a unitary view of schizophrenia and schizotypy. However, there are moves away from this unitary idea. For example, Siever and Gunderson (1983) advocated the division of DSM-III schizotypal symptoms into "cognitive–perceptual" and "social–interpersonal" aspects, whereas Kendler, Gruenberg, and Tsuang (1983) suggested a division of schizotypy into positive schizotypal symptoms, which would include magical thinking and illusions and negative schizotypal symptoms, including suspiciousness and social isolation.

Prior to that, much work on schizophrenia questioned its unitary nature, and the idea of "positive" versus "negative" symptomatology (e.g., Andreasen & Olsen, 1982) has become common coinage, although, as Berrios (1985) has shown, the concept has a long history. Furthermore, Crow (1980) has suggested that these two different symptom clusterings (his type 1 and type 2) are based on different etiological foundations: biochemical in the case of type 1, where positive symptoms predominate, and structural in type 2, where negative symptoms are the main characteristic. Taking this bidimensional view of schizophrenia, one could suggest that Meehl's "schizotaxia" may have at least two versions.

Other work has, however, suggested that even the binary division of schizophrenia outlined above is not sufficient. (see below). It is therefore the purpose of this chapter to examine how plausible it is to extend the multidimensional view of schizophrenia, which is gaining credence, into the concept of schizotypy.

The multidimensionality of schizophrenia

Strauss, Carpenter, and Bartko (1974), in a theoretical review, proposed a three-dimensional view of schizophrenia and, with particular relevance to this chapter, stated that "the symptoms of schizophrenia are not specific only to schizophrenia but are related to other human behaviors through continua" (p. 64). They suggested that symptoms could be grouped into three categories: positive symptoms, negative symptoms, and disorders of relating. Subsequent studies all tend to agree on the nature of the first two categories but are less than unanimous on the nature of the third. However, this may be due to the content of the measures entered into the factor analyses that have been carried out to back up this three-dimensional view. Table 6.1 summarizes the findings from those studies to be reviewed which can conveniently be shown together, insofar as they nearly all make use of the Scale for the Assessment of Negative Symptoms (SANS) and, although less consistently, the Scale for the Assessment of Positive Symptoms (SAPS) measures. The exceptions are those of Bilder, Mukherjee, Rieder, and Pandurangi (1985), who use the Schedule for Affective Disorders and Schizophrenia (SADS; Endicott & Spitzer, 1978) scale to derive measures of positive symptoms; and Liddle (1987), who used the Comprehensive Assessment of Symptoms and History (CASH) scale (Andreasen, 1983), which contains the SANS, to measure negative symptoms, and the Present State Examination (PSE; Wing, Cooper, & Sartorius, 1974) to measure positive symptoms. In addition, Liddle and Barnes (1990) used the Manchester scale (Krawiecka, Goldberg, & Vaughan, 1977) to measure positive symptoms.

There is no disagreement among the studies about the existence of a "positive symptom" factor, with the content being centered on the presence of hallucinations and delusions. Although thought disorder and bizarre behavior have loadings on the first factor in Bilder et al.'s analysis, these are low and the major loadings for these items are on the third factor. Thought disorder does not appear as a symptom having a loading on the positive-symptom fac-

Table 6.1. *Summary of results of studies showing a three-factor grouping of schizophrenic symptoms*

	Factors/clusters			
Author(s)	Positive symptom	Negative symptom	Disorganization/ Social impairment	Scale
Strauss et al. (1974)	Delusions, hallucinations, catatonia	Blocking, apathy, blunting of affect	Disorders of relating	See text
Bilder et al. (1985)	Delusions, hallucinations, bizarre behavior, thought disorder	Avolition/apathy, anhedonia, alogia, affective flattening, attentional impairment	Bizarre behavior, thought disorder, alogia, attentional impairment	SADS SANS
Kulhara, Kota, & Joseph (1986)	Delusions, hallucinations	Avolition, anhedonia, alogia, affective flattening, attentional impairment	Bizarre behavior, formal thought disorder, alogia	SANS SAPS
Liddle (1987); Liddle & Barnes (1990)	Delusions of persecution, delusions of reference, voices speak to patient	Poverty of speech, increased speech latency, decreased movement, unchanging facial expression, affective nonresponsivity, lack of vocal inflection, poverty of expressive gesture, poor eye contact	Inappropriate affect, poverty of speech content, tangentiality, derailment, pressure of speech, distractibility	CASH SANS SAPS
Arndt et al. (1991)	Delusions, hallucinations	Avolition, anhedonia, alogia, affective flattening, attentional deficit	Alogia, bizarre behavior, positive thought disorder	SANS SAPS
Lenzenweger et al. (1991)	Positive symptoms	Negative symptoms	Premorbid social impairment	See text
Peralta et al. (1992)[a]	Delusions, hallucinations	Avolition, anhedonia, alogia, affective flattening, poverty of speech content	Inappropriate affect, poverty of speech content, attentional impairment, formal thought disorder	SANS SAPS

[a]Peralta et al. show bizarre behavior as loaded on a fourth factor.

tor in any of the other studies. The second, "negative symptom" factor is consistently characterized by avolition, anhedonia, and affective flattening. There are inconsistencies in the loadings on alogia and attentional impairment, which sometimes appear as loadings on the third "disorganization" factor, which is consistently loaded on thought disorder. In the Bilder et al. (1985) study, the greatest amount of variance is explained by the third factor shown in Table 6.1, and it is this factor that has the highest correlations with scores on neuropsychological tests. The most significant correlations were with tests that measured language and memory performance. It is also to be noted that alogia has a very high loading on this factor. The position of "alogia" is partly but not completely resolved by its division by Liddle (1987) into "poverty of speech" and "poverty of speech content" (see Table 6.1). Miller, Arndt, and Andreasen (1993), however, show clearly that poverty of speech is a negative-symptom item whereas poverty of speech content loads on the disorganization factor.

In contrast to the work reviewed above, a study by Lenzenweger et al. (1991) used scales developed from the SANS and PSE and the Venables–O'Connor Scale for rating paranoid schizophrenia (Venables & O'Connor, 1959). Most importantly, Lenzenweger et al. used the Zigler and Phillips (1960) Social Competence and Premorbid Sexual Adjustment scales to test which of the following views was more appropriate: that embodied in the paper by Strauss et al. (1974), which assumes that disordered social relations characterized a third factor independent of those characterizing positive and negative symptoms; or the alternative, exemplified for instance by Walker and Lewine (1988), that social impairment is associated with negative symptoms. The outcome of testing the data by a latent structure model is that the data are best fitted by a three process model, with disordered premorbid relationships as the third process.

Thus, the problem posed by the material reviewed is whether the third factor exemplified by "disorders of relating" in the theory of Strauss et al. (1974) and the data of Lenzenweger et al. (1991) can be aligned with the "disorganization" characterization of the third factor in the data reviewed in Table 6.1.

One study that directly shows a conjunction between thought disorder and lack of social competence is that of Dworkin et al. (1990). These authors showed that adolescents at risk for schizophrenia had significantly poorer social competence and greater formal thought disorder than controls.

One suggestion for a mechanism linking the two aspects comes from a study by Caplan, Perdue, Tanguay, and Fish (1990), who found that both childhood schizophrenics and children with a diagnosis of schizotypal personality disorder had high thought disorder scores; following Rochester and

Martin (1979), they hypothesized that those with thought disorder have difficulty in taking listeners' needs into consideration, and this difficulty results in social impairment.

The multidimensionality of schizotypy

Although the material from studies on schizophrenia is comparatively easy to organize in a summary fashion, that from studies using schizotypy scales is less so, particularly because in different studies, different selections of scales are analyzed factorially, and as a result, the makeup of factors in any one study can be biased by the common variance available. The comparison of these different studies demonstrates the old issue that the outcome of a factor analysis is determined by the variables that are entered into it. Another problem with all but two studies in the literature is that they are concerned with the factor analysis of scales rather than of items. Thus the analyses inevitably reflect the biases that went into the construction of the scales that may not themselves be unidimensional.

Five relatively recent studies factor-analyze schizotypal scale scores. Of these, three produce results that are not comparable to those from the factor analysis of material from studies of schizophrenics outlined above, whereas the remaining two studies produce results that are comparable. The results of these studies are outlined in Table 6.2; the codes used for the various scales are given at the bottom of the table.

In this table four factors are shown. It is worthwhile dealing with the fourth before continuing with consideration of the remainder, as this is concerned with the position of a dimension whose relation to schizotypy may be seen as controversial. This factor is labeled psychoticism/nonconformity since, in the three studies where it appears, Eysenck's "psychoticism" (P); (Eysenck & Eysenck, 1976) is the identifying variable. Roger and Morris (1991) examined the structure of the EPQ (Eysenck & Eysenck, 1975) and found that the P scale could be broken down into two factors, one concerned with callousness, paranoia, and intolerance, the other with impulsiveness and nonplanning. If one bears in mind this heterogeneity of the P scale, one is not surprised that the factor in the Kendler and Hewitt (1992) study labeled as psychoticism/nonconformity in Table 6.2 should be loaded on impulsive nonconformity (P, NC; Chapman, Chapman, Numbers, Edell, Carpenter, & Beckfield, 1984), physical anhedonia (PA); (Chapman, Chapman, & Raulin, 1976), and finally social anhedonia (SA), possibly reflecting the aspect of P concerned with callousness and intolerance in interaction with people. A similar loading of P and SA together is found in the study by Raine and Allbutt (1989). Less clear is

Table 6.2. *Summary of results of studies factorizing measures of aspects of schizotypy*

	Factors			
	Positive schizotypy (Cognitive–perceptual)	Negative schizotypy (Introverted anhedonia)	Social anxiety aspects of schizotypy	Psychoticism/ Nonconformity
Muntaner et al. (1988)	STA, STB, MI, PAB, N	SA, PA, -E		P, -L STB
Raine & Allbutt (1989)	STA, STB, PAB, LSHS, SZPH			P, SA
Bentall et al. (1989)	STA, STB, MI, PAB, HOP, LSHS, P, -L	SA, PA, -E	STA, STB, PAB, N, SZPH, SZD, -E.	
Kendler & Hewitt (1992)	MI, PAB, LSHS, -PA, CMI, CPAB	SA, CPI, -E	CPAB, CPI, NC, CMI, N.	P, NC, PA, SA
Kelley & Coursey (1992)	STA, MI, PAB, NC, SZPH, 278, SZD, IA, CS, SF	PA, -PAB -MI		

Key: STA & STB, Schizotypy and Borderline scales (Claridge & Brcks, 1984). E, N, P, L, Extraversion, Neuroticism, Psychoticism, and Lie scales (Eysenck & Eysenck, 1975). MI, Magical Ideation Scale (Eckblad & Chapman, 1983). PAB, Perceptual Aberration Scale (Chapman et al., 1978). HOP, Hypomanic Personality Scale (Eckblad & Chapman, 1986). SA, Social Anhedonia Scale; PA, Physical Anhedonia Scale (Chapman et al., 1976). NC, Impulsive Nonconformity Scale (Chapman et al., 1984). SZPH, Schizophrenism Scale (Nielsen & Petersen, 1976). SZD, Schizoidia Scale (Golden & Meehl, 1979). 278, MMPI scales 2, 7, and 8 (Kincannon, 1968). IA, Intense Ambivalence Scale (Raulin, 1984). CS, Cognitive Slippage Scale (Miers & Raulin, 1985). SF, Social Fear Scale (Raulin & Wee 1984). CPAB, CMI, & CPI, Claridge Perceptual Aberration, Magical Ideation, and Paranoid Ideation; subscales of the STA resulting from the analysis of that scale by Hewitt and Claridge (1989); see text.

the conjunction in the study of Muntaner, Garcia-Sevilla, Fernandez, and Torrubia (1988) of P, L (the lie scale from the EPQ), and STB.

In all the five studies shown in Table 6.2, the first factor has loadings on Perceptual Aberration (PAB; Chapman, Chapman, & Raulin, 1978) and Magical Ideation (MI; Eckblad & Chapman, 1983) (except for the Raine & Allbutt, 1989, study, where it was not used). These two scales, combined together as the Per–Mag Scale, have been shown to be most promising for the identification of psychosis-prone individuals (see Chapman, Chapman, & Kwapil, Chapter 5, this volume). It might be noted *en passant* however, that Kendler and Hewitt (1992) have shown in their twin study that MI has a substantial genetic loading whereas PAB does not.

The other scale that appears in the first factor in all but one of the studies (Kendler & Hewitt, 1992, in which it was not used in its unitary form) is the STA scale of Claridge and Broks (1984). This scale was devised to cover the areas of dysfunction outlined in the DSM-III (1980) as schizotypal personality disorder (SPD). However, as the original paper of Spitzer, Endicott, and Gibbon (1979), which led to the definition of SPD, shows, some of the items that can be taken to define SPD are "positive symptom" items whereas others are more concerned with social anxiety. Thus, if the SPD definition is used to produce a single scale, the outcome is likely to be a mixture of these types of items. Thus, it is not surprising that scales, such as the STA, have a mixed content and that in the Bentall, Claridge, and Slade (1989) study, STA has loadings on the first and third factors in Table 6.2.

Three subscales derived from the STA are the results of a factor analysis of the STA carried out by Hewitt and Claridge (1989). This analysis was carried out on the *items* of the STA scale, and produced three factors which the authors name (1) Magical thinking, (2) Unusual perception experiences, and (3) Paranoid ideation and suspiciousness. These three factors are used by Kendler and Hewitt (1992) and are labeled by them as Claridge Magical Ideation (CMI), Claridge Perceptual Aberration (CPAB), and Claridge Paranoid Ideation (CPI).

Returning, therefore, to consideration of the first factor shown in Table 6.2, we note that the scale scores CMI and CPAB are also part of the content of this factor in the Kendler and Hewitt (1992) study.

The other scale that helps with the identification of the first factor is that of Launay and Slade (1981) (LSHS), measuring the tendency to experience hallucinations.

If we take MI, PAB, STA, CMI, CPAB, and LSHS as marker variables, then it would seem reasonable to identify the first factor as embodying cognitive and perceptual disorder or, paralleling the work on schizophrenia, "positive-symptom schizotypy." It should be noted that the factor analysis of Kelley and Coursey (1992) produces virtually only a single factor, and it could be asserted that this first factor is the only factor and represents a unitary schizotypy. It can, however, be argued that this is a result of the set of variables that they choose to analyze – in particular, their use of only a single anhedonia scale, and the omission of the Eysenck and Eysenck (1975) EPQ scale (which they correctly say does not measure schizotypy, per se) – which, in other studies, help to produce variance in common with schizotypy scales in the second, third, and fourth factors in Table 6.2.

There would seem to be little doubt that the second factor may be labeled introverted anhedonia, in that it has negative loadings on E and positive loadings on SA. The position of PA is more equivocal, possibly because, as argued above, it has some relation to P. Insofar as Kirkpatrick and Buchanan (1990) showed that schizophrenics with deficit syndrome had higher scores on PA and SA than nondeficit schizophrenics, and Kendler and colleagues (1991) showed that a factor defined by PA and SA was related to a factor of negative-symptom schizotypy defined by a wider range of clinically rated symptoms, it may be legitimate to label the second factor in Table 6.2 as "negative-symptom schizotypy."

So far, there is probably little controversy about the differential identification of factors 1 and 2. As examples, Chapman, Chapman, and Miller (1982) showed that PAB and MI are strongly intercorrelated and weakly negatively correlated to PA; Asarnow, Nuechterlein, and Marder (1983) showed that good and poor performers on the Span of Apprehension test were differentiated on MI and PAB but not on PA; Haberman, Chapman, Numbers, and McFall (1979) showed that PA-defined subjects were less socially skilled than controls, whereas PAB-defined subjects did not show this deficit; and Bernstein and Riedel (1987) showed that PA-defined subjects were electrodermally hyporesponsive compared to controls, whereas PAB-defined subjects were not.

The more controversial aspect of this review is thus concerned with the third factor. The data derived from schizophrenic patients, which were reviewed in Table 6.1, showed that in addition to positive-symptom and negative-symptom schizophrenia, the studies allowed for the identification of a third component, labeled "disorganization/social impairment," with concern about whether this dual labeling was appropriate. The question that arises, therefore, is whether, in the analysis of schizotypic material, a third factor can be identified which corresponds to that derived from the analysis of data on schizophrenics.

Two papers cited in Table 6.2 – Bentall et al. (1989) and Kendler and

Hewitt (1992) – suggest the existence of a third factor. Bentall et al. say of this factor that it "appears to refer to the social anxiety aspects of schizotypy. This is indicated by the especially high loading for Eysenck's N scale and other scales that have items of this nature." "It might also be argued that this factor reflects a degree of cognitive disorganization as the scales loading on this factor also tend to include items pertaining to attentional difficulties and distractibility (e.g., the STA and the Nielsen–Petersen scale)" (p. 369). Thus as quoted here, Bentall et al.'s description of this factor matches fairly closely that of the third, "disorganization/social impairment" factor shown in Table 6.1, which was derived from the analysis of patient data. Bentall et al. include this factor as a component of schizotypy, and draw attention to the parallel nature of this factor to the disorganization factor produced by Liddle's (1987) work. On the other hand, Kendler and Hewitt (1992) call their comparable factor "neuroticism–paranoid ideation" and appear to think of it primarily as neuroticism (?, and hence not part of schizotypy). It is worthwhile noting here that the Claridge Paranoid Ideation (CPI) scale, which has a high loading on this factor, contains items for which a broader definition of "social anxiety" could be considered, which would make the definition of this factor more comparable to that of Bentall et al. [However, it should be noted that Eckblad, Chapman, Chapman, and Mishlove (1982), in their revision of the Chapman et al. (1976) Social Anhedonia scale, removed social anxiety items, in order that the scale might better reflect schizoid asociality, which they view as an important part of the schizotypal personality.] Discussing the status of neuroticism (N) in their results, Kendler and Hewitt (1992) point out that if an oblique rotation is carried out on their data, their "positive trait schizotypy" and "neuroticism–paranoid ideation" factors are correlated ($r = +0.47$). They make the point that "although 'positive trait schizotypy' and neuroticism are clearly separable, they are in the general population significantly intercorrelated," a view that is probably not supported by Eysenck (1992) when he states that "schizotypy scales usually show high correlations with N; indeed these are sometimes so high as to suggest that what is being measured is N rather than P" (p. 769).

Finally it is important to review a self-report scale that aims to provide a closer match to the clinically defined category SPD than do other scales that are available. This is the SPQ scale of Raine (1991), which taps each of the nine aspects of DSM-III-R, SPD (DSM-III-R, 1987). Raine and colleagues (1994) used confirmatory factor analysis to show that this scale had a three-factor structure. The first factor, identified by "ideas of reference," "magical thinking," "unusual perceptual experiences," and "paranoid ideation," has the same content as that labeled as positive-symptom schizophrenia in the review above. The second factor is loaded on "social anxiety," "no close friends," "blunted affect," and also "paranoid ideation" and is labeled by Raine et al. as an "interpersonal" factor." The third factor is loaded on "odd behavior" and "odd speech" and is labeled as "disorganized." The second and third factors resulting from this analysis thus pose some problems in relation to the earlier discussion insofar as the second factor might appear to contain some of the content of the third factor in Table 6.2, were it not for the inclusion of blunted affect. Furthermore, the third factor in this analysis, with loadings on odd behavior and odd speech, might also be seen as having some of the content of the third factor in Table 6.2. Thus this material does suggest some differentiation between "disorganization" and "social impairment" which lump together in other analyses.

In summary, the provisional standpoint that can be reached is the following: (1) that positive-symptom schizophrenia and positive-symptom schizotypy have something in common; (2) that negative-symptom schizophrenia and negative-symptom schizotypy also have something in common, although we are placing much weight on anhedonia, in making this statement in the absence of other measures of schizotypy, which tap in a parallel fashion some of the other characteristics of negative schizophrenia; (3) that there is a degree of comparability in the disorganization/social impairment factor in work on schizophrenic patients and the factor labeled in Table 6.2 as social anxiety aspects of schizotypy, but this is more controversial.

Some empirical data

The work described below measures schizotypy by means of a scale that is short, and that has items not immediately identifiable as tapping abnormality (see Venables et al., 1990; and Venables, 1990, for details). The Mauritius High-Risk study (Venables, 1978; Venables et al., 1978) was the major initial user of this scale, although the original development was made on a less exotic population.

In earlier papers (Venables, 1990; Venables et al., 1990) the pattern of responses to this questionnaire was described as two-dimensional. One dimension, following Nielsen and Petersen (1976), was labeled as "schizophrenism" and was at that time considered equivalent to positive-symptom schizophrenia; the other, "anhedonia," having partial relations to negative-symptom schizophrenia. However, in these analyses, the adoption of a two-factor solution was dictated by the attempt to provide the most parsimonious solution where the data were derived from a diverse set of samples. One of the data sets used in the analysis was a large sample of British subjects with a wide age range (Sample 4; Venables et al., 1990, and the material presented here arises from the independent analysis of that data set. Details of subjects, scoring, and analysis are presented in Venables and Bailes (1994).

The 30 items in the questionnaire are presented in Table 3 of Venables et al. (1990). The items are shown in factor groupings in Table 6.3 of this chapter.

The total number of subjects was 770, consisting of 389 males and 381 females. The mean age of the subjects was 27.24 (S.D. ± 14.65), range 15–69 years.

A principal factor analysis was conducted, after which an oblique rotation was performed. Cattell's (1966) Scree test suggested the presence of four factors. The highest correlation between factors was that between factors 1 and 2 ($r = 0.20$) (see Table 6.3), which suggested that for the purpose of initial presentation an orthogonal rotation could be carried out. The results are presented in Table 6.3. Only loadings greater than 0.3 are shown, and because no item had a loading on any factor other than the one shown which was greater than 0.3, all items are "pure" representatives of their respective factors.

Factors 3 and 4 (F3 and F4) may be interpreted as Physical and Social Anhedonia, respectively. Their original derivation from the Chapman et al. (1976) scales is shown in the final column of the table. Factor 3 is made up of PA items, except for items 6 and 9, both of which are SA items in the Chapman scales. It may be noted that the activities that make up these items – that is, letter writing and hugging – both involve physical action, although of course this is carried out in a social context, and the absence of loading of these items on F4 indicates that they may be considered as PA items. Factor 4 is loaded mainly on SA items. The only exception is item 28 – "listening to music" – which, although defined as a PA item, is an activity, perhaps particularly in this sample, that is carried out in a social context, and hence appears as an SA item.

Factors 1 and 2 (F1 and F2) load on items that, in the two-factor solution published in Venables et al. (1990), loaded on a single factor, labeled "schizophrenism," and was considered "positive" factor.

The item content of the two factors is rather different. Factor 1 (F1) contains items that are concerned with unusual perceptual experiences and models of paranoid and magical ideation. The original derivation of the highest loading items is from the Chapman PAB and MI scales. On the other hand, factor 2 (F2) contains no MI or PAB items; their original derivation is from the Nielsen and Petersen (1976) scale or the items listed in Browne and Howarth (1977). The items loading on this factor appear to indicate a mixture of disorganization and social impairment.

Thus it would appear that the result of the factor analysis of this short scale is to produce a set of factors that show some parallels with the clustering of symptoms shown in schizophrenia (Table 6.1) and in part in the clustering of scales shown in schizotypic data (Table 6.2). Factor (F1) appears to correspond to the positive-symptom schizophrenia factor. The separation of this factor from (F2), which has loadings on both items measuring social anxiety and items measuring distractibility and thought disorder, appears to indicate that these aspects of positive schizotypy should be split off from the aspects loaded on hallucinations and delusions, as they are in the data from schizophrenics shown in Table 6.1. Furthermore, the doubts raised about the inclusion, in the analysis of schizophrenic data, of "disorganization" and "social impairment" in the same factor (when one considers the third factor in Table 6.1) may, on the basis of these findings, be resolved at a premorbid level. The fact that F3 (PA) and F4 (SA) appear as separate factors indicates that the two measures do, in some instances, appear to behave differently, as for instance in the Kendler and Hewitt (1992) data.

Another way of probing the parallelism of dimensions of schizophrenia and of schizotypy is to examine how far sex differences in aspects of schizophrenia are repeated in schizotypy. As examples, several researchers (Goldstein & Link, 1988; Lewine, 1981; Mueser, Bellack, Morrison, & Wade, 1990) provide examples of sex differences which show that schizophrenic men show more negative-symptom attributes, whereas schizophrenic women tend to show positive-symptom characteristics. These findings on schizophrenic patients are, in general, supported by work on schizotypy (Claridge & Hewitt, 1987; Muntaner et al., 1988; Young, Bentall, Slade, & Dewey, 1986) which shows that women score higher on MI, PAB, LSHS, and STA scales – that is, those that appear in the positive schizotypy cluster in Tablc 6.2 – whereas males score higher on PA and SA scales (see Chapman et al., 1976; Kendler & Hewitt, 1992; Muntaner et al., 1988).

In the present study, females, as expected, scored higher on factor 1, identified as exemplifying magical and paranoid ideation and unusual perceptual experiences, [$F(1/758) = 11.56$, $p < .001$]. In the case of factors 3 and 4, PA and SA, men scored higher than women, [$F(1/758) = 53.29$; $p < .0001$] and [$F(1/758) = 8.94$; $p < .003$], respectively. In the case of these three factors there was no interaction of sex with age. In the case of factor 2, the social anxiety and disorganization factor, there was a significant interaction between sex and age, showing that older men scored significantly lower than all other groups, and older females had lower scores than younger females. Thus based on the analyses carried out, this factor is assumed to be a positive-symptom factor, and its relationship with gender to move in the expected direction.

Table 6.3. *Rotated (varimax) factor loadings for four-factor solution for total sample, adolescents, and adults*

	Factors	ALL	ADOL	ADUL	SCE
Factor 1	(Unusual perceptual experiences / Paranoid and magical ideation)				
25	Sometimes people I know well begin to look like strangers.	.53	.48	.44	PAB
16	Now and then when I look in a mirror, my face seems quite different from usual.	.52	.47	.43	PAB
15	When introduced to strangers, I often wonder if I have seen them before.	.47	.39	.47	MI
29	I have sometimes felt that strangers were reading my mind.	.46	.42	.39	MI
27	Good luck charms don't work.	.43	.25	.40	MI
7	I often get a restless feeling that I want something but do not know what.	.43	.39	.42	SC
4	I often change between positive and negative feelings towards the same person.	.40	.31	–	SZ
Factor 2	(Social anxiety / Disorganization)				
10	I suddenly feel shy when I talk to a stranger.	.45	.46	.46	BH
24	I prefer others to make decisions for me.	.45	.39	.47	SZ
17	People can easily influence me even though I thought my mind was made up on a subject.	.45	.33	.56	BH
19	I often have great difficulties controlling my thoughts when I am thinking.	.44	.39	.51	SZ
1	I am not easily confused if a number of things happen at the same time.	.36	.37	.36	SZ
14	I find it difficult to concentrate, irrelevant things seem to distract me.	.35	.27	.43	SZ
13	I am not usually self-conscious.	.33	.21	.52	BH
5	I am not much worried by humiliating experiences	.31	.33	.33	SZ
Factor 3	(Physical anhedonia)				
11	Beautiful scenery has been a great delight to me.	.61	.63	.22	PA
18	A brisk walk has sometimes made me feel good all over.	.57	.49	.31	PA
2	When I pass flowers, I often stop to smell them.	.49	.33	.45	PA

		ALL	ADOL	ADUL	SCE
22	I have been fascinated with the dancing of flames in the fireplace.	.43	.42	.26	PA
30	I don't understand why people enjoy looking at the stars at night.	.37	.42	.35	PA
9	When I have been extremely happy I have sometimes felt like hugging someone.	.34	–[b]	.28	SA
6	Writing letters to friends is more trouble than it's worth.	.31	.35	.29	SA
Factor 4 (Social anhedonia)					
20	When anticipating a visit from a friend I have often felt happy and excited.	.52	.57	.43	SA
28	I get a lot of pleasure from listening to music.	.44	.68	.00	PA
3	I attach little importance to having close friends.	.40	.39	.42	SA
12	Getting together with close friends has been one of my greatest pleasures.	.38	.33	.57	SA
26	I have thoroughly enjoyed laughing at jokes with other people.	.37	.44	.00	SA
23	The idea of going out and mixing with people at parties has always pleased me.	.31	.27	.31	SA

Notes: Factor loadings are shown when loadings for the total sample (ALL) are greater than 0.3; for all these items there are no loadings on other factors that are greater than 0.3. Items omitted from the results above are: 8 (It is not possible to harm people merely by thinking bad thoughts about them) – this item was not loaded on any of the factors; and 21 (I would like other people to be afraid of me) – this item performed erratically in other analyses. Loadings for items 21 (see text) and 8 (no loading greater than 0.3) have been omitted.

Key: ALL, total sample; ADOL, adolescent sample; ADUL, adult sample; SCE, source codes. The final column (SCE) shows the source codes for the items: PAB, Perceptual Aberration Scale (Chapman et al., 1978); MI, Magical Ideation Scale (Eckblad & Chapman, 1983); SC, MMPI Schizophrenia Scale; SZ, Schizophrenism Scale (Nielsen & Petersen, 1976); BH, Brown and Howarth (1977); PA, Physical Anhedonia Scale (Chapman et al., 1976); SA, Social Anhedonia Scale (Chapman et al., 1976).

[a]The loading for this item had the value of 0.31 on factor 2.

[b]The loading for this item had the value of 0.36 on factor 4.

The relation of factor 1 with factor 2 needs to be delineated. As stated earlier, when an oblique rotation was carried out on the principal factor analysis of the data, the correlation between factor 1 and factor 2 was 0.20. If scale scores are calculated by the addition of scores on the items loading on each of the two factors, the correlation between the two scales is 0.31. Kendler and Hewitt (1992) also carried out an oblique rotation on their data and reported a correlation of 0.47 between the factors they called "positive trait schizotypy" and "neuroticism/paranoid-ideation," which have close analogy to factors 1 and 2 in the present work.

Thus, although gender relations suggest some similarity between factors 1 and 2 (which is supported by the correlation between the two factors outlined in the paragraph above), the common variance between the two factors is only some 9%; and as Kendler and Hewitt (1992) say (perhaps controversially), although these factors are related in the general population, they are "clearly separable."

In the construction of the scale, using a British sample, Venables et al. (1990) reported that some items were selected for inclusion on the basis of their relationship to skin conductance responsivity. These items are identified in table 3 of Venables et al. (1990). Of these seven items, only one, item 7, appears in the first factor, which, as has been pointed out, is identified mainly by Chapman PAB and MI items. However, 6 of the 7 items (1, 5, 10, 13, 17, 24) appear in the second factor, whose items are drawn preponderantly from the Nielsen and Petersen (1976) schizophrenism scale.

This finding is in line with data in the literature. Simons (1981) showed no difference in electrodermal orienting in subjects with high scores on the PAB scale and controls. This finding was replicated by Bernstein and Riedel (1987). In contrast, Nielsen and Petersen (1976) showed that high scores on their schizophrenism scale (from which the items in factor 2 are largely drawn) were related to electrodermal hyperresponsivity.

Data from the Mauritius High-Risk study may be used to reinforce this distinction further. Venables (1993) reported that those subjects who showed electrodermal hyperresponsivity to intense (but not orienting) stimuli at age 3 had higher scores ($p < .05$) on the factor (labeled as schizophrenism), when measured at age 16/17 years, which appeared as the positive-symptom factor in the two-factor solution of the analysis of the present 30-item questionnaire. This schizophrenism factor contained the items now split among the first and second factors in the present analysis. The hypothesis that can now be drawn on the basis of the findings outlined above is that if scores on the schizophrenism scale, as used in Mauritius, are broken down into scales representing factors 1 and 2 in the present analysis, then there should be no relation of the first factor scores to early electrodermal responsivity, but the second factor should show such a relationship.

The findings are that groups of subjects, divided into nonresponders, median responders, and hyperresponders on the basis of their skin conductance responses to intense (90 db) stimuli, were significantly different on scores on the second factor [$F(2/378) = 3.21$; $p = .042$], but not on the first factor [$F(2/378) = 1.38$; $p = .253$].

Work on the Continuous Performance Test (CPT) suggests that poor performance is associated with high scoring on the PAB (see Lencz & Raine, Chapter 18, this volume).

Data are available from the Mauritius High-Risk study on a degraded stimulus version of the CPT (Nuechterlein, 1991) measured at age 14/15 years. The correlation between F1 and number of hits on the CPT is −.18 ($p = .027$, $N = 692$), and between F2 and CPT performance −.01 ($p = .743$, $N = 692$). Although neither of these correlations accounts for much variance, the difference between the two is in accord with expectation.

Further data are available from the Span of Apprehension Test (SOA; Asarnow, Granholm, & Sherman, 1991), which were obtained at the same time as those from the CPT above. The correlation between performance on the most difficult version and F1 is −.13 ($p < .0001$, $N = 688$), whereas that for F2 is −.06 ($p = .11$, $N = 688$).

These results, both of which involve measures of attention, tend to reinforce the label given to the first factor in Table 6.2 as involving cognitive/perceptual aspects of schizotypy.

Earlier, it was suggested that it was the positive aspects of schizophrenia that led to a person being labeled as a patient. If factor F1 can be thought of exemplifying the positive, externally evident, aspects of schizotypy, then it would be expected that this variable, rather than F2, would be related to external assessments of the subject by other persons. In the Mauritius study, ratings by teachers and employers on the subjects are available at ages 16–17 years on the Revised Behavior Problem Checklist (Quay & Peterson, 1987). Factor analysis of scores from this instrument indicated a single factor that might be labeled “abnormal behavior.” The correlation between this factor and F1 is 0.14 ($p < .0001$ $N = 771$) and between the “abnormal behavior” factor and F2 is 0.05 ($p = .13$, $N = 771$). Again the size of this correlation is small, but it is notable that the questionnaire factor (F1) designated as positive-symptom schizotypy is related to abnormal behavior that can be detected by members of the general public, whereas the self-reported behavior (F2) designated as social anxiety / disorganization is not.

In summary, these data support the division of the positive aspect of schizotypy into two parts, labeled in this instance as "unusual perceptual experiences/ paranoid and magical ideation," and "social anxiety / disorganization," and suggest that there may be reasons to view anhedonia as not a unitary concept.

Discussion

In the opening section of this chapter, the question was posed whether there was a similarity between the schizophrenic symptoms shown by the patient and the schizotypal characteristics shown premorbidly, which could suggest that they could be seen as arising as primary results of the original predisposition. If the position is that a particular type of predisposition gives rise to schizotypic and schizophrenic characteristics that can be seen as related, then this results in a set of hypotheses different from those arising from a "vulnerability" perspective, which assumes the premorbid condition to bear no necessary similarity to the schizophrenic characteristics eventually seen in the patient. Thus, for instance, measures such as those of attention or of psychophysiological status, which distinguish schizophrenic patients from normal subjects, would not distinguish subjects scoring high on a schizotypy scale from those scoring low, if schizotypic status were no more than a vulnerability measure unrelated to schizophrenia. That this is not the case is shown by many studies (e.g., Asarnow et al., 1983; Drewer & Shean, 1993; Lencz et al., 1993; Lenzenweger, Dworkin, & Wethington, 1991; Simons, 1981; Simons, MacMillan, & Ireland, 1982; Wilkins & Venables, 1992), which indicate that schizotypal subjects are distinguished from normals (those low on the schizotypy scale) on the same measures that distinguish schizophrenics from normals. However, it should be pointed out that the ubiquitous relation of neuroticism (N) to schizotypy does raise the possibility that N might be considered to be a "vulnerability" variable of the type proposed by Zubin and Steinhauer (1981).

The review of currently available studies suggested a tripartite division of schizophrenic symptomatology. Thus to support the view of the direct relation between schizotypy and schizophrenia, there should be a similar trichotomy of schizotypy. The literature reviewed and the data produced suggest that trichotomy of schizotypy is not unreasonable. However, at the level of behavior and psychophysiology, only rather weak data are available to suggest that there is a trichotomy of the underlying predisposition or schizotaxia.

Two sorts of data appear to be required to provide support in this area. The first type suggests that there may be continua within the types of schizotaxia, so that the minor aspects of schizotypy seen in the otherwise normal person might be produced by minor anomalies in the structural aspects of the brain. These are the features that, when more major, and in interaction with external stressors, produce schizophrenia. (Alternatively, the structural defects may be relatively gross, but the external stressors on the person relatively weak.) The second requirement is that different types of schizotaxia may have to be present to produce the different types of schizotypy and schizophrenia that have been the focus of this chapter. As the investigation of structural and consequent functional anomalies in schizophrenia is a major area of study at the present time, to attempt to provide any substantial coverage here is out of the question. However, data do provide some answers to questions that are particularly relevant when one considers the relation between schizophrenia and schizotypy, especially in the context of high-risk studies. One is concerned with the extent to which a particular form of schizotaxia may be considered to be a deficit existing at or before birth [see Mednick, Cannon, Barr, & Lyon (1991) for a review of data which suggests that events occurring in the second trimester of pregnancy produce disturbances in the developing brain in those areas which in scanning (CAT, MRI, and PET) or postmortem studies have shown to be particularly involved in the production of schizophrenic symptoms], or whether it is a result of disorders later in the developmental process. If the latter, it does of course invalidate any attempt to seek a direct parallel between schizotypic behavior measured in childhood and later schizophrenia.

One of the areas particularly vulnerable to disturbance in fetal development is the hippocampus (Conrad & Scheibel, 1987). Venables (1992) has reviewed the psychological evidence that implies the involvement of the hippocampus in schizophrenia. It was noted that the same tests (e.g., of latent inhibition), which evidence from animals shows to be related to hippocampal dysfunction, produce abnormal response both in schizophrenics and in those with high schizotypal scores. Of specific interest in the present context is a study by Weinberger, DeLisi, Perman, Targum, and Wyatt (1982), in which ventricle size is measured in chronic schizophrenics, in patients with schizophreniform disorder, in patients with other psychiatric disorders, and controls. The patients with schizophreniform disorders and the chronic schizophrenics did not differ in mean ventricular brain ratio (VBR), but both groups had significantly larger VBRs than patients with other psychiatric disorders and controls. What is notable, however, is the overlap in range of VBRs in the schizophreniform and schizophrenic patients, and the fact that many of the VBRs of these patients were within the range of values produced by the other groups.

Reviews of the data on ventricular enlargement (e.g., Goetz & van Kammen, 1986; Seidman, 1983) point to the relation of this enlargement to negative symptomatology. Thus, if ventricular enlargement, as suggested above, is present from birth, this would imply that negative symptoms are primary and not, as suggested as a possibility in the introduction, a secondary reaction to the onset of positive symptoms. Their primary nature is implied by the results of a study by Dykes, Mednick, Machon, Praestholm, and Parnas (1992) which shows that those subjects who are at genetic risk for schizophrenia and who show a widened third ventricle are more likely to show signs of behavioral underarousal as infants. However, as pointed out by Goldberg (1985), negative symptoms do respond to neuroleptics, and possibly may not thus be the result of a structural defect. We are thus left with the possibility that there may be two kinds of negative symptoms. Perhaps, those that are most closely related to what have been defined as negative characteristics in schizotypy may be those that should be considered to be primary. However, as negative symptoms in schizotypy are almost exclusively defined by measures of anhedonia, it is important to explore this area further by studies that extend measurement to other negative characteristics.

Of particular importance, the questions as to when before adolescence the measurement of schizotypic characteristics should be carried out with the aim of relating this to later schizophrenia, and when this schizotypic measurement is to be theoretically related to a type of schizotaxia, are explored in the work of Benes (1989), who showed that it is only in late adolescence that the myelination of the subiculum and presubiculum might allow the completion of the central corticolimbic circuitry of those areas of the brain whose malfunction is implicated in schizophrenia. Thus it might be assumed, as suggested above, that if aspects of schizotypy have direct parallels to those exhibited in schizophrenia, they might not present themselves until adolescence, as the "schizotaxia" is latent until that time.

In summary, the work reviewed in this chapter suggests (1) that there are three dimensions on which schizophrenic symptoms may be arranged; (2) that these are paralleled by dimensions of schizotypic characteristics; and (3) that this tridimensional structure may have an underlying tridimensionality of etiology. Because a three-dimensional structure is advocated, the coexistence of symptoms or characteristics of the three dimensions is by definition possible and does not conflict with the positing of disorders in different areas of the brain, which, because they must be considered as part of a total system, necessarily interact.

References

Andreasen, N. C. (1983). *Comprehensive Assessment of Symptoms and History (CASH)*. University of Iowa, College of Medicine.

Andreasen, N. C., & Olsen, S. (1982). Negative v. positive schizophrenia. *Archives of General Psychiatry, 39,* 789–794.

Arndt, S., Alliger, R. J., & Andreasen, N. C. (1991). The distinction of positive and negative symptoms: The failure of a two-dimensional model. *British Journal of Psychiatry, 158,* 317–322.

Asarnow, R. F., Granholm, E., & Sherman, T. (1991). Span of apprehension in schizophrenia. In S. R. Steinhauer, J. H. Gruzelier, & J. Zubin (Eds.), *Neuropsychology, psychophysiology and information processing* (pp. 335–370). Amsterdam: Elsevier.

Asarnow, R. F., Nuechterlein, K. H., & Marder, A. R. (1983). Span of apprehension performance, neuropsychological functioning, and indices of psychosis proneness. *Journal of Nervous and Mental Disease, 171,* 662–669.

Benes, F. M. (1989). Myelination of cortical–hippocampal relays during late adolescence. *Schizophrenia Bulletin, 15,* 585–593.

Bentall, R. P., Claridge, G. S., & Slade, P. D. (1989). The multidimensional nature of schizotypal traits: A factor analytic study with normal subjects. *British Journal of Clinical Psychology, 28,* 363–375.

Bernstein, A. S., & Riedel, J. A. (1987). Psychophysiological response patterns in college students with high physical anhedonia: Scores appear to reflect schizotypy rather than depression. *Biological Psychiatry, 22,* 829–847.

Berrios, G. E. (1985). Positive and negative symptoms and Jackson: A conceptual history. *Archives of General Psychiatry, 42*(1), 95–97.

Bilder, R. M., Mukherjee, S., Rieder, R. O., & Pandurangi, A. K. (1985). Symptomatic and neuropsychological components of defect states. *Schizophrenia Bulletin, 11,* 409–419.

Browne, J., & Howarth, E. (1977). A comprehensive factor analysis of personality questionnaire items: A test for twenty putative factor hypothesis. *Multivariate Behavioral Research, 12,* 399–427.

Caplan, R., Perdue, S., Tanguay, P. E., & Fish, B. (1990). Formal thought disorder in childhood onset schizophrenia and schizotypal personality disorder. *Journal of Child Psychology and Psychiatry, 31,* 1103–1114.

Cattell, R. B. (1966). The Scree Test for number of factors. *Multivariate Behavioral Research, 1,* 245–266.

Chapman, L. J., Chapman, J. P., & Miller, E. N. (1982). Reliabilities and intercorrelations of eight measures of proneness to psychosis. *Journal of Consulting and Clinical Psychology, 50,* 187–195.

Chapman, L. J., Chapman, J. P., Numbers, J. S., Edell, W. S., Carpenter, B. N., & Beckfield, D. (1984). Impulsive nonconformity as a trait contributing to the prediction of psychotic-like and schizotypal symptoms. *Journal of Nervous and Mental Disease, 172,* 681–691.

Chapman, L. J., Chapman, J. P., & Raulin, M. L. (1976). Scales for physical and social anhedonia. *Journal of Abnormal Psychology, 85,* 374–382.

Chapman, L. J., Chapman, J. P., & Raulin, M. L. (1978). Body-image aberration in schizophrenia. *Journal of Abnormal Psychology, 87,* 399–407.

Claridge, G., & Broks, P. (1984). Schizotypy and hemisphere function – I. Theoretical considerations and the measurement of schizotypy. *Personality and Individual Differences, 5,* 633–648.

Claridge, G. S., & Hewitt, J. K. (1987). A biometrical study of schizotypy in a normal population. *Personality and Individual Differences, 8,* 303–312.

Conrad, A. J., & Scheibel, A. B. (1987). Schizophrenia and the hippocampus. *Schizophrenia Bulletin, 13,* 577–588.

Crow, T. J. (1980). Molecular pathology of schizophrenia: More than one disease process? *British Medical Journal, 280,* 66–68.

Drewer, H. B., & Shean, G. D. (1993). Reaction time crossover in schizotypal subjects. *Journal of Nervous and Mental Disease, 181*(1), 27–30.

DSM-III (1980). *Diagnostic and statistical manual of mental disorders* (3rd ed.). Washington, D.C.: American Psychiatric Association.

DSM-III-R (1987). *Diagnostic and statistical manual of mental disorders – revised* (3rd revised ed.). Washington D.C.: American Psychiatric Association.

Dworkin, R. H., Green, S. R., Small, N. E., Warner, M. L., & Erlenmeyer-Kimling, L. (1990). Positive and negative symptoms and social competence in adolescents at risk for schizophrenia and affective disorder. *American Journal of Psychiatry, 147*(9), 1234–1236.

Dykes, K. L., Mednick, S. A., Machon, R. A., Praestholm, J., & Parnas, J. (1992). Adult third ventricle width and infant behavioral arousal in groups at high and low risk for schizophrenia. *Schizophrenia Research, 7,* 13–18.

Eckblad, M., & Chapman, L. J. (1983). Magical ideation as an indicator of schizotypy. *Journal of Consulting and Clinical Psychology, 51,* 215–225.

Eckblad, M., & Chapman, L. J. (1986). Development and validation of a scale for hypomanic personality. *Journal of Abnormal Psychology, 95,* 214–222.

Eckblad, M., Chapman, L. J., Chapman, J. P., & Mishlove, M. (1982). The Revised Social Anhedonia Scale, University of Wisconsin, Madison, Wis. (unpublished test).

Endicott, J., & Spitzer, R. L. (1978). A diagnostic interview: The Schedule for Affective Disorders and Schizophrenia. *Archives of General Psychiatry, 35,* 837–844.

Eysenck, H. J. (1992). The definition and measurement of psychoticism. *Personality and Individual Differences, 13,* 757–785.

Eysenck, H. J., & Eysenck, S. B. G. (1975). *Manual of the Eysenck Personality Questionnaire.* London: Hodder and Stoughton.

Eysenck, H. J., & Eysenck, S. G. B. (1976). *Psychoticism as a dimension of personality.* London: Hodder and Stoughton.

Goetz, K. L., & van Kammen, D. P. (1986). Computerized axial tomography scans and subtypes of schizophrenia. *Journal of Nervous and Mental Disease, 174,* 31–41.

Goldberg, S. C. (1985). Negative and deficit symptoms of schizophrenia do respond to neuroleptics. *Schizophrenia Bulletin, 11,* 453–456.

Golden, R. R., & Meehl, P. E. (1979). Detection of the schizoid taxon with MMPI indicators. *Journal of Abnormal Psychology, 84,* 217–233.

Goldstein, J. M., & Link, B. G. (1988). Gender and the expression of schizophrenia. *Journal of Psychiatric Research, 22,* 141–155.

Haberman, M. C., Chapman, L. J., Numbers, J. S., & McFall, R. M. (1979). Relation of social competence to scores on two scales of psychosis proneness. *Journal of Abnormal Psychology, 88,* 675–677.

Hewitt, J. K., & Claridge, G. (1989). The factor structure of schizotypy in a normal population. *Personality and Individual Differences, 10,* 323–330.

Kelley, M. P., & Coursey, R. D. (1992). Factor structure of schizotypy scales. *Personality and Individual Differences, 13*(6), 723–731.

Kendler, K. S., Gruenberg, A. M., & Tsuang, M. T. (1983). The specificity of DSM-III schizotypal symptoms. In *136th annual meeting of the American Psychiatric Association.* Washington, D.C.: APA.

Kendler, K. S., & Hewitt, J. (1992). The structure of self-report schizotypy in twins. *Journal of Personality Disorders, 6,* 1–17.

Kendler, K. S., Ochs, A. L., Gorman, A. M., Hewitt, J. K., Ross, D. E., & Mirsky, A. F. (1991). The structure of schizotypy: A pilot multitrait twin study. *Psychiatry Research, 36,* 19–36.

Kincannon, J. C. (1968). Prediction of the standard MMPI scale scores from 71 items: The Mini-Mult. *Journal of Consulting and Clinical Psychology, 32,* 319–325.

Kirkpatrick, B., & Buchanan, R. W. (1990). Anhedonia and the deficit syndrome in schizophrenia. *Psychiatry Research, 31,* 25–30.
Krawiecka, M., Goldberg, D., & Vaughan, M. (1977). A standardized psychiatric assessment for rating chronic psychiatric patients. *Acta Psychiatrica Scandinavica, 55,* 299–308.
Kulhara, P., Kota, S. J., & Joseph, S. (1986). Positive and negative subtypes of schizophrenia: A study from India. *Acta Psychiatrica Scandinavica, 74,* 353–359.
Launay, G., & Slade, P. (1981). The measurement of hallucinatory predisposition in male and female prisoners. *Personality and Individual Differences, 2,* 221–234.
Lencz, T., Raine, A., Scerbo, A., Redmon, M., Brodish, S., Holt, L., & Bird, L. (1993). Impaired eye tracking in undergraduates with schizotypal personality disorder. *American Journal of Psychiatry, 150*(1), 152–154.
Lenzenweger, M. F., Dworkin, R. H., & Wethington, E. (1991). Examining the underlying structure of schizophrenic phenomenology: Evidence for a three-process model. *Schizophrenia Bulletin, 17,* 515–524.
Lewine, R. R. J. (1981). Sex differences in schizophrenia: Timing or subtypes? *Psychological Bulletin, 90,* 432–444.
Liddle, P. F. (1987). The symptoms of schizophrenia; a re-examination of the positive–negative dichotomy. *British Journal of Psychiatry, 151,* 145–151.
Liddle, P. F., & Barnes, T. R. E. (1990). Syndromes of chronic schizophrenia. *British Journal of Psychiatry, 157,* 558–561.
Mednick, S. A. (1958). A learning theory approach to research in schizophrenia. *Psychological Bulletin, 55,* 316–327.
Mednick, S. A., Cannon, T. D., Barr, C. E., & Lyon, M. (1991). *Fetal neural development and adult schizophrenia.* Cambridge: Cambridge University Press.
Meehl, P. E. (1962). Schizotaxia, schizotypy and schizophrenia. *American Psychologist, 17,* 827–838.
Miers, T. C., & Raulin, M. L. (1985). The development of a scale to measure cognitive slippage. Paper presented at the Eastern Psychological Association convention. Boston:
Miller, D. D., Arndt, S., Andreasen, N. C. (1993). Alogia, attentional impairment, and inappropriate affect: Their status in the dimensions of schizophrenia. *Comprehensive Psychiatry, 34,* 221–226.
Mueser, K. T., Bellack, A. S., Morrison, R. L., & Wade, J. H. (1990). Gender, social competence and symptomatology in schizophrenia: A longitudinal analysis. *Journal of Abnormal Psychology, 99,* 138–147.
Muntaner, C., Garcia-Sevilla, L., Fernandez, A., & Torrubia, R. (1988). Personality dimensions, schizotypal and borderline personality traits and psychosis proneness. *Personality and Individual Differences, 9,* 257–268.
Nielsen, T. C., & Petersen, K. E. (1976). Electrodermal correlates of extraversion, trait anxiety and schizophrenism. *Scandinavian Journal of Psychology, 17,* 73–80.
Nuechterlein, K. H. (1991). Vigilance in schizophrenia and related disorders. In S. R. Steinhauer, J. H. Gruzelier, & J. Zubin (Eds.), *Neuropsychology, psychophysiology and information processing* (pp. 397–433). Amsterdam: Elsevier.
Peralta, V., de Leon, J., & Cuesta, M. J. (1992). Are there more than two syndromes in schizophrenia? A critique of the positive–negative dichotomy. *British Journal of Psychiatry, 161,* 335–343.
Quay, H. C., & Peterson, D. R. (1987). *Manual for the Revised Behavior Problem Checklist.* Coral Gables, Fla.: H. C. Quay & D. R. Peterson.
Raine, A. (1991). The SPQ: A scale for the assessment of schizotypal personality disorder based on DSM-III-R criteria. *Schizophrenia Bulletin, 17,* 555–564.

Raine, A., & Allbutt, J. (1989). Factors of schizoid personality. *British Journal of Clinical Psychology, 28,* 31–40.

Raine, A., Reynolds, C., Lencz, T., Scerbo, A., Triphon, N., & Kim, D. (1994). Cognitive–perceptual, interpersonal, and disorganized features of individual differences in schizotypal personality in the general population. *Schizophrenia Bulletin, 21,* 191–201.

Raulin, M. L. (1984). Development of a scale to measure intense ambivalence. *Journal of Consulting and Clinical Psychology, 52,* 63–72.

Raulin, M. L., & Wee, J. L. (1984). The development and initial validation of a scale of social fear. *Journal of Clinical Psychology, 40,* 780–784.

Rochester, S. R., & Martin, J. R. (1979). *Crazy talk: A study of the discourse of schizophrenic speakers.* New York: Plenum Press.

Roger, D., & Morris, J. (1991). The internal structure of the EPQ scales. *Personality and Individual Differences, 12,* 759–764.

Seidman, L. J. (1983). Schizophrenia and brain dysfunction: An integration of recent neurodiagnostic findings. *Psychological Bulletin, 94*(2), 195–238.

Siever, L. J., & Gunderson, J. G. (1983). The search for a schizotypal personality: Historical origins and current status. *Comprehensive Psychiatry, 24*(3), 199–212.

Simons, R. F. (1981). Electrodermal and cardiac orienting in psychometrically defined high-risk subjects. *Psychiatry Research, 4*(3), 347–356.

Simons, R. M., MacMillan, F. W., & Ireland, F. B. (1982). Reaction-time crossover in preselected schizotypic subjects. *Journal of Abnormal Psychology, 91,* 414–419.

Spitzer, R. L., Endicott, J., & Gibbon, M. (1979). Crossing the border into borderline personality and borderline schizophrenia. *Archives of General Psychiatry, 36,* 17–24.

Strauss, J. S., Carpenter, W. T., & Bartko, J. J. (1974). The diagnosis and understanding of schizophrenia, Part III. Speculations on the processes that underlie schizophrenic symptoms and signs. *Schizophrenia Bulletin* (11), 61–69.

Venables, P. H. (1978). Psychophysiology and psychometrics. *Psychophysiology, 15*(4), 302–315.

Venables, P. H. (1990). The measurement of schizotypy in Mauritius. *Personality and Individual Differences, 11*(9), 965–971.

Venables, P. H. (1992). Hippocampal function and schizophrenia: Experimental psychological evidence. In D. Friedman & G. Bruder (Eds.), *Psychophysiology and experimental psychopathology* (pp. 111–127). New York: The New York Academy of Sciences.

Venables, P. H. (1993). Electrodermal indices as markers for the development of schizophrenia. In J.-C. Roy, W. Broucseir, D. C. Fowles, & J. H. Gruzelier (Eds.), *Electrodermal activity: From physiology to psychology.* New York: Plenum.

Venables, P. H., & Bailes, K. (1994). The structure of schizotypy, its relation to subdiagnoses of schizophrenia and to sex and age. *British Journal of Clinical Psychology, 33,* 277–294.

Venables, P. H., Mednick, S. A., Schulsinger, F., Raman, A. C., Bell, B., Dalais, J. C., & Fletcher, R. P. (1978). Screening for risk of mental illness. In G. Serban (Ed.), *Cognitive defects in the development of mental illness* (pp. 273–303). New York: Brunner/Mazel.

Venables, P. H., & O'Connor, N. (1959). A short scale for rating paranoid schizophrenia. *Journal of Mental Science, 105,* 815–818.

Venables, P. H., Wilkins, S., Mitchell, D. A., Raine, A., & Bailes, K. (1990). A scale for the measurement of schizotypy. *Personality and Individual Differences, 11,* 481–495.

Walker, E., & Lewine, R. J. (1988). The positive/negative symptom distinction in schizophrenia: Validity and etiological relevance. *Schizophrenia Research, 1*(5), 315–328.

Weinberger, D. R., DeLisi, L. E., Perman, G. P., Targum, S., & Wyatt, R. J. (1982). Computed tomography in schizophreniform disorder and other acute psychiatric disorders. *Archives of General Psychiatry, 39,* 778–783.

Wilkins, S., & Venables, P. H. (1992). Disorder of attention in individuals with schizotypal personality. *Schizophrenia Bulletin, 18,* 717–723.

Wing, J. K., Cooper, J. E., & Sartorius, N. (1974). *The measurement and classification of psychiatric symptoms.* London: Cambridge University Press.

Young, H. F., Bentall, R. P., Slade, P. D., & Dewey, M. E. (1986). Disposition towards hallucination, gender and EPQ scores: A brief report. *Personality and Individual Differences, 7,* 247–249.

Zigler, E., & Phillips, L. (1960). Social effectiveness and symptomatic behaviors. *Journal of Abnormal and Social Psychology, 61,* 231–238.

Zubin, J. (1985). Negative symptoms: Are they indigenous to schizophrenia? *Schizophrenia Bulletin, 11,* 461–470.

Zubin, J., & Steinhauer, S. (1981). How to break the logjam in schizophrenia: A look beyond genetics. *Journal of Nervous and Mental Disease, 169*(8), 477–492.

PART IV

Categorical versus dimensional approaches

7

Tracking the taxon: on the latent structure and base rate of schizotypy

MARK F. LENZENWEGER and LAUREN KORFINE

The study of schizotypic psychopathology is likely to advance our understanding of the nature of schizophrenia. One possible route of such advancement concerns clarification of the basic nature and structure of the common liability[1] that appears to underlie both schizophrenia and schizotypic psychopathology. We shall discuss briefly the need for a latent liability construct in this area, general substantive and methodological issues relevant to the search for latent taxa (classes) in psychopathology, and our own taxometric work directed specifically toward illuminating the *structure* of the liability for

[1] In this context we wish to distinguish our conceptualization of liability from two related but different concepts, namely "vulnerability" and "risk factor." As defined by Holzman (1982), vulnerability refers to "a perceivable, palpable, and measurable variation in structure or function that represents a predisposition to a specific disease process" (p. 19); however, vulnerability per se is not the same as the disease, albeit detectable prior to the onset of a disease. Holzman (1982) defines "risk factor" as a factor (e.g., a behavior) that increases one's statistical likelihood that one will in fact develop a disease (e.g., cigarette smoking increases the risk for coronary artery disease). Vulnerability traits represent necessary but not sufficient conditions for disease development, whereas risk factors are neither necessary nor sufficient for disease development (see Holzman, 1982, p. 20). Our view of "liability" is much more akin, though narrower in definition, to vulnerability; we consider liability to be nearly isomorphic with the disease process (though not necessarily isomorphic with clinical expression of the disease). In the case of schizophrenia, vulnerability implies the need for environmental stressors for disease expression; that is, one could be vulnerable to schizophrenia yet never develop the illness in full form. Our view of liability suggests that the schizophrenia disease process will always manifest itself in some manner regardless of environmental stressors; that is, some aspect of the latent liability for schizophrenia will always manifest itself in some (perhaps not obvious) form – no triggering is needed. We do not suggest, however, that schizophrenia liability always shows up as clinically diagnosable schizophrenia; rather it will manifest itself across a range of compensation and in alternative forms. Our view of liability represents a partial synthesis of Meehl's (1990) model of schizotypy and the latent trait model of Holzman and Matthysse (Holzman et al., 1988; Matthysse et al., 1986).

schizophrenia. Our research in this area will be cast within the context of Meehl's (1962, 1990) model of schizotypy and schizophrenia.

We note that the terms "schizoid," "schizotypal," "schizotypy," and "schizotype" have been used in a variety of ways and therefore, we provide here some orienting remarks to clarify our usage of these terms, which are by no means synonymous. In the present discussion, the term "schizotypy" refers to an underlying personality organization; it is essentially a hypothetical latent construct that cannot be observed directly. Moreover, our view is that schizotypy, by definition, embodies the fundamental liability for schizophrenia. We do not view schizotypy as a syndrome consisting of those phenotypic (directly observable) manifestations such as mildly disordered thought, peculiar use of language, interpersonal aversiveness, anxiety, odd–eccentric behavior and appearance, and so on. Rather, we prefer the term "schizotypic" (see Meehl, 1964) or "schizotypal" to describe such observable phenotypic manifestations. One can speak of a "schizotype" or a "schizotypal individual" to describe a particular person, whereas schizotypy per se is a latent hypothetical construct. Our conceptualization of schizotypy has been guided by Meehl's (1962, 1990) model of the development of schizophrenia (see below) as well as influenced by the "latent trait" model of Holzman and Matthysse (Holzman et al., 1988; Matthysse, Holzman, & Lange, 1986).

Theoretical excursus: Rado, Meehl, and schizotypy

Descriptions of schizotypic psychopathology have a long history in the clinical psychopathology literature. Both Kraepelin (1919/1971, p. 234) and Bleuler (1911/1950, p. 239) made note of what they termed "latent schizophrenia," a form of personality aberration thought to be, in essence, a quantitatively less severe expression of schizophrenia. Early depictions of schizotypic psychopathology were primarily descriptive and lacked any detailed consideration of the etiology and development of schizotypic pathology. Although there was often speculation about an association with schizophrenia and a possible "hereditary connection," the precise pathway(s) leading from the underlying liability for schizophrenia-related pathology to the phenotypic expression of a clinical disorder was absent. Even though the current American psychiatric nomenclature (DSM-III-R) contains a variant of these valuable clinical insights in the form of schizotypal personality disorder (SPD), the DSM-III-R criteria for SPD, however, remain merely descriptive and atheoretical in nature, reflecting but a clustering of symptoms (i.e., etiology and development are unspecified). One must turn elsewhere for models of pathogenesis.

Perhaps one of the most heuristically valuable models of schizotypic psychopathology and schizophrenia that moves considerably beyond the descriptive level is P. E. Meehl's (1962, 1990) theoretical model. The roots of Meehl's model can be found in the observations of Sandor Rado (1960). Working within the psychodynamic clinical tradition, Rado made initial strides toward an integrative model that sought to link genetic influences for schizophrenia and observed schizotypic personality functioning. Rado (1960) argued, from a psychodynamic position informed by an appreciation for genetics, that schizotypal behavior derived from a fundamental liability to schizophrenia. Rado, in fact, coined the term "schizotype" to represent a condensation of "schizophrenic phenotype" (Rado, 1960, p. 87). Rado (1960) was careful to point out that the individual who possessed the schizophrenic phenotype was a schizotype, whereas the correlated traits deriving from this "type" were termed "schizotypal organization," and the overt behavioral manifestations of the schizotypal traits were termed "schizotypal behavior" (see his p. 87).

For Rado, the causes of schizotypal "differentness" were to be found in two core psychodynamic features of such patients, both of which were thought to be driven by "mutated genes." The two core defects present in the schizotype were (1) a diminished capacity for pleasure, or pleasure deficiency (Rado, 1960, p. 88); and (2) a proprioceptive (kinesthetic) diathesis that resulted in an aberrant awareness of the body (a feature giving rise to schizotypic body-image distortions (Rado, 1960; see his pp. 88 and 90). A most important concept in Rado's model concerned what he termed "developmental stages of schizotypal behavior," by which he suggested that a common schizophrenia diathesis could lead to a variety of phenotypic outcomes ranging from compensated schizotypy to deteriorated schizophrenia; thus an etiologic unity was proposed as underlying a diversity of clinical manifestations.

Unlike earlier workers (including Rado), Meehl (1962, 1964, 1990) conjectured a complex integrative developmental model that set him apart from other clinical researchers. Meehl (1962, 1990) conjectured that clinically diagnosable schizophrenia is the result of a complex developmental interaction among several crucial factors: (1) a "schizotaxic" brain characterized by a genetically determined hypothetical neural integrative defect at the level of the synapse, a defect termed "hypokrisia" (Meehl conjectures a single major locus – the "schizogene" – to cause hypokrisia); (2) environmentally mediated social learning experiences (that bring about a schizotypal personality organization); and (3) the polygenic potentiators (anxiety, hypohedonia). The "modal" schizotype does not decompensate into diagnosable schizophrenia; however, Meehl suggested that all schizotypes reveal the influence of their latent liability for schizophrenia through some degree of aberrant psychological and social functioning. Meehl (1962, 1964) described what he believed to be the four fundamental signs and symptoms of schizotypy: (1) cognitive slippage (or mild associative loosening), (2) interpersonal aversiveness (social fear), (3) anhedonia (pleasure capacity deficit), and (4) ambivalence. All aspects of the core clinical phenomenology and psychological functioning seen in the schizotype were hypothesized to derive fundamentally from aberrant CNS-based synaptic functioning (Meehl terms this deficit "hypokrisia") as determined by a "schizogene," which acts against a background of polygenic effects (a "mixed model") as well as social learning contexts. For example, "primary slippage" (at the level of the synapse) gave rise to observable "secondary cognitive slippage" in thought, speech, affective integration, and behavior, whereas primary aversive drift (i.e., the steady developmental progression toward negative affective tone in personality functioning across the life-span) gave rise to the signs and symptoms of social fear, ambivalence, and anhedonia – features seen commonly among schizotypes and individuals with schizophrenia.

According to Meehl's model, schizotypy, as a personality organization reflective of a latent liability for schizophrenia, can manifest itself behaviorally and psychologically in various degrees of clinical compensation. Thus, similarly to Rado (1960), Meehl (1962, 1990, p. 25) argued that the schizotype may be highly compensated, or may reveal transient failures in compensation, or may be clinically schizophrenic. Schizotypes, therefore, can range clinically from apparent normality through psychosis, yet all share the schizogene and resultant schizotypic personality organization. According to Meehl (1962, 1990), not all schizotypes develop diagnosable schizophrenia; however, all schizotypes will display some evidence, albeit sometimes subtle, of their underlying liability in the form of aberrant psychobiologic and/or psychological functioning, and all schizophrenic individuals must first have been schizotypes.

Thus, in summary, Meehl (1962, 1990) theorized that schizophrenia is the complex developmental result of the interaction of a single major genetic factor relatively specific for schizophrenia with other genetically determined potentiators (e.g., anxiety, hedonic potential, social introversion) and environmental stressors. He hypothesized that the single major gene (schizogene) codes for a functional CNS synaptic control aberration termed *hypokrisia,* which results in *schizotaxia,* extensive synaptic slippage throughout the brain. Through social learning experiences, essentially all schizotaxic individuals develop *schizotypy,* a personality organization that harbors the latent liability for schizophrenia (cf. Meehl, 1990, p. 35). As a personality organization, schizotypy cannot be observed directly per se; however, this latent personality organization gives rise to schizotypic psychological and behavioral manifestations (Meehl, 1964) and is also reflected in deviance on laboratory measures (e.g., eye tracking dysfunction, sustained attention deficits). Schizotypic individuals (though not necessarily diagnosable as having DSM-III-R SPD) exhibit cognitive slippage, interpersonal aversiveness, pan-anxiety, and mild depression. The majority remain only schizotypic throughout the life-span with only a subset going on to develop diagnosable schizophrenia.

Finally, Meehl conjectures that the base rate of schizotaxia (and, by definition, the schizotypy taxon) in the general population is approximately 10%. Meehl's (1990, 1993) base rate estimate is founded on a dominant-gene formulation which posits that every schizophrenic person must, by definition, have a parent who is a schizotype – namely, a parent carrying the schizophrenia-producing genotype (whether clinically expressed or not). The specific base rate estimate derives empirically from the combined observations that

1. Only 10% of individuals affected with schizophrenia have a similarly affected parent (i.e., 5% of the parents are clinically schizophrenic). Meehl argues that this 10% figure suggests a "clinical penetrance" of the gene for clinical schizophrenia is roughly 10% (i.e., 90% of known carriers go unexpressed).
2. The population prevalence of schizophrenia is approximately 1% (cf. Meehl, 1993, p. 5).

Thus, a reasonable schizotypy taxon base rate estimate would be 10% for the general unselected population.

On the need for a latent liability construct

Much of the discussion above has assumed a common underlying liability for these illnesses. What is the empirical basis for such an assumption? We believe there is ample evidence in support of a latent liability conceptualization in schizophrenia that includes schizotypic psychopathology among other things. First, schizotypic psychopathology is linked, presumably via genetics (Torgersen, 1985), to schizophrenia (Kendler, 1985). Perhaps the most influential evidence that helped to establish a link between schizotypic phenomenology and clinical schizophrenia came from the Danish Adoption Study of Schizophrenia (Kety, Rosenthal, Wender, & Schulsinger, 1968). Kety and colleagues (1968), using a clinically based definition of "borderline schizophrenia," found elevated rates of borderline or latent schizophrenia in the biological relatives of schizophrenic adoptees. These results provided compelling evidence for a genetically transmitted component underlying both manifest schizophrenia and the less severe schizophrenia-like disorders. The hypothesized continuity between the conditions was thus not merely phenomenological, but also genetic. Moreover, confirming the early Kety et al. findings, numerous family studies have found an excess of schizotypic disorders in the biological relatives of schizophrenic individuals (see Kendler, McGuire, Gruenberg, O'Hare, Spellman, & Walsh, 1993). Clearly, the boundaries of the phenotypic expression of schizophrenia liability extend beyond manifest psychosis. Thus, liability manifestations are not isomorphic with expressed psychosis.

Second, the existence of a clinically unexpressed liability for schizophrenia has been confirmed (Gottesman & Bertelsen, 1989; Lenzenweger & Loranger, 1989a). Thus, liability can exist without obvious phenotypic, or symptomatic, manifestations. Third, a well-established biobehavioral marker, namely eye tracking dysfunction (Holzman et al., 1988; Levy, Holzman, Matthysse, & Mendel, 1993), which bears no immediately discernible phenotypic connection to overt schizophrenia, is known to be associated with a latent diathesis for the illness. Thus, liability can manifest itself in an alternative phenotypic form. Finally, if the base rate of schizophrenia liability (or the schizotypy taxon) is, in fact, 10% as conjectured by Meehl (1990), then perhaps well over 50% of those carrying liability for schizophrenia may go clinically "undetected" across the life-span (i.e., an estimate derived from combined prevalence of schizophrenia, schizotypal PD, and paranoid PD is roughly 5%; cf. Loranger, 1990). Taken together, both theoretical and empirical considerations argue strongly for the plausibility of a complex latent liability construct in schizophrenia.

Given that most persons vulnerable to schizophrenia may never show flagrant psychosis or easily detectable signs and symptoms of shizotypic personality functioning, researchers have sought ways to detect schizotypy using more sensitive detection approaches (i.e., various laboratory and psychometric measures). Efforts have been made to discover valid objective indicators of schizotypy that function efficiently across a range of clinical compensation as well as mental state and are capable of detecting liability even in clinically unexpressed (nonsymptomatic) cases. Such indicators, psychometric and otherwise, are thought to assess an "endophenotype" (a feature not visible to the unaided, naked eye; see Gottesman, 1991), and their inclusion in research investigations of the genetics and familiality of schizophrenia is likely to enhance those efforts even when the putative indicators are only modestly correlated with the latent liability (Smith & Mendell, 1974).

On the structure of the latent liability

Assuming that schizotypy, as conceptualized by Meehl (1962, 1990), represents a defensible latent-liability construct and the potential research utility of valid schizotypy indexes is evident, a basic question about the fundamental structure of schizotypy remains. Is it continuous (i.e., "dimensional") or truly discontinuous ("qualitative") in nature? For example, at the level of the gene, both Meehl's (1962, 1990) model and the "latent trait" model (Holzman et al., 1988; Matthysse et al., 1986) conjecture the existence of a qualitative discontinuity, whereas the polygenic multifactorial threshold model (Gottesman, 1991) predicts a continuous distribution of levels of liability.[2] Clarification of the structure of schizotypy may help to resolve ambiguous issues that remain in discussions concerning appropriate genetic models for schizophrenia, and such information may aid in planning future studies in this area. Nearly all investigations of the structure of schizophrenia liability done to date have relied exclusively on fully expressed, diagnosable schizophrenia (see Gottesman, 1991), and the results of these studies have left unresolved the question of liability structure. Moreover, one surely cannot reason with confidence that a unimodal distribution of phenotypic schizotypic traits supports the existence of a continuum of liability (e.g., Kendler, Ochs, Gorman, Hewitt, Ross, & Mirsky, 1991). In recent years, however, it has been proposed that a possible "expansion" of the schizophrenia phenotype to include other schizophrenia-related phenomena, such as eye tracking dysfunction (Holzman et al., 1988), might be helpful in efforts to illuminate the latent structure of liability in schizophrenia. We have pursued an approach, complementary to the "expanded phenotype" proposal, through the application of a psychometric approach to the detection of schizotypy (see Lenzenweger, 1993). Thus, we have undertaken over the past several years a series of studies that begin to explore the latent structure of schizotypy. Our work has drawn extensively upon the theoretical formulations of Rado and Meehl, and we have used a well-validated measure of schizotypy, namely the Chapmans'

[2] We note that the polygenic multifactorial threshold model predicts an essentially qualitative discontinuity at the phenotypic level, or the level of clinical expression. In this report, we are concerned with assumptions concerning the latent structure of schizotypy, or schizophrenia liability.

Perceptual Aberration Scale (Chapman, Chapman, & Raulin, 1978) in these efforts.

Discontinuities in psychology and psychopathology: a detour on biases and methods

Before moving on, we believe it important to take a brief detour on the issue of continuity versus discontinuity in connection with psychological and/or psychopathological constructs. When one speaks of a taxon (latent class or "nonarbitrary" natural subgroup), one is concerned with a difference of type or kind, rather than a difference of degree or intensity. Hypothesizing the existence of discrete types in psychological science, especially within the realm of personality and psychopathology, has been the object of lively debate (see Gangestad & Snyder, 1985; Meehl, 1992). Many psychologists seem opposed to the very existence of types, though the reasons for such opposition may have more to do with one's point of view (or ideology) on the conduct of science and structure of nature rather than otherwise. It has been argued (Gangestad & Snyder, 1985; Meehl, 1992) that looking for "types" in the psychological realm is unpopular and runs counter to the thinking (biases?) of most psychological theorists (see Eysenck, 1986, for an example of a prominent dimensional approach to personality).

Although the dimensionality of many variables in psychology seems plausible and well established (e.g., sociability, impulsivity), it is important to bear in mind that the act of "measuring" a variable continuously does not necessarily "make" the latent construct continuous in nature. There are striking examples of graded or continuous measurement that illustrate difficulties with an assumption that, somehow, continuity in measurement implies continuity in structure. To take a crude comparison, for example, the temperature of water can be measured continuously; however, temperatures above 212°F or below 32°F are associated with qualitative changes of organizational state (or "type") – namely, transitions to a vapor or solid, respectively. In a more closely related vein, we regard body temperature as a reflection of "health," and we can measure reliably the temperature of the human body in a continuous fashion. Once body temperature passes 98.6°F, however, we typically speak of the presence of "illness" (i.e., we recognize a meaningful discontinuity in continuous data). Perhaps closer still to our subject matter, although intelligence is routinely measured in a continuous manner in the form of IQ scores, we speak of retardation as we descend into the lower tail of the population distribution of IQ in recognition of a readily apparent qualitative change. The basic point we seek to make is relatively straightforward: One's approach to measurement should not determine one's views of the structure of nature; one should not be persuaded that nature is structured in a dimensional manner merely because one has relied on continuous measurement approaches. One's views of the structure of nature must be open to empirical confirmation or disconfirmation. As Meehl (1992) argues, "Whether or not the entities, properties, and processes of a particular domain (such as psychopathology or vocational interest patterns) are purely dimensional, or are instead a mix of dimensional and taxonic relations, *is an empirical question,* not to be settled by a methodological dogma about how science works" (p. 119).

Finding compelling evidence for the existence of a discontinuity in the realm of personality is not an easy task, partly because many workers have relied on methods for the detection of latent taxa that are either largely inadequate for the task (i.e., group contrasts, factor analysis) or are potentially misleading [e.g., bimodality in the distribution of scores on a variable of interest (Grayson, 1987; Murphy, 1964; see also Levy et al., 1993) or cluster analysis (Golden & Meehl, 1980)]. Factor-analytic approaches will always yield continuous factors, yet a dimensional latent structure to the data is not necessarily ensured; cluster analysis will always yield qualitative clusters, yet a typological latent structure to the data is not ensured. Furthermore, the existence of bimodality in a distribution of scores for a phenomenon under study does not ensure the existence of a latent discontinuity (see Grayson, 1987), and bimodality may fail to surface in a score distribution when, in fact, it should be apparent. For example, major gene effects on a quantitative character may not reveal themselves in an easy discernible manner (e.g., "bimodality" in a metric character distribution), yet a major gene (a latent taxonic entity) is active nonetheless (e.g., Falconer, 1989). Moreover unimodality does not ensure the presence of a continuum at the latent level. Finally, to complicate matters further, a qualitative phenotypic character (e.g., extra toes in guinca pigs or cats) can be the result of an underlying system that is quantitative (e.g., polygenic) in nature (see Gottesman, 1991).

The very nature of variability in human behavior, coupled with the multitude of facets of human psychological functioning worthy of scientific study, makes the task of finding a discontinuity in an aspect of personality organization, trait structure, or behavior a relatively daunting undertaking. Whereas certain observable human traits or behaviors are likely to be truly discontinuous in structure (Meehl, 1992), many will not be so. Further, many "continuous" human characters, though not all, will be expressions of continuously distributed genetic determinants. Indeed, as Falconer (1989) so aptly notes, "One has only to consider one's fellow men and women to realize that they all differ in countless ways, but that these differences are nearly all matters of degree and seldom present clear-cut distinctions attributable to the segregation of major genes" (p. 104). In other instances, however, a complex behavioral or trait phenotype will be an expression of a major gene(s). How then best to proceed? We argue that the search for a qualitative break in some human behavior or trait must first be founded on solid observation and theoretical conjecture (cf. Meehl, 1990, 1992; see also Matthysse, 1993), and appropriate statistical procedures that are "up to the job," so to speak, must be used. Fortunately, statistical techniques have been developed that can be used to discern discontinuities in human traits and behaviors [e.g., admixture analysis (Everitt & Hand, 1981), latent class analysis (Lazarsfeld & Henry, 1968), complex segregation analysis (Lalouel, Rao, Morton, & Elston, 1983), and taxometric analysis (Golden & Meehl, 1978; Meehl, 1973; Meehl & Golden, 1982; Meehl & Yonce, 1994; Meehl & Yonce, in preparation)]. We shall proceed with our discussion of schizotypy with two notions in mind: that (1) qualitative "types" (or taxa) of human behavior (traits, conditions) can exist, and (2) their accurate detection requires the use of appropriate statistical procedures.

Body image and perceptual aberrations in schizotypy

In theoretical discussions of schizotypy a great deal of importance has been attached to body image and perceptual distortions in schizotypy as defined by both Rado and Meehl. Rado (1960) described body-image distortions and perceptual anomalies thought to characterize the psychological experience of the schizotype. Meehl identified body-image aberrations as a schizotypic sign in his (1964) *Manual,* providing rich descriptions of the clinical manifestations of such phenomena (see his pp. 24–27). Further, Meehl (1990) refers to body-image distortions several times in his revised theory of schizotypy (see pp. 9, 19, and 23). Perceptual and body-image distortions as phenomenological manifestations of a liability for (or expression of) schizophrenia (and other psychoses) have a long history in descriptive psychopathology (Chapman et al., 1978).

The Perceptual Aberration Scale: a valid index of schizotypy

Loren and Jean Chapman (Chapman et al., 1978) developed the Perceptual Aberration Scale (PAS) to operationalize the rich clinical observations of body-image distortion and perceptual aberrations abounding in the schizophrenia literature (e.g., Meehl, 1964). The PAS is a 35-item true–false self-report measure of disturbances and distortions in perceptions of body image as well as other objects. The PAS item content and the details of its construction can be found elsewhere (Chapman & Chapman, 1985; Chapman, Chapman, & Kwapil, Chapter 5, this volume).

Although space constraints preclude an extensive review of the literature on the PAS, it is useful to highlight several critical linkages between the PAS and other indicators of validity in schizophrenia. In the tradition of construct validation (Cronbach & Meehl, 1955) as well as the operational approach to the validation of diagnostic entities suggested subsequently by Robins and Guze (1970), we briefly review three kinds of evidence supportive of the validity of the PAS: (1) family history of schizophrenia, (2) performance on established laboratory tests on which schizophrenic patients are known to be deviant, and (3) clinical phenomenology. Evidence regarding the predictive validity of the PAS is promising and is reviewed extensively by Chapman, Chapman, and Kwapil (Chapter 5, this volume), and other newer criterion validation data can be found in Holzman et al. (Chapter 15, this volume). Finally, we discuss our recent taxometric effort (below) in connection with Robins and Guze's (1970) fifth validity criterion – namely, "delimination from other disorders."

Family history of schizophrenia

If the PAS is a valid schizotypy index, then it should detect a latent liability for schizophrenia in compensated (nonpsychotic) persons, who, in turn, should display an elevated rate of schizophrenia among their first-degree biological relatives. To examine this possibility, Lenzenweger and Loranger (1989a) examined the lifetime expectancy (morbid risk) of treated schizophrenia, unipolar depression, and bipolar disorder in the biological first-degree relatives of 101 nonpsychotic psychiatric patients (probands) who were classified as either "schizotypy-positive" or "schizotypy-negative" according to the PAS. The relatives of schizotypy-positive probands were significantly more likely to have been treated for schizophrenia than the relatives of schizotypy-negative probands; the morbid risk for treated unipolar depression or bipolar disorder among the relatives of the two proband groups did not differ. Consistent with the Lenzenweger and Loranger (1989a) results, Miller and Chapman (1993) have demonstrated recently that the PAS has a substantial heritable component, and Kendler and Hewitt (1992) have found that "positive trait schizotypy" (of which perceptual aberration is a component) is substantially heritable. Furthermore, Battaglia et al. (1991), in a study of the relatives of schizotypal patients, found that recurrent illusions (akin to perceptual aberrations) were present in every schizotypal personality disorder (SPD) patient with a positive family history of schizophrenia.

Deviance on laboratory tests

A deficit in sustained attention, a leading biobehavioral indicator of a possible schizophrenia liability, has been found to be associated with elevated PAS scores. Lenzenweger and associates (1991), using a low a priori signal-probability, high-processing-load Continuous Performance Test (Cornblatt, Lenzenweger, & Erlenmeyer-Kimling, 1989), found deficits in sustained attention in a group of compensated schizotypic subjects relative to normal controls. Replication results, using the same measure of sustained attention, have been reported recently by Obiols and colleagues (1993). Grove et al. (1991) have also replicated Lenzenweger et al. (1991), in finding a significant association between high PAS scores and poor sustained attention performance among the first-degree biological relatives of individuals with diagnosed schizophrenia.

Additional work exploring associations between PAS deviance and other putative indicators of liability for schizophrenia also support the validity of the measure. Studies examining indicators such as eye tracking dysfunction (e.g., Simons & Katkin, 1985), dorsolateral prefrontal cortex–related executive memory functions and abstraction ability (Lenzenweger & Korfine, 1994), spatial working memory (cf. Park & Holzman, 1992; Park, Holzman, & Lenzenweger, in press), and antisaccade performance (O'Driscoll, Holzman, & Lenzenweger, in preparation) have provided supportive and intriguing results (see Holzman et al., Chapter 15, this volume, for a synopsis of these studies).

PAS deviance is also closely associated with schizophrenia-related deviance on the Minnesota Multiphasic Personality Inventory (MMPI) (Lenzenweger, 1991), schizophrenia-related personality disorder features (Lenzenweger & Korfine, 1992b), and thought disorder (Coleman, Levy, Lenzenweger, & Holzman, in preparation; Edell & Chapman, 1979; Holzman et al., Chapter 15, this volume).

Clinical phenomenology

Lenzenweger and Loranger (1989b) used the Personality Disorder Examination (PDE) and other established measures of psychopathology to document the associations between the PAS and both DSM-III-R Axis II personality pathology as well as anxiety, depression, premorbid adjustment, global functioning, and other indexes. In brief, and consistent with Meehl's model of schizotypy, elevations on the PAS were most closely associated with SPD symptoms and clinically assessed anxiety. This pattern of data provided additional criterion validity linking high PAS scores with schizotypic and "psychotic-like" phenomenology outside university settings (cf. Chapman, Edell, & Chapman, 1980; see also Chapman et al., Chapter 5, this volume).

Summary

Given the supportive array of both criterion and construct validity data associated with the PAS, we have argued that the measure could be plausibly considered a schizotypy index. Furthermore, as a measure of body image distortions and perceptual aberrations (a content domain reflective of experiences at the heart of both Rado and Meehl's models of schizotypy), we view the PAS as a reasonably well-validated indicator of liability (schizotypy) as distinguished from a measure of Meehl's polygenic potentiators (e.g., social introversion). The long-range predictive validity and specificity of the PAS in relation to schizophrenia and closely related conditions remains to be established firmly. The available intermediate-term (i.e., 10-year) follow-up data of the Chapmans (Chapter 5, this volume) are encouraging in this regard, although the issue is by no means closed. We await long-term follow-up data (20–25 yr) from the Chapman study as well as the Cornell series being followed in our laboratory. Any thoughtful consideration of the PAS as a schizotypy index must bear in mind that the instrument is likely to generate some unspecified rate of false positives in regard to final outcome (e.g., schizophrenia-related diagnoses), just as any screening device is expected to. On the other hand, the false negative rate of the PAS in the prediction of clinical outcome (e.g., schizophrenia-related diagnoses at follow-up) must also be considered. Both false positive and false negative classification on the basis of the PAS will only serve to minimize group differences on any outcome measures such as clinical phenomenology, family history of schizophrenia, and laboratory measures (e.g., sustained attention, eye tracking).

The MAXCOV-HITMAX taxometric method: a conceptual introduction

Meehl introduced MAXCOV-HITMAX as a data-analytic technique for use in detecting latent taxa in his seminal volume of selected papers, *Psychodiagnosis* (1973), and has discussed the approach in several subsequent papers (Meehl, 1990, 1992; Meehl & Golden, 1982; Meehl & Yonce, in preparation). We have used the MAXCOV-HITMAX procedure in our taxometric explorations of schizotypy and offer a brief nontechnical overview of the technique.

The core idea of MAXCOV-HITMAX is elegant, although simple, drawing on logically anticipated relations among psychometric indicators (or, behavioral signs) when assessed in a population composed of an admixture of individuals belonging to one of two latent classes, or a taxon and its complement. In short, MAXCOV-HITMAX is a procedure that is sensitive to the fact that the association (i.e., covariance) between two indicators will be greatest (hence, MAXCOV) when evaluated in a sample that consists of nearly balanced rates of two "types" of members (i.e., a mixed population) and will be smallest in a population made up of individuals who share membership in the same single class, either the taxon or its complement. Stated somewhat differently, the maximum covariance method looks at the covariance of two output indicators as a function of successive intervals on a third, input, indicator. If the latent structure is taxonic, then covariance increases in the vicinity of greater taxon–complement mixture; if the latent structure is nontaxonic, the covariance across intervals is flat (Meehl, 1973; Meehl & Golden, 1982).

An example is perhaps a good way to demonstrate the conceptual basis of MAXCOV-HITMAX. Imagine an investigator has three continuous psychometric (or behavioral) indicators (x, y, z) of a putative latent taxon (i.e., a discontinuous or qualitative latent entity). Imagine, too, that values are available for each of these indicators for a large sample of individuals (e.g., $n > 1{,}000$), preferably sampled randomly from a large unselected population. Ideally, the three indicators should be as statistically independent as possible (both within and outside the taxon), however, the MAXCOV-HITMAX technique appears robust even in the face of relatively high degrees of interindicator covariance (Meehl & Golden, 1982; Meehl & Yonce, in preparation). One conducts MAXCOV-HITMAX by examining the covariances (associations) between each possible pairing of the three indicators as a function of the remaining third, or "input," indicator – that is, the one left out of the pairing under examination. More specifically, one examines the covariance between x and y (cov_{xy}) for that subsample of persons falling in the lowest 10% of scores on z, then the covariance for x and y for that subsample of persons in the next 10% of scores on z, and so on until all levels of z have been covered. In practical terms, one is studying the covariance of x and y in "minisamples" drawn from the larger overall study sample, with specific "minisample" membership defined by score on z. The cuts taken on z need not necessarily be in deciles; standard deviation units or some other increment could also be used to define mini-samples.

If one is dealing with a latent taxon underlying scores on *z,* then one will observe that the covariances between *x* and *y* will be minimal in the minisamples that contain only complement or taxon members, and greater in samples where there is a mix of complement and taxon members. Meehl (1973; Meehl & Golden, 1982; Meehl & Yonce, in preparation) argued this pattern will emerge because at the latent level, the individuals falling at the low end of *z* constitute a class (i.e., are essentially alike) and have comparable values on *x* and *y* (i.e., minimal variance on each in the minisample), and consequently, *x* and *y* will display minimal covariance; the same pattern should emerge for the *x* and *y* covariance for the high end of the *z* indicator (those individuals belong to a different class). We could speak of one of the classes being constituted of taxon "members" and the other constituted of "nonmembers." Furthermore, and quite interestingly, since one is dealing with an imperfect indicator in *z,* there will be some persons obtaining a middle range score on *z* who are actually members of the latent class found at the "low end" of *z* and some persons obtaining a middle score on *z* who are actually members of the latent class defined by the "high end" of *z;* thus an admixture of taxon members and nonmembers exists "beneath" (i.e., at the latent, unobservable level) middle values of *z.* A latent mixture of taxon members and nonmembers in terms of *z* then creates a situation where variation can exist on the observed indicators *x* and *y,* and therefore, the covariance for *x* and *y* in this minisample will increase, being maximized when the mixture of taxon members and nonmembers is approximately equal (i.e., the so-called HITMAX interval used to estimate a taxon base rate; see Meehl, 1973; Meehl & Golden, 1982). When depicted graphically, the plot of the covariances of *x* and *y* as a function of *z,* when one is dealing with a taxonic latent entity, will appear as an inverted "V," with a peak at the midpoint of the *z* values (Figure 7.1). It is important to note that simple visual inspection of the distribution of scores on *z* will not necessarily provide any clues as to whether or not a taxon (or class) underlies *z;* however, systematic MAXCOV analysis of the covariance of *x* and *y* in relation to *z* will illuminate the latent situation. This is the heart of the MAXCOV-HITMAX approach.[3]

When one is dealing with a relatively common latent taxon (e.g., base rate = .40 to .50), the peak of the covariance curve will fall predictably in the midrange of an input indicator (*z* in the present example) as this is where an even (i.e., 50/50) or balanced latent mixture of taxon members and nonmem-

[3] See also Gangestad and Snyder (1985, pp. 348–349) for a succinct, though slightly more technical, discussion of the rationale underlying the conjecture that a "peaked" covariance curve will obtain from a MAXCOV-HITMAX analysis of indicators tapping a latent taxonic entity.

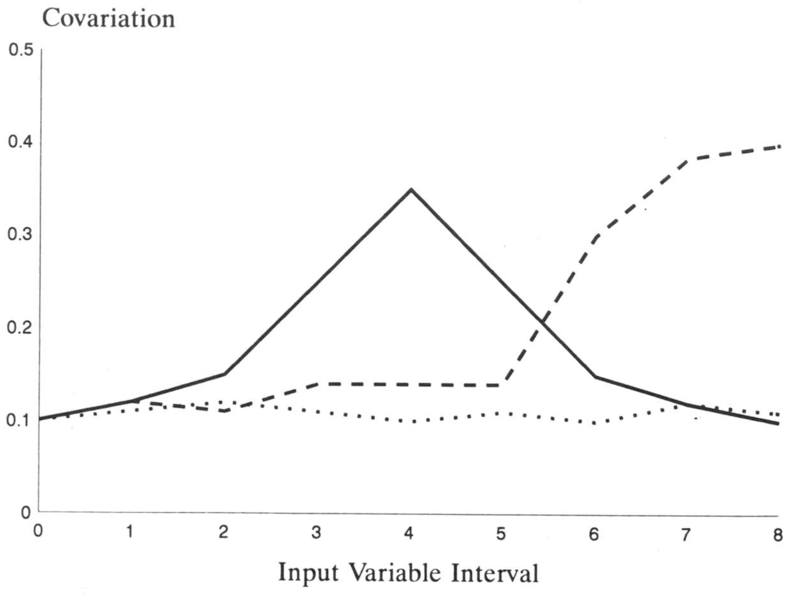

Fig. 7.1. Hypothetical covariation curves for a MAXCOV-HITMAX taxometric analysis of a tonic latent entity with a base rate of approximately .50, a taxonic latent entity with a low base rate (e.g., < .20), and a nontaxonic "dimensional" latent construct.

bers occurs. When the base rate of the taxon under investigation drops to .25 or less, the "peak" of the curve moves, predictably, along toward the right (high values on the input indicator keyed in the direction of taxon membership) as that is where, logically, the greatest mixing of taxon members and nonmembers can occur at the latent level (see Meehl & Yonce, in preparation; see also Figure 7.1). Finally, to complete the present example, we note that the same covariance analyses would be carried out for the x and z pairing as well as the y and z pairing as functions of the y and x indicators, respectively. The three resulting covariance curves may be averaged and, if desired, smoothed using established techniques (see Tukey, 1977).

One might ask, How does MAXCOV-HITMAX "behave" when one is dealing with indicators not tapping a latent taxon but, rather, tapping a truly dimensional construct? If a latent construct that is continuous in nature and the hypothesized indicators x, y, and z are tapping that construct, then the results of the analysis described above will be quite discernibly different. A "peaked" or "taxonic" covariance curve should not have emerged. Rather cov_{xy} will be approximately equal across all of the "minisamples," and the resulting covariance curve essentially flat (Figure 7.1). The flatness of the covariance curve obtained from the analysis of a truly dimensional latent construct is due to the fact that individuals falling within a given interval (e.g., lowest 10% of *z*) are just as much like one another as those falling within any of the other nine remaining deciles, and therefore, the observed covariances for *x* and *y* across *z* must be, by definition, nearly equal or, at least, highly comparable. The reason is that in the dimensional latent situation there are no classes to mix, so to speak, and persons differ only in degree; those persons falling in each minisample of the input indicator (*z* in our example) are highly comparable to one another and therefore yield little variance on indicators *x* and *y*. An example, adapted from Trull's excellent discussion (Trull, Widiger, & Guthrie, 1990) of MAXCOV-HITMAX, will serve us well here. Imagine our investigator had been doing a taxometric analysis of indicators of physical height, a known dimensional construct, and each of the three indicators (*x, y, z* again) was coded 0–9, yielding a 10-point scale for each indicator. Those persons obtaining a 5 on the 10-point scale *z* for height would be just as much like one another with respect to height as would those within the subsamples defined by, say, a 0 or 9 on *z*. A group of persons having a score of 5 on *z* would *not* consist of two classes (e.g., taxon members & nonmembers; or giants & midgets) but, rather, would merely include persons whose height varies somewhat around the value of 5 on *z*. As a result the covariation for *x* and *y* for the "5" group on indicator *z* should be no greater or less than that obtained from the other groups defined by *z*, and the resulting covariance curve for *x* and *y* across *z* would be flat. Gangestad and Snyder (1985) have actually conducted a MAXCOV-HITMAX analysis of impulsivity using real data, and the results of their analysis were as predicted, a relatively "nonpeaked" covariance curve indicating a dimensional latent construct. Trull et al. (1990) obtained similar results for the continuous latent dimension of dysthymia, whereas MAXCOV-HITMAX results for indicators known to tap biological sex produced a markedly peaked covariance curve.

The MAXCOV-HITMAX approach just described is comparable to the original description presented by Meehl (1973) and assumed the use of three continuous indicators. The approach can be applied to data structured differently as well. The technique can be applied to a *set* of dichotomous indicators selected from a single, though well-validated, indicator. MAXCOV-HITMAX can also be conducted on three "subscales" composed of items taken from a larger scale.[4] In the first instance, one might be particularly interested in, say, eight true–false items derived from a 35-item measure of a

[4] The three-"subscale" approach was suggested to us by Dr. Loren Chapman (personal communication, May 1993).

particular construct, or one might want to conduct a MAXCOV-HITMAX analysis of the sets of dichotomous diagnostic criteria that define any of the DSM-III-R personality disorders. A MAXCOV-HITMAX analysis using this "dichotomous indicator" approach is described in detail below (see also Gangestad & Snyder, 1985; Trull et al., 1990). In the second instance, one could assemble randomly three "subscales" from an original single, but longer, measure and proceed essentially as detailed above.

Taxometric exploration on schizotypy using the PAS

To explore the latent structure of the PAS and, thereby, address an aspect of validity associated with the PAS [namely Robins & Guze's (1970) "delimitation from other disorders"] as well as to examine Meehl's (1962, 1990) hypotheses concerning the likelihood of a discontinuous entity underlying schizotypy, we conducted two studies of the PAS, using Meehl's MAXCOV-HITMAX procedure ("dichotomous indicator data" application).

Taxometric study #1 (Lenzenweger & Korfine, 1992a)

Subjects

For our first study (Lenzenweger & Korfine, 1992a), we selected subjects from two samples of first-year undergraduates from Cornell University who voluntarily completed a 200-item objective psychological inventory entitled "Attitudes, Feelings, and Experiences Questionnaire" that included the PAS. Both samples were collected using a rigorous epidemiological-type data collection procedure described in detail elsewhere (Lenzenweger & Korfine, 1992a), which resulted in excellent response rates and representative sampling. The data from the two samples were checked for pseudorandom responding and invalid test-taking attitudes, and the final sample consisted of 1,093 individuals (see Lenzenweger & Korfine, 1992a).

Taxometric procedure

In the case of dichotomous indicator data, following Meehl's (1973) MAXCOV-HITMAX taxometric model, Gangestad and Snyder (1985) reasoned that if one assumes a latent class variable to be influencing the items on a measure, then any item that can discriminate between the classes (i.e., the taxon and its complement) should correlate strongly with the overall scale. Guided by this reasoning, we conducted an item analysis to select eight PAS items that correlated highly with the rest of the scale (total score minus the item under consideration). We excluded a highly correlated item if it was very similar in content to another item under consideration, so as to minimize any existing correlation between two items within the putative classes.

Given the predicted low base rate and hypothesized taxonic structure of schizotypy, we anticipated our MAXCOV analysis would reveal a covariance curve with a marked "right end peak" that would be comparable to Monte Carlo simulations conducted by Meehl and Yonce (in preparation) as well as logically consistent with the mathematical assumptions defining covariance in the HITMAX interval. To perform the MAXCOV analysis, we removed two PAS items (*i* and *j*) from the eight we selected and calculated a score for each subject based on the remaining six items, thus obtaining seven subsamples of individuals. That is, all subjects obtained a score on a 7-point scale such that those with a total score of zero on the six items composed (or made) one subsample, and the same was true for those with a total score of one, and so on through a total possible score of six. We then calculated the covariance for *i* and *j* for each subsample and repeated this procedure for all possible (28) pairs of selected PAS items (i.e., all possible *i* and *j* combinations) (see Gangestad & Snyder, 1985; Trull et al., 1990). Taking the means across all 28 pairs for each interval on the scale (i.e., for each subsample), we constructed an averaged covariance curve. We smoothed the curve using Tukey's (1977) medians of three procedures, repeated it twice, and copied on the endpoints (cf. Meehl, 1973; see also Gangestad & Snyder, 1985; Trull et al., 1990). Here we note that Meehl (1992) suggests that continuous variables function best as output indicators in MAXCOV. He acknowledges, however, the necessity for work using dichotomous indicators (Meehl, 1992, p. 134).

We estimated the schizotypy taxon base rate (*P*) by applying the method described by Meehl and Golden (1982) to the mean unsmoothed covariances for each interval as well as the smoothed covariances. Furthermore, we estimated the taxon base rate for each individual PAS item derived from the covariance values averaged across the seven pairings involving a given item for each item and calculated a median schizotypy base rate estimate across the eight items (see Lenzenweger & Korfne, 1992, for more detail).

Results

Table 7.1 contains the eight PAS items that were identified through item analysis as candidate items for our taxometric analyses. We report on the observed endorsement frequencies for each of the eight items (see Table 7.1). Figure 7.2 contains the covariance curve (both unsmoothed and smoothed)

Table 7.1. *Perceptual Aberration Scale endorsement frequencies and taxon base-rate estimates*

	Study #1		Study #2	
Item	Endorsement frequency	Taxon base rate	Endorsement frequency	Taxon base rate
1. Parts of my body occasionally seem dead or unreal. (T)	.105	.084	.061	.027
2. I have had the momentary feeling that my body has become misshapen. (T)	.177	.110	.036	.066
3. Now and then when I look in the mirror, my face seems quite different than usual. (T)	.457	.067	.183	.026
4. I have sometimes felt that some part of my body no longer belonged to me. (T)	.071	.287	.024	.067
5. Sometimes part of my body has seemed smaller than it usually is. (T)	.249	.086	.108	.080
6. Sometimes when I look at things like tables and chairs, they seem strange. (T)	.265	.188	.081	.017
7. The boundaries of my body always seem clear. (F)	.242	.303	.081	.033
8. Occasionally I have felt as though my body did not exist. (T)	.112	.037	.050	.106
Median taxon base rate	—	.098	—	.050
Averaged unsmoothed curve	—	.096	—	.034
Averaged smoothed curve	—	.088	—	.032

Note: Taxon base rates calculated following Meehl and Golden (1981). T = true; F = false; T or F indicates scoring direction for item. Median = median taxon base-rate estimate across the eight item-based estimates.
Source: Adapted from Lenzenweger and Korfine (1992a) and Korfine and Lenzenweger (1995).

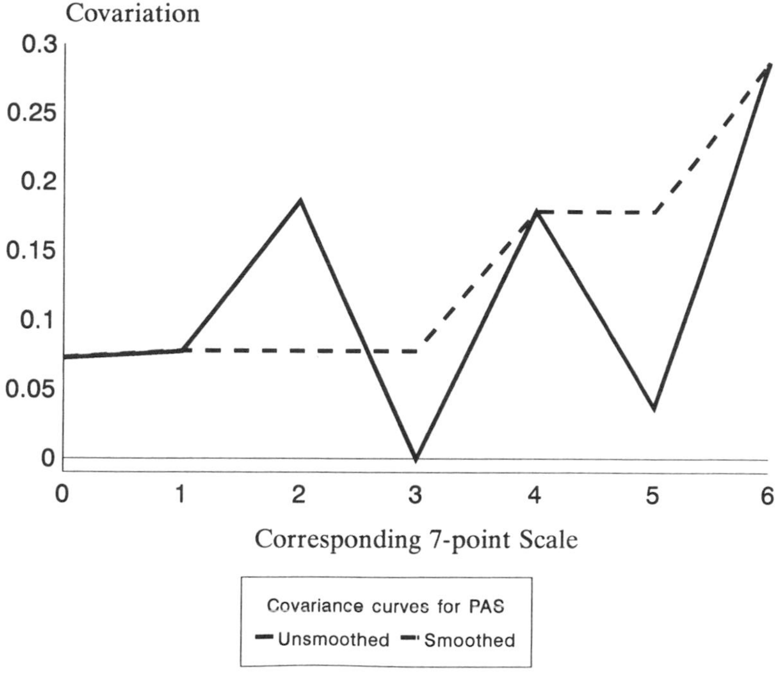

Fig. 7.2. Study #1. MAXCOV-HITMAX covariation curves for the Perceptual Aberration Scale (PAS) based on the average correlations across all 28 pairings for each interval on the corresponding 7-point scale for both the smoothed and unsmoothed data ($N = 1{,}093$). (Adapted from Lenzenweger & Korfine, 1992.)

based on the average covariances across all 28 pairings for each interval on the corresponding 7-point scale (i.e., each subsample). Inspection of Figure 7.2 reveals that both curves display a marked "right end peak." The unsmoothed curve shows marked peaks in several intervals ending with the right end peak, whereas the smoothed curve shows a pattern characterized by flatness over lower intervals, and an upward sweep toward the right end (i.e., higher intervals). A purely dimensional construct would have yielded a flat covariance curve across the 7-point scale indicating the absence of a taxon (i.e., all intervals would yield comparable covariances). The curves are consistent with the existence of a low base-rate taxon (cf. Meehl & Yonce, in preparation).

The taxon base-rate results are presented in Table 7.1. The P estimate (base rate) for the unsmoothed average covariance curve is 9.6% and for the smoothed curve P = 8.8%. The median base rate observed across all eight items analyzed separately is 9.8%. The base rates we observed do not simply reflect endorsement frequencies of the items (see Table 7.1). In fact, the correlation between the endorsement frequencies and taxon base-rate estimates across the eight items is –.18. These results are essentially identical to the 10% base rate of the schizotypy taxon in the general population as hypothesized by Meehl (1990).

Taxometric study #2 (Korfine & Lenzenweger, 1995)

Subjects

In order to determine the stability of our findings for the PAS from Study #1 (Lenzenweger & Korfine, 1995), we conducted a replication study using PAS data gathered during a recent fall term. Using identical survey distribution and collection methods, we assembled a second representative randomly ascertained sample of university students (n = 1,684; 51.3% women, 48.7% men) with a response rate of 84.2%. The final sample size for analysis was 1,646 cases.

Results

An item analysis conducted prior to the MAXCOV analysis revealed that the eight PAS items examined in Study #1 were also excellent candidate items for our second MAXCOV analysis, thereby ensuring a straightforward replication effort. The observed endorsement frequencies for each of the eight PAS items from Study #2 are also in Table 7.1. Figure 7.3 contains the covariance curves (both unsmoothed and smoothed) based on the average covariances across all 28 pairings for each interval on the corresponding 7-point scale (i.e., each subsample). Inspection of Figure 7.3 reveals that both curves display a marked "right end peak." As noted previously, a purely dimensional (or, factorial) construct would, by definition, have yielded a flat covariance curve across the 7-point scale, indicating the absence of a taxon (i.e., all intervals would yield comparable covariances). The curves we observed are consistent with the existence of a low base-rate taxon.

We again estimated the taxon base rates, and the results for Study #2 are also presented in Table 7.1 The P estimate (base rate) for the unsmoothed average covariance curve is 3.4%, and for the smoothed curve P = 3.2%. The median base rate observed across all eight items analyzed separately is 5.0%. Once again, we note that the item-derived taxon base rates we observed clearly do not simply reflect the endorsement frequencies (i.e., difficulty levels) of the items (see Table 7.1). In fact, the correlation between the endorse-

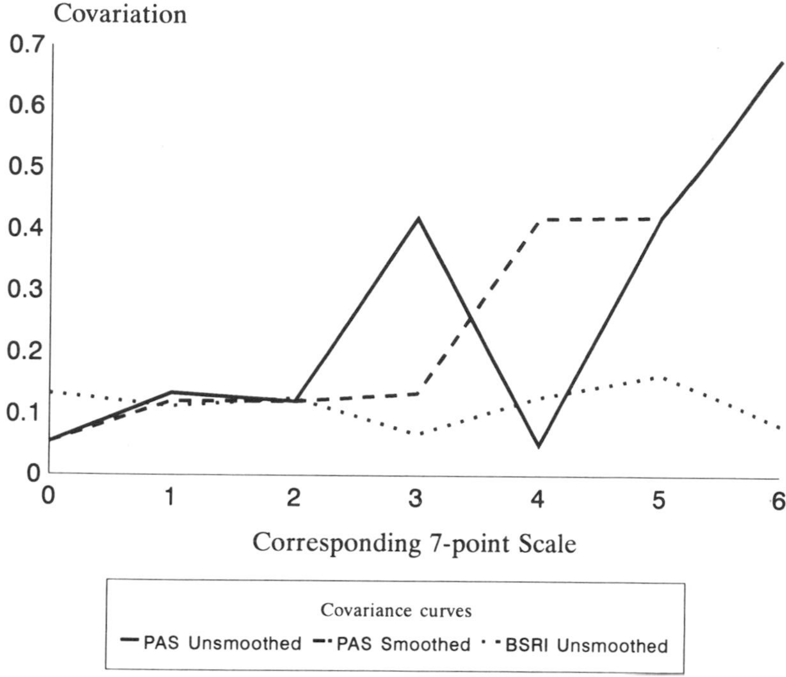

Fig. 7.3. Study #2. MAXCOV-HITMAX covariation curves for the Perceptual Aberration Scale (PAS) and the Bem Sex Role Inventory (BSRI) Femininity scale based on the average correlations across all 28 pairings for each interval on the corresponding 7-point scale (N = 1,646). PAS data presented both smoothed and unsmoothed; BSRI data presented unsmoothed only. (Adapted from Korfine & Lenzenweger, 1995.)

ment frequencies and taxon base-rate estimates across the eight items is –.41. These results are somewhat less than the base rate of the schizotypy taxon in the general population estimated by Meehl (1990), but nevertheless are compatible with his estimate.

Summary

The results of both of these taxometric studies suggest that a latent discontinuity may underlie scores on the PAS and the general population taxon base-rate estimate is in accord with the estimate conjectured by Meehl (1990). We readily acknowledge that the median taxon base-rate estimates for studies #1 (P = 9.8%) and #2 (P = 5.0%) are somewhat different; however, the means of the two figures (i.e., 7.4%) most likely represents a more stable estimate of the base rate. Our results are clearly consistent with Meehl's (1990) conjectures.[5] Moreover, the median taxon base-rate estimate for the replication study falls within the 95% confidence interval surrounding our initial 1992 taxon base-rate estimate of 9.8%. In this context we emphasize that finding a discontinuity underlying PAS scores using MAXCOV-HITMAX does not necessarily tell us a great deal about the members of the taxon that was detected. To explore this issue further, we examined the personality disorder features, assessed via a new self-report measure ("Personality Disorder Examination Screen," A. W. Loranger, unpublished manuscript), of the probable taxon members in Study #2 in contrast to nonmembers and found that probable taxon members were most characterized by schizotypic phenomenology (see Korfine & Lenzenweger, in press). This pattern of results strongly suggested that we had detected a schizotypic taxon. In sum, we believe our studies highlight the utility of MAXCOV-HITMAX for exploring the latent structure of a conjectured schizophrenia liability indicator in search of a taxon, particularly when the observed distribution of psychometric values provides few clues to latent structure.

Taxometric analysis: questions and challenges

Meehl's (1973) MAXCOV-HITMAX technique is but one procedure he has developed to search for latent taxa, and clearly, other approaches exist for addressing comparable aims (e.g., admixture analysis; latent class analysis). With respect to MAXCOV-HITMAX the question can arise, Why should we trust this approach? We should like to discuss this and related questions briefly. To begin, we are currently unaware of any published analytic position that has faulted the mathematical underpinnings of the method, and a large number of Monte Carlo simulations (see Meehl & Yonce, in preparation) support the validity of the method for detecting taxa as currently implemented. Furthermore, at this time the technique has been applied in over a dozen published studies (see Meehl, 1992) that have addressed genuine classification problems using real data derived from empirical studies. The performance of the approach in these studies appears to have been nonproblematic.

How well does the method perform in detecting a real latent class whose boundaries are not as "fuzzy" as, say, schizotypy? The data for the detection of biological sex in Trull et al. (1990) speak to this issue rather well. In their report, Trull and colleagues present a sharply peaked covariance curve for

[5] We are reliably informed that other workers have obtained comparable, though unpublished, results for the PAS (see Lowrie & Raulin, 1990, unpublished manuscript).

results obtained from fallible indicators of maleness/femaleness, a pattern of results unambiguously supportive of taxonicity where a taxon is known to exist. A related issue (or question) concerns what Meehl (1992) has termed the "pseudotaxa" situation, or the possibility that MAXCOV may suggest a taxon to be present when in reality no genuine taxon exists. In other words, will (or, how often will) the method mislead us into thinking that a taxonic latent structure exists, when in reality no such discontinuity is truly there? Data available to date do not suggest that the MAXCOV-HITMAX method falsely generates evidence for taxonicity; we are unaware of any published report that demonstrates such a "false positive" tendency for the method. Clearly, if one applies a taxometric procedure to a data set that has been derived from a population where an artificial taxonic situation has been "artificially created" (e.g., MAXCOV analysis of height conducted on a sample of people consisting only of giants and midgets), then pseudotaxa can indeed result. However, we argue the method per se is not at fault in such situations; rather its application has been artifactually affected by sampling bias. Meehl's position on this issue is perhaps more clearly stated: "No statistical method should ever be applied blindly, unthinkingly, paying no attention to anything else about the situation than the way the numbers behave" (Meehl, 1992, p. 143). Finally, we explore a related question, Will MAXCOV analysis, somehow, always suggest that a latent taxon is present? The answer to this extreme challenge is clearly, no. Evidence supporting the ability of the technique for finding a latent dimension is available for dimensions such as impulsivity (Gangestad & Snyder, 1985) and dysthymia (Trull et al., 1990).

Along the lines of challenges to the taxometric approach – MAXCOV in particular – another question strikes us as relevant here, namely: Does item format lead one falsely to infer taxonicity in the application of MAXCOV-HITMAX? For example, does MAXCOV analysis of true–false psychometric inventory data somehow interact with the MAXCOV procedure to generate, artifactually, "taxonic" results? Gangestad and Snyder (1985) and Trull et al. (1990) both analyzed data that were structured in a dichotomous format and found evidence for latent continua; the structure of their data did not drive the MAXCOV procedure to generate taxonic results (see original reports for additional detail). In our work with MAXCOV, we have sought to address this issue as well by posing the question, Will MAXCOV detect a latent continuum even when the data have been forced into a dichotomous format? To answer this question, we drew upon data available from our subjects in Study 2 described above for the psychological dimension of femininity as assessed by the Bem Sex Role Inventory (BSRI; Bem, 1974).

In brief, the BSRI is a 60-item self-report questionnaire that assesses masculinity and femininity as two dimensions. Subjects are asked to rate how well each adjective or phrase describes themselves on a scale that ranges from 1 ("Never or almost never true") to 7 ("Always or almost always true"). The items on the masculinity and femininity scales were selected on the basis of their sex-typed social desirability. On the BSRI, each subject receives two total scores, a masculinity score and a femininity score (each an average of the relevant ratings for each dimension). For present taxometric purposes, we conducted an internal consistency analysis to identify eight femininity scale items that had high item–total correlations with the femininity total scale score (minus item under consideration). We sought items that were not unduly similar or synonymous so as to avoid elevated interitem correlations (cf. Meehl & Golden, 1982). We identified eight femininity items as candidate items for MAXCOV-HITMAX analysis. In order to ensure that item format of these items was consistent with that of the PAS (i.e., true–false), the eight BSRI items were all dichotomized at the median for each item (recalling that they were rated from 1 to 7). Unlike biological sex (cf. Trull et al., 1990), we argue that psychological femininity as a construct is best conceptualized as a dimension; therefore, scores on the BSRI-F are phenotypic expressions of a continuous latent construct. As a result, we anticipated that the covariance curve resulting from the MAXCOV analysis would be relatively flat, suggesting a latent continuum. Our MAXCOV analysis was conducted on data available for the 1,646 subjects in Study #2 for the following BSRI items: "affectionate," "sympathetic," "sensitive to the needs of others," "compassionate," "eager to soothe hurt feelings," "warm," "tender," and "gentle." For comparison purposes the data from this examination of femininity are also plotted in Figure 7.3. Inspection of the figure reveals, even without smoothing, an essentially flat covariance curve. These data clearly support the fact that MAXCOV can detect a known latent continuum, even in the face of dichotomously structured input data.

Should one "settle for" data derived from a MAXCOV-HITMAX analysis to resolve the taxonomic question of taxonicity for a given construct, such as schizotypy as we have discussed? Clearly no single taxometric analysis can provide a definitive answer to such a taxonomic question. We agree with Meehl (1992) in advocating that any investigation of the latent structure of a theoretical construct must rely on multiple corroboration and consistency tests. Namely, replication efforts are essentially in this type of work, and investigators should employ different taxometric methods, especially ones that are nonredundant in terms of their mathematical underpinnings, to analyze any given data set (see Meehl, 1992). Ideally taxometric findings should be replicated using additional unselected populations as well, thus ensuring that one is indeed exploring the natural latent structure of a construct in a population uninfluenced by any a priori selection (i.e., distortion), however subtle.

At this juncture we note that the MAXCOV-HITMAX procedure continues to be refined and questions concerning its application and relation to other latent class techniques arise naturally. For example, can the MAXCOV-HITMAX formalism give rise to a null model against which an alternative model of "taxonicity" can be contrasted? Additionally, in its present form the technique is designed to detect a single latent class (a taxon and its complement); what would one expect from the procedure if one were dealing with a latent structure that consisted of three or more classes rather than two? We raise these questions as they have come to us while using this technique within a context of discovery, and we should like to pursue them further.

Substantive issues and implications for understanding schizotypy

In this chapter we have discussed a prominent model of schizotypy as well as an approach to testing one of the model's primary assumptions, namely the latent structure of schizotypy. In outlining the taxometric approach advocated by Meehl (Meehl, 1973, 1992; Meehl & Golden, 1982), we have also sought to highlight the utility of the general approach for researching latent class questions in psychopathology. Despite the robust nature of the taxometric approach and the relatively specific case of schizotypy, one could ask the question, What difference does it make? (cf. Meehl, 1992). In other words, why should psychopathologists be concerned with whether or not something is taxonic at the latent level? Here we consult Meehl (1992), who addressed this challenge in a recent discussion of taxonomic issues. He argues that there are at least four reasons for determining whether or not a construct in psychology or psychopathology is structured qualitatively. If genuine taxa exist, then, according to Meehl (adapted from Meehl, 1992, pp. 161–2):

1. Theoretical science should come to know them.
2. The construction of assessment devices will proceed differently, given that the goal would be the assignment of individuals to a category versus location of individuals on a dimension.
3. We could determine whether the classification of patients, as in organic medicine, is justified in terms of both improved treatment and prognosis.
4. Causally oriented researchers will often proceed differently if a taxonic conjecture has initially been taxometrically corroborated.

We believe the fourth issue raised by Meehl is particularly important. For example, in the study of the genetics of schizophrenia (and, by default, schizotypy), the debate over the precise mode of transmission has continued for decades without resolution. Any approach that might shed light on the latent structure of liability for schizophrenia could only advance the field, and results favoring one model over others (i.e., single major locus vs. mixed vs. multifactorial polygenic threshold transmission) would help to bring clarity and greater momentum to a research area seeking such. For example, taxometric evidence supporting the existence of a latent discontinuity in the liability for schizophrenia clearly provides important support for models that hypothesize the existence of a single major gene influence (e.g., mixed model; the Holzman–Matthysse "latent trait" model). In short, knowing that the latent liability for schizophrenia is taxonic in nature will increase the likelihood that we shall pursue empirically genetic models holding such an assumption.

We conclude by highlighting a critical issue that remains in this particular research area, but one that extends broadly in its implications. In conducting taxometric work on schizotypy, we have been struck by the importance of how one conceptualizes a liability indicator in relation to the specific genetic influences for schizophrenia. In other words, how close is one's indicator to the genetic factors responsible for schizophrenia? The answer to this question not only affects how one interprets taxometric results, but also influences decisions regarding the placement (and causal importance) of indicators in models of schizotypy.

If we maintain an endophenotype conceptualization (Gottesman, 1994) – namely, where the endophenotype lies between the genotype and phenotype (i.e., genotype → endophenotype → phenotype) but is not visible to the unaided (or "naked") eye – and if we assume that a putative indicator assesses an endophenotypic manifestation of schizotypy with a reasonable degree of validity, then the following predictions obtain vis-à-vis taxometric explorations: If the indicator assesses a psychological (or other biobehavioral) aberration that is relatively "close" to (or highly influenced by) the gene(s), and if schizophrenia liability is, in fact, influenced by a major gene, then taxometric analysis should reveal that a taxon underlies indicator scores, thereby providing evidence for a major gene (or, "latent trait") model. If the indicator assesses an aberration relatively "close" to the gene(s) causally responsible for schizophrenia and if the genetic underpinnings of schizophrenia are truly polygenic in nature, then a latent taxon should not be found underlying the PAS scores. If the indicator assesses an aberration that is relatively "far" from the gene(s) (i.e., closer to phenotype) and if the genetic structure is influenced by either a polygenic system or single major locus, then we would expect to find evidence for a latent taxon underlying the PAS scores, but it may represent a "threshold effect" in a polygenic model or a major gene influence in a single major locus model.

For us, this series of questions growing out of our taxometric efforts requires careful future analytical work and additional empirical investigations to clarify the precise distance that exists between our candidate indicators and the genetic factors in schizotypy and schizophrenia. We emphasize that these issues pertain to all putative indicators of liability such as eye tracking dysfunction, sustained attention deficits, and other psychometric measures. Furthermore, taxometric techniques may have utility in research on other forms of psychopathology (e.g., affective illness, personality disorders). In our work, we have found compelling evidence for a latent discontinuity underlying the scores on a subset of items from the PAS – results clearly consistent with Meehl's conjectures regarding a schizogene as well as the central tenet of the "latent trait" model of Holzman and Matthysse. The relation of our results to the multifactorial polygenic threshold model (Gottesman, 1991; McGue & Gottesman, 1989) is less clear, depending considerably on the "distance" between the genetic determinants of schizotypy and what the PAS measures as noted above. We encourage others to undertake taxometric explorations of additional candidate liability indicators and to address the substantive issues we have discussed above. Clearly, once one finds a reliable discernible break in the structure of schizotypy, it would be reasonable then to proceed with additional genetic investigations using techniques such as segregation analysis (Cavalli-Sforza & Bodmer, 1971) as well as other approaches (e.g., the "latent trait" model; Matthysse et al., 1986). We do not consider the latent structure of schizotypy to be entirely clarified by any means, though our results are encouraging, and they raise additional questions; thus we shall continue to track the taxon.

Acknowledgments

We thank Loren J. Chapman, Jean P. Chapman, Philip S. Holzman, Deborah L. Levy, and Steven Matthysse for their comments on this chapter. We thank also Paul E. Meehl and Leslie J. Yonce for both their generous ongoing consultations concerning taxometric methods as well as their comments on this chapter. Finally, we are grateful to Hal Stern and Donald B. Rubin for useful discussions concerning latent class techniques.

This research was supported in part by Grant MH-45448 from the National Institute of Mental Health to Mark F. Lenzenweger. Computing resources were provided by the Cornell Institute for Social and Economic Research, which is funded jointly by Cornell University and the National Science Foundation.

References

Battaglia, M., Gasperini, M., Sciuto, G., Scherillo, P., Diaferia, G., & Bellodi, L. (1991). Psychiatric disorders in the families of schizotypal subjects. *Schizophrenia Bulletin, 17,* 659–668.

Bem, S. L. (1974). The measurement of psychological androgyny. *Journal of Consulting and Clinical Psychology, 47,* 155–162.

Bleuler, E. (1911/1950). *Dementia praecox or the group of schizophrenias.* (J. Zinkin, trans.). New York: International Universities Press.

Cavalli-Sforza, L. L., & Bodmer, W. F. (1971). *The genetics of human populations.* New York: W. H. Freeman.

Chapman, L. J., & Chapman, J. P. (1985). Psychosis proneness. In M. Alpert (Ed.), *Controversies in schizophrenia: Changes and constancies* (pp. 157–172). New York: Guilford Press.

Chapman, L. J., Chapman, J. P., & Raulin, M. L. (1978). Body-image aberration in schizophrenia. *Journal of Abnormal Psychology, 87,* 399–407.

Chapman, L. J., Edell, W. S., & Chapman, J. P. (1980). Physical anhedonia, perceptual aberration, and psychosis proneness. *Schizophrenia Bulletin, 6,* 639–653.

Coleman, M., Levy, D. L., Lenzenweger, M. F., & Holzman, P. S. (in preparation). Thought disorder among psychometrically identified schizotypes.

Cornblatt, B. A., Lenzenweger, M. F., & Erlenmeyer-Kimling, L. (1989). The Continuous Performance Test, Identical Pairs Version: II. Contrasting attentional profiles in schizophrenic and depressed patients. *Psychiatry Research, 29,* 65–85.

Cronbach, L. J., & Meehl, P. E. (1955). Construct validity in psychological tests. *Psychological Bulletin, 52,* 281–302.

Edell, W. S., & Chapman, L. J. (1979). Anhedonia, perceptual aberration, and the Rorschach. *Journal of Consulting and Clinical Psychology, 51,* 215–255.

Everitt, B. S., & Hand, D. J. (1981). *Finite mixture distributions.* New York: Chapman & Hall.

Eysenck, H. J. (1986). A critique of contemporary classification and diagnosis. In T. Millon & G. L. Klerman (Eds.), *Contemporary directions in psychopathology* (pp. 73–78). New York: Guilford.

Falconer, D. S. (1989). *Introduction to quantitative genetics* (3rd ed.). New York: Wiley.

Gangestad, S., & Snyder, M. (1985). "To carve nature and its joints": On the existence of discrete classes in personality. *Psychological Review, 92,* 317–349.

Golden, R. R., & Meehl, P. E. (1978). Testing a single dominant gene theory without an accepted criterion variable. *Annals of Human Genetics (London), 41,* 507–514.

Golden, R. R., & Meehl, P. E. (1980). Detection of biological sex: An empirical test of cluster methods. *Multivariate Behavioral Research, 15,* 475–496.

Gottesman, I. I. (1991). *Schizophrenia genesis: The origins of madness.* New York: W. H. Freeman.

Gottesman, I. I., & Bertelsen, A. (1989). Confirming unexpressed genotypes for schizophrenia: Risks in the offspring of Fischer's Danish identical and fraternal discordant twins. *Archives of General Psychiatry, 46,* 867–872.

Grayson, D. A. (1987). Can categorical and dimensional views of psychiatric illness be distinguished? *British Journal of Psychiatry, 151,* 355–361.

Grove, W. M., Lebow, B. S., Clementz, B. A., Cerri, A., Medus, C., & Iacono, W. G. (1991). Familial prevalence and coaggregation of schizotypy indicators: A multitrait family study. *Journal of Abnormal Psychology, 100,* 115–121.

Holzman, P. S. (1982). The search for a biological marker of the functional psychoses. In M. J. Goldstein (Ed.), *Preventive intervention in schizophrenia: Are we ready?* DHHS Publication No. ADM 82-1111, pp. 19–38. Washington, D.C.: U.S. Government Printing Office.

Holzman, P. S., Kringlen, E., Matthysse, S., Flanagan, S. D., Lipton, R. B., Cramer, G., Levin, S., Lange, K., & Levy, D. L. (1988). A single dominant gene can account for eye tracking dysfunctions and schizophrenia in offspring of discordant twins. *Archives of General Psychiatry, 45,* 641–647.

Kendler, K. S. (1985). Diagnostic approaches to schizotypal personality disorder: A historical perspective. *Schizophrenia Bulletin, 11,* 538–553.

Kendler, K. S., & Hewitt, J. (1992). The structure of self-report schizotypy in twins. *Journal of Personality Disorders, 6,* 1–17.

Kendler, K. S., McGuire, M., Gruenberg, A. M., O'Hare, A., Spellman, M., & Walsh, D. (1993). The Roscommon Family Study: III. Schizophrenia-related personality disorders in relatives. *Archives of General Psychiatry, 50,* 781–788.

Kendler, K. S., Ochs, A. L., Gorman, A. M., Hewitt, J. K., Ross, D. E., & Mirsky, A. F. (1991). The structure of schizotypy: A pilot multitrait twin study. *Psychiatry Research, 36,* 19–36.

Kety, S. S., Rosenthal, D., Wender, P. H., & Schulsinger, F. (1968). The types and prevalence of mental illness in the biological and adoptive families of adopted schizophrenics. *Journal of Psychiatric Research, 6,* 345–362.

Korfine, L., & Lenzenweger, M. F. (1995). The taxonicity of schizotypy: A replication. *Journal of Abnormal Psychology, 104,* 26–31.

Kraepelin, E. (1919/1971). *Dementia praecox and paraphrenia* (R. M. Barclay, trans.; G. M. Robertson, ed.). Huntington, N.Y.: Krieger.

Lalouel, J. M., Rao, D. C., Morton, N. E., & Elston, R. L. (1983). A unified model for complex segregation analysis. *American Journal of Human Genetics, 35,* 816–826.

Lazarsfeld, P. F., & Henry, N. W. (1968). *Latent structure analysis.* New York: Houghton Mifflin.

Lenzenweger, M. F. (1991). Confirming schizotypic personality configurations in hypothetically psychosis-prone university students. *Psychiatry Research, 37,* 81–96.

Lenzenweger, M. F. (1993). Explorations in schizotypy and the psychometric high-risk paradigm. In Chapman, L. J., Chapman, J. P., & Fowles, D. (Eds.), *Progress in experimental personality and psychopathology research* (Vol. 16, pp. 66–116). New York: Springer.

Lenzenweger, M. F., Cornblatt, B. A., & Putnick, M. E. (1991). Schizotypy and sustained attention. *Journal of Abnormal Psychology, 100,* 84–89.

Lenzenweger, M. F., & Korfine, L. (1992a). Confirming the latent structure and base rate of schizotypy: A taxometric approach. *Journal of Abnormal Psychology, 101,* 567–571.

Lenzenweger, M. F., & Korfine, L. (1992b). Identifying schizophrenia-related personality disorder features in a nonclinical population using a psychometric approach. *Journal of Personality Disorders, 6,* 264–274.

Lenzenweger, M. F., & Korfine, L. (1994). Perceptual aberrations, schizotypy, and Wisconsin Card Sorting Test performance. *Schizophrenia Bulletin, 20,* 345–357.

Lenzenweger, M. F., & Loranger, A. W. (1989a). Detection of familial schizophrenia using a psychometric measure of schizotypy. *Archives of General Psychiatry, 46,* 902–907.

Lenzenweger, M. F., & Loranger, A. W. (1989b). Psychosis proneness and clinical psychopathology: Examination of the correlates of schizotypy. *Journal of Abnormal Psychology, 98,* 3–8.

Levy, D. L., Holzman, P. S., Matthysse, S., & Mendell, R. (1993). Eye tracking dysfunction and schizophrenia: A critical perspective. *Schizophrenia Bulletin, 19,* 461–536.

Lowrie, G. S., & Raulin, M. L. (1990). Search for schizotypic and nonschizotypic taxonomies in a college population. Presented at the 61st annual convention of the Eastern Psychological Association, Philadelphia, March, 1990.

McGue, M., & Gottesman, I. I. (1989). Genetic linkage in schizophrenia: Perspectives from genetic epidemiology. *Schizophrenia Bulletin, 13,* 453–464.

Matthysse, S. (1993). Genetics and the problem of causality in abnormal psychology. In P. B. Sutker & H. E. Adams (Eds.), *Comprehensive handbook of psychopathology* (pp. 178–186). New York: Springer-Verlag.

Matthysse, S., Holzman, P. S., & Lange, K. (1986). The genetic transmission of schizophrenia: Application of Mendelian latent structure analysis to eye tracking dysfunctions in schizophrenia and affective disorder. *Journal of Psychiatric Research, 20,* 57–67.

Meehl, P. E. (1962). Schizotaxia, schizotypy, schizophrenia. *American Psychologist, 17,* 827–838.

Meehl, P. E. (1964). *Manual for use with checklist of schizotypic signs.* Minneapolis, Minn: University of Minnesota.

Meehl, P. E. (1973). MAXCOV-HITMAX: A taxonomic search method for loose genetic syndromes. In P. E. Meehl, *Psychodiagnosis: Selected papers* (pp. 200–224). Minneapolis, Minn.: University of Minnesota Press.

Meehl, P. E. (1990). Toward an integrated theory of schizotaxia, schizotypy, and schizophrenia. *Journal of Personality Disorders, 4,* 1–99.

Meehl, P. E. (1992). Factors and taxa, traits and types, differences of degree and differences in kind. *Journal of Personality, 60,* 117–174.

Meehl, P. E. (1993). The origins of some of my conjectures concerning schizophrenia. In L. J. Chapman, J. P. Chapman, & D. Fowles (Eds.), *Progress in experimental personality and psychopathology research* (Vol. 16, pp. 1–10). New York: Springer.

Meehl, P. E., & Golden, R. R. (1982). Taxometric methods. In P. C. Kendall & J. N. Butcher (Eds.), *Handbook of research methods in clinical psychology* (pp. 127–181). New York: Wiley.

Meehl, P. E., & Yonce, L. J. (1994). Taxometric analysis: I. Detecting taxonicity with two quantitative indicators using means above and below a sliding cut (MAMBAC procedure). *Psychological Reports* (Monograph Supplement 1-V74).

Meehl, P. E., & Yonce, L. J. (in preparation). Taxometric analysis: II. Detecting taxonicity using covariance of two quantitative indicators in successive intervals of a third indicator (MAXCOV procedure).

Miller, M. B., & Chapman, J. P. (1993). *A twin study of schizotypy in college-age males.* Presented at the Eighth Annual meeting of the Society for Research in Psychopathology, Chicago, October 7–10.

Murphy, E. A. (1964). One cause? Many causes? The argument from the bimodal distribution. *Journal of Chronic Diseases, 17,* 301–324.

Obiols, J. E., Garcia-Domingo, M., de Trincheria, I., & Domenech, E. (1993).

Psychometric schizotypy and sustained attention in young males. *Personality and Individual Differences, 14,* 381–384.

O'Driscoll, G., Holzman, P. S., & Lenzenweger, M. F. (in preparation). Schizotypy and antisaccade performance in a nonclinical sample.

Park, S., & Holzman, P. S. (1992). Schizophrenics show working memory deficits. *Archives of General Psychiatry, 49,* 975–982.

Park, S., Holzman, P. S., & Lenzenweger, M. F. (in press). Individual differences in spatial working memory in relation to schizotypy. *Journal of Abnormal Psychology.*

Rado, S. (1960). Theory and therapy: The theory of schizotypal organization and its application to the treatment of decompensated schizotypal behavior. In S. C. Scher & H. R. Davis (Eds.), *The outpatient treatment of schizophrenia* (pp. 87–101). New York: Grune & Stratton.

Robins, E., & Guze, S. (1970). Establishment of diagnostic validity in psychiatric illness: Its application to schizophrenia. *American Journal of Psychiatry, 126,* 983–987.

Simons, R. F., & Katkin, W. (1985). Smooth pursuit eye movements in subjects reporting physical anhedonia and perceptual aberrations. *Psychiatry Research, 14,* 275–289.

Smith, C., & Mendell, N. R. (1974). Recurrence risks from family history and metric traits. *Annual of Human Genetics, 37,* 275–286.

Torgersen, S. (1985). Relationship of schizotypal personality disorder to schizophrenia: Genetics. *Schizophrenia Bulletin, 11,* 554–563.

Trull, T. J., Widiger, T. A., & Guthrie, P. (1990). Categorical versus dimensional status of borderline personality disorder. *Journal of Abnormal Psychology, 99,* 40–48.

Tukey, J. W. (1977). *Exploratory data analysis.* Reading, Mass.: Addison-Wesley Publishing.

8

Detection of a latent taxon of individuals at risk for schizophrenia-spectrum disorders

AUDREY R. TYRKA, NICK HASLAM, and TYRONE D. CANNON

Family, twin, and adoption studies have demonstrated that there is a substantial genetic component to the etiology of schizophrenia (Gottesman & Shields, 1982; Tsuang, Gilbertson, & Faraone, 1991). Genetic factors cannot fully explain transmission of schizophrenia, however, because concordance in monozygotic twins, who are genetically identical, is on the order of 50% (Gottesman & Shields, 1982; Kendler, 1983). These observations have led several investigators to propose diathesis – stress models of schizophrenia (Cannon & Mednick, 1993; Meehl, 1962, 1989, 1990; Nuechterlein et al., 1992; Shields et al., 1975). In its most general form, this model predicts that schizophrenia results from the interaction of genetic liability with particular environmental stressors; neither genetic nor environmental factors alone are believed to be sufficient to give rise to the disorder. Paul Meehl (1962, 1989, 1990), following Rado (1953), has further proposed that genetic vulnerability to schizophrenia is expressed in a variety of subpsychotic signs (i.e., cognitive slippage, social aversiveness, anhedonia, and ambivalence) that are unified in the construct "schizotypy." In this framework, schizotypy is thought to be the basic genetic condition; schizophrenia is an environmentally provoked complication of schizotypy.

In this chapter we review recent empirical findings from a prospective, longitudinal study of offspring of schizophrenic parents which support and further specify the hypotheses summarized above. Specifically, we report on a series of taxometric analyses that attempt to discern whether schizotypal symptoms and signs assessed during childhood, young adulthood, and middle age define a latent class of individuals with high risk for developing schizophrenia-spectrum disorders, and we examine the stability of schizotypal class membership across the life-span. In presenting the background for this work, we review (1) the genetic relationship between schizophrenia and schizotypal personality disorder (SPD); (2) the contributions of environmental factors to the development of schizophrenia in genetically at-risk individuals; (3) premorbid behavioral antecedents of the schizophrenia spectrum; and (4) stability of schizotypal symptoms and signs over time.

Genetic relationship between schizophrenia and SPD

A substantial body of evidence supports the notion that genetic risk for schizophrenia encompasses a behavioral syndrome that we shall refer to as "schizotypy." In the Danish adoption studies, subpsychotic schizophrenia-like symptoms were more common in the biological relatives of schizophrenic adoptees than in the biological relatives of control adoptees (Kety, 1987, 1988). Furthermore, the frequency of schizophrenia-spectrum disorders (i.e., schizophrenia and "schizophrenic personalities") in biological offspring of schizophrenic parents was three to five times higher for those subjects who had, in addition to one schizophrenic parent, a second parent with "schizophrenic personality," than for subjects who did not have a second parent with "schizophrenic personality" (Rosenthal, 1975). These traits were developed into criteria for the DSM-III [American Psychiatric Association (APA), 1980] and DSM-III-R (APA, 1987) diagnostic category, schizotypal personality disorder. In addition, many of the same traits are included in the list of prodromal and residual symptoms of schizophrenia (APA, 1987). According to the DSM-III-R, schizotypal signs and symptoms include ideas of reference, social anxiety, odd beliefs, unusual perceptual experiences, odd behavior, no close friends, odd speech (e.g., impoverished or digressive speech), inappropriate or constricted affect, and suspiciousness (APA, 1987).

Several recent family studies have found that SPD and schizotypal traits appear more frequently among the biological relatives of schizophrenics than among members of the general population (Baron, Gruen, Rainer, Kane, Asnis, & Lord, 1985; Grove, Lebow, Clementz, Cerri, Medus, & Iacono, 1991; Parnas, Cannon, Jacobsen, Schulsinger, Schulsinger, & Mednick, 1993; Squires-Wheeler, Skodol, Bassett, & Erlenmeyer-Kimling, 1989; Stephens, Atkinson, Kay, Roth, & Garside, 1975); there is also an elevated prevalence of schizophrenia and SPD in families of individuals diagnosed with SPD (Baron et al., 1985; Battaglia, Gasperini, Sciuto, Scherillo, & Bellodi, 1991; Schulz, Schulz, Goldberg, Ettigi, Resnick, & Friedel, 1986; Siever et al., 1990; Stone, 1977; Thaker, Adami, Moran, Lahti, & Cassady, 1993). Two other putative schizophrenia-spectrum diagnostic categories, schizoid and paranoid personality disorders, are defined by subsets of SPD criteria (i.e., social and affective withdrawal, and paranoia, respectively). The evidence concerning the possible genetic relationship between schizophrenia and these disorders is less substantial than that between schizophrenia and SPD; recent work suggests that in offspring of schizophrenic mothers, paranoid and schizoid personality disorder diagnoses are in large part coextensive with SPD diagnoses (Parnas et al., 1993).

Environmental contributions to the schizophrenia spectrum

In view of the evidence indicating a common genetic basis for schizophrenia and schizotypy, there must be other factors that explain why some individuals with the genetic predisposition develop schizophrenia, some develop SPD, and some do not meet diagnostic criteria for mental illness. High-risk and twin studies have found evidence consistent with the notion that environmental stressors increase the risk of overt schizophrenia among those genetically predisposed. We have previously reported that among the offspring of schizophrenic mothers, a larger percentage of individuals who became schizophrenic had a history of familial instability or birth complications than did individuals who developed SPD or who did not develop mental illness (Cannon & Mednick, 1993; Cannon, Mednick, & Parnas, 1990; Parnas, Schulsinger, Teasdale, Schulsinger, Feldman, & Mednick, 1982; Parnas, Teasdale, & Schulsinger, 1985). These environmental variables were not associated with an increase in schizophrenia among a matched group of low-risk offspring (i.e., children of parents who were free of mental illness). Thus, genetic liability was required for environmental factors to influence the development of schizophrenia (i.e., there was a gene–environment interaction). In addition, several studies have found that in monozygotic twins discordant for schizophrenia, the affected twin tends to have experienced more difficulties during delivery (Mednick, Cannon, & Barr, 1991).

Premorbid behavioral antecedents of the schizophrenia spectrum

If schizophrenia and SPD are unified by a common genetic diathesis, with schizophrenia occurring primarily among genetically vulnerable individuals who experience environmental stressors and with SPD occurring primarily among genetically vulnerable individuals who escape environmental stressors, then it seems reasonable to hypothesize that the symptoms and signs of

SPD represent the primary behavioral manifestations of the genetic diathesis and may therefore precede the development of overt psychosis among those who eventually become schizophrenic. Consistent with this notion, in a 15-year follow-up study of subjects who were hospitalized with SPD and/or borderline personality disorder features, Fenton and McGlashan (1989) found that 67% of the subjects who went on to develop schizophrenia had three or more DSM-III SPD features at initial admission. This result suggests that SPD traits may precede the onset of schizophrenia by several years. However, since the initial assessment occurred during a hospital admission, it is unclear whether the SPD symptoms were truly present "premorbidly" or whether they represented prodromal manifestations of a psychotic episode.

Some retrospective studies have identified a premorbid history of behavioral deviance during childhood in about half of schizophrenics studied (Hanson, Gottesman, & Heston, 1976). The interpretability of these studies is limited, however, by possible reporting biases (Hanson et al., 1976; Hanson, Gottesman, & Meehl, 1977; Mednick & McNeil, 1968).

Prospective studies eliminate some major sources of reporting bias (i.e., recall errors, reports that are confounded by awareness of diagnostic status) since data are collected prior to the onset of illness. These investigations have typically compared the childhood and adolescent behavior of offspring of schizophrenics (high-risk group) and offspring of normals (low-risk group). A problem with this approach is that offspring of schizophrenics are a genetically heterogeneous group, and only a subgroup is actually at risk for schizophrenia (Gottesman & Shields, 1982; Hanson et al., 1977). Such within-group heterogeneity is likely to dilute the differentiating features of the at-risk group. One solution is to follow the samples through the risk period for developing a schizophrenia-spectrum disorder (i.e., ages 18 to 40) and then search for premorbid characteristics that differentiate those who become spectrum-disordered from those who develop other psychiatric disorders or do not develop a psychiatric disorder. While it is important to note that not all individuals with the predisposing gene(s) would necessarily be expected to meet criteria for a psychiatric diagnosis (Meehl, 1990; Tsuang et al., 1991), features that do precede diagnosable spectrum disorders should bear the strongest relationship with genetic liability.

Deficits in the performance of high-risk subjects relative to low-risk subjects have been reported for the following domains: (1) attention (Asarnow, 1988; Asarnow, Steffy, MacCrimmon, & Cleghorn, 1978; Nuechterlein & Dawson, 1984; Cornblatt & Erlenmeyer-Kimling, 1985), (2) memory and information processing (Syzmanski, Kane, & Lieberman, 1991; Nuechterlein & Dawson, 1984), (3) motor coordination and IQ (Asarnow, 1988;

Erlenmeyer-Kimling, Golden, & Cornblatt, 1989), (4) smooth pursuit eye movement and event-related potentials (Syzmanski et al., 1991), (5) psychophysiological responding (Syzmanski et al., 1991; Nuechterlein et al., 1992), (6) affective rapport and interpersonal relationships (Asarnow, 1988; Hanson et al., 1976), and (7) achievement in school (Asarnow, 1988).

None of these putative indicators, however, has been shown to be necessary or sufficient in defining liability for schizophrenia (Hanson et al., 1976, 1977; Meehl, 1973; Moldin, Rice, Gottesman, & Erlenmeyer-Kimling, 1990). Meehl has proposed that the aggregation of deviant scores on a cluster of indicators may better serve to indicate liability for schizophrenia. Several statistical techniques have been used to determine whether sets of indicator variables define distinct subclasses of a given population, including admixture analysis (Lenzenweger & Moldin, 1990; Moldin et al., 1990) and taxometric analysis (Erlenmeyer-Kimling et al., 1989; Golden & Meehl, 1979; Haslam, 1994; Haslam & Beck, 1994; Meehl, 1973). The latter technique was developed specifically for determining the nature of the latent liability distribution (e.g., dichotomous, continuous) in schizophrenia. The approach has been validated on both simulated and actual data sets of continuous and discontinuous distributions (Golden, 1982; Golden & Meehl, 1979; Lenzenweger & Korfine, Chapter 7, this volume).

Results consistent with a dichotomous latent liability distribution have been found in taxometric analyses examining the base rate of schizotypy in college students (Lenzenweger & Korfine, 1992) and nonpsychotic inpatients (Golden & Meehl, 1979), and an admixture analysis of perceptual aberration items revealed three subgroups in a sample of college students (Lenzenweger & Moldin, 1990). However, the relevance of these studies to the genetics of the schizophrenia spectrum awaits demonstration of a greater frequency of spectrum disorder outcomes in these groups than in the general population.

Results of several studies of high-risk children have also been consistent with a dichotomous distribution of liability for schizophrenia. In the New York High Risk Project, a taxometric analysis of cognitive and neuromotor variables (Erlenmeyer-Kimling et al., 1989) and an admixture analysis of MMPI items (Moldin et al., 1990) each yielded two subgroups, one composed of deviant scorers and the other composed of nondeviant scorers. Using simple frequency analysis, Hanson and colleagues (1976) identified a subgroup of HR children who had deviant scores on measures of motor skills, cognitive performance, and "schizoid" behavior, and Asarnow et al. (1978) found a subgroup of HR foster children who scored in the bottom third of the distributions of three attentional tasks.

All of these studies, however, utilized data from a small number of subjects (*n*'s of the HR samples ranged from 9 to 55). Small sample sizes are particularly problematic in the studies using behavioral measures, as these involve a relatively large amount of measurement error. In addition, none of these investigations performed definitive analyses regarding whether premorbid schizotypy classification is a sensitive and specific predictor of the later emergence of schizophrenia-spectrum disorders. Hanson, Gottesman, and Heston (1990) conducted a preliminary follow-up investigation of much of their sample (four of the five subjects identified as deviant in childhood) into their early twenties, and failed to find evidence of major psychiatric disturbance in the four identified subjects. The report by Erlenmeyer-Kimling and colleagues (1989) included an analysis of the prediction of future psychiatric hospitalization on the basis of cognitive and neuromotor deviance in childhood, but data regarding the prediction of specific diagnoses were not provided.

Further, no high-risk study has investigated whether the behavioral abnormalities associated with the criteria for SPD define a latent class of subjects at high risk for schizophrenia-spectrum disorders, as would be predicted on the basis of the Danish Adoption study findings and the other work reviewed above.

Longitudinal stability of schizotypy

Finally, as might be expected of behavior that is largely genetically determined, schizotypy has been found to be fairly stable from childhood to adulthood. In the New York High-Risk Project, 70% of high-risk subjects who had four or more SPD features at an average age of 16 years also had a schizophrenia-spectrum disorder outcome and/or four or more SPD features at an average age of 25 years (Squires-Wheeler, Skodol, & Erlenmeyer-Kimling, 1992). A follow-up study of schizoid/schizotypal children who were referred to a psychiatric hospital at a mean age of 10 years found that 75% of subjects met DSM-III criteria for SPD at a mean age of 27 years (Wolff, Townshend, McGuire, & Weeks, 1991).

Taken together, the findings that SPD features are genetically related to schizophrenia, precede the development of schizophrenia among those genetically predisposed, and show continuity from childhood to young adulthood suggest that the aggregation of such signs and symptoms may serve as a longitudinally stable marker of genetic liability for the schizophrenia spectrum across the life-span. To our knowledge, this hypothesis has never before been tested empirically.

The Copenhagen high-risk study

We have recently conducted taxometric analyses of putative schizotypy indicators from the Copenhagen schizophrenia high-risk project. Detailed descriptions of the samples and methods have been provided elsewhere (Mednick & Schulsinger, 1965; Parnas et al., 1993; Schulsinger, 1976; Tyrka, Cannon, Haslam, Mednick, Schulsinger, Schulsinger, & Parnas, 1995), and only brief summaries are given here.

Subjects

In 1962, Mednick and Schulsinger began following 207 offspring of mothers with schizophrenia (high-risk group, HR) and 104 controls with no family history of mental illness (low-risk group, LR) who were matched to the HR group with respect to age, sex, social class, institutional rearing during childhood, and urban/rural residence. In 1962 the subjects were a mean age of 15.1 years and none had a psychiatric illness (Mednick & Schulsinger, 1965). From a later diagnostic evaluation of the subjects' biological fathers, it was determined that 62 HR subjects had a schizophrenia-spectrum-disordered father in addition to a schizophrenic mother and were thus at "super-high-risk" (SHR) for schizophrenia (Parnas, 1985).

Diagnostic follow-up assessments of offspring

Major follow-up assessments were conducted on two occasions, first in 1972–4, when the subjects were a mean age of 25 years, and most recently in 1986–9, when subjects were a mean age of 39 years, and were thus nearly through the risk period for schizophrenia-spectrum disorders (Parnas et al., 1993). The diagnostic procedures in 1972–4 included two structured psychiatric interviews, the Present State Examination (PSE; Wing, Cooper, & Sartorius, 1974) and the Current and Past Psychopathology Scales (Endicott & Spitzer, 1972), and an additional set of items. The 1986–9 diagnostic procedure included the Schedule for Affective Disorders and Schizophrenia – lifetime version (SADS-L; Spitzer & Endicott, 1978), the PSE, the PSE lifetime ratings of psychotic symptoms, the PSE Syndrome Checklist for current and lifetime psychopathology, the Scales for the Assessment of Positive and Negative Symptoms (Andreasen, 1983, 1984), and the Personality Disorder Examination (Loranger, Sussman, Oldham, & Russakoff, 1985). Information thus collected was used in determining Axis I and II DSM-III-R diagnoses for each subject at each assessment. A single lifetime diagnosis was determined that reflected the most severe DSM-III-R diagnosis the subject had been assigned over the course of the study. Lifetime diagnoses were categorized in the following way: (1) schizophrenia, (2) spectrum personality disorders (i.e., schizotypal, paranoid, and schizoid), (3) other Axis I and Axis II disorders, and (4) no psychiatric disorder.

Schizotypy indicators

Measures of schizotypal signs and symptoms were constructed independently for each of the three measurement points (i.e., 1962, 1972–4, and 1986–9). The 1962 indicators were derived from behavioral and psychological assessment items including a school behavior scale, a psychiatric interview, and a word association test (Tyrka et al., 1995). Items from these sources that pertained to the diagnostic criteria for SPD were used to form 10 candidate indicators: social withdrawal, social anxiety, flat affect, passivity, poor prognosis, peculiarity, acting out, positive thought disorder, negative thought disorder, and rated thought disorder.

The 1972–4 schizotypy indicators were composed of items from the PSE, CAPPS, and additional items from a clinical interview. The 1986–9 scales were composed of items from the PSE and PDE. The compositions of the indicators from these two assessment periods were very similar; both represented the nine schizotypal personality disorder criteria noted above (Cannon, Haslam, Tyrka, Medrick, Schulsinger, Schulsinger, & Parnas, (1995).

Hypotheses

Based on the foregoing empirical and theoretical work, it was hypothesized that:

1. The aggregation of schizotypal indicators at each measurement point will be consistent with an underlying dichotomous liability distribution. One class of subjects will be characterized by deviant indicator scores (i.e., the hypothesized taxon or "schizotypal" class); the other class will be characterized by nondeviant indicator scores (i.e., the complement).
2. Membership in the schizotypal class will be systematically related to level of genetic risk for schizophrenia as determined by maternal and paternal schizophrenia-spectrum diagnoses.

3. Membership in the schizotypal class at each measurement point will be associated with a higher risk for both schizophrenia and spectrum personality disorders, but not for nonspectrum psychopathology.
4. Membership in the schizotypal class will be stable across the life-span.

Results

Latent subgroup detection

Item analyses

The taxometric method described by Golden and Meehl (1979; see also Lenzenweger & Korfine, Chapter 7, this volume) is based on the assumption that a set of indicators is available, each of which discriminates between the taxon and complement, and is relatively independent of the other indicators within each taxonomic class. Consistency tests, derived from Monte Carlo simulations and based on the internal consistency of the indicators in defining the taxon, are used to determine whether or not these assumptions have been met; only those indicators that satisfy the criteria are selected for further analysis.

Four of the ten indicators from the 1962 assessment failed to fulfill the criteria of the method. Social withdrawal, social anxiety, passivity, flat affect, peculiarity, and poor prognosis were retained. All of the nine DSM-III-R schizotypal personality disorder symptoms from the 1972 and 1986 assessments passed the exclusion criteria.

A note is in order regarding the poor prognosis indicator from the 1962 assessment. This indicator did not assess prognosis in the sense of predicting the course of an illness since none of the subjects had diagnosable mental illness at or before 1962. Rather, the variable involved judgments regarding the likelihood of future illness status on the basis of present and past behavior. Thus, although this indicator was less specific than the other variables in terms of the behavioral domain assessed, it was theoretically comparable to the other indicators in that it was a measure of deviant premorbid behavior. Empirically, this indicator aggregated with the other indicators and was not rejected on the basis of the exclusion criteria.

Covariance curve

In the taxometric procedure, covariance among items is examined to determine if the aggregation of the indicators is consistent with an underlying dichtomous liability distribution. The average covariance of all possible indicator pairs is plotted at each level of a scale formed by the sum of the remaining indicators. If the indicators are intercorrelated only to the extent that they define a latent taxon and complement, substantial covariance between any two indicators will occur only at the point of intersection of the latent distributions (i.e., toward the middle of the scale of the remaining indicators), and not within each latent class (i.e., at the ends of this scale). Covariance within a taxon and a complement is minimal because there is little variance within each group: Subjects in the taxon tend to have positive scores on most indicators, whereas subjects in the complement tend to have negative scores on most indicators; there is substantial covariance in the middle region of the scale where taxon and complement intersect because there is variance due to the mixture of the two distributions. It is important to note that this covariance procedure does not yield a frequency distribution; rather, it yields a parametric covariance curve that is used to test for the presence of a dichotomous liability distribution on the basis of the degree of correlation among indicators at the high and low ends of the scale of indicators. In a later step, a frequency distribution is derived from Bayes's theorem to determine whether the aggregation of the observed indicators is bimodally distributed.

In the covariance procedure, a plot with a single peak and near-zero points at the ends of the scale is consistent with a dichotomous liability distribution. A curve with more than one region of high covariance could be indicative of three or more distributions or of excessive intrataxon correlation. Conversely, a single distribution of a dimensional, rather than categorical, construct would correspond to a flat covariance curve (see Lenzenweger & Korfine, Chapter 7, this volume; Trull, Widiger, & Guthrie, 1990).

Figure 8.1 presents the obtained covariance functions for the 1962, 1972–4, and 1986–9 schizotypy indicators. Each function has a region of elevated covariance near the middle of the scale, with near-zero points at the ends of the scale, and is thus indicative of a dichotomous liability distribution. That the 1962 covariance curve peaks across a few scale values indicates that the taxon and complement distributions overlap across more than one value of the scale; thus, the boundary between taxon and complement in the 1962 analysis is not as sharp as that obtained with the 1972–4 and 1986–9 data.

Bayesian probabilities

The model-based probability that a subject is a member of the taxon is calculated for the sample according to Bayes's theorem. A U-shaped probability distribution, with most of the probabilities close to zero or one, has been shown in Monte Carlo analyses to be indicative of the presence of two categorically distinct groups (i.e., taxon and complement).

Figure 8.2 shows the probability distributions for the 1962, 1972–4, and

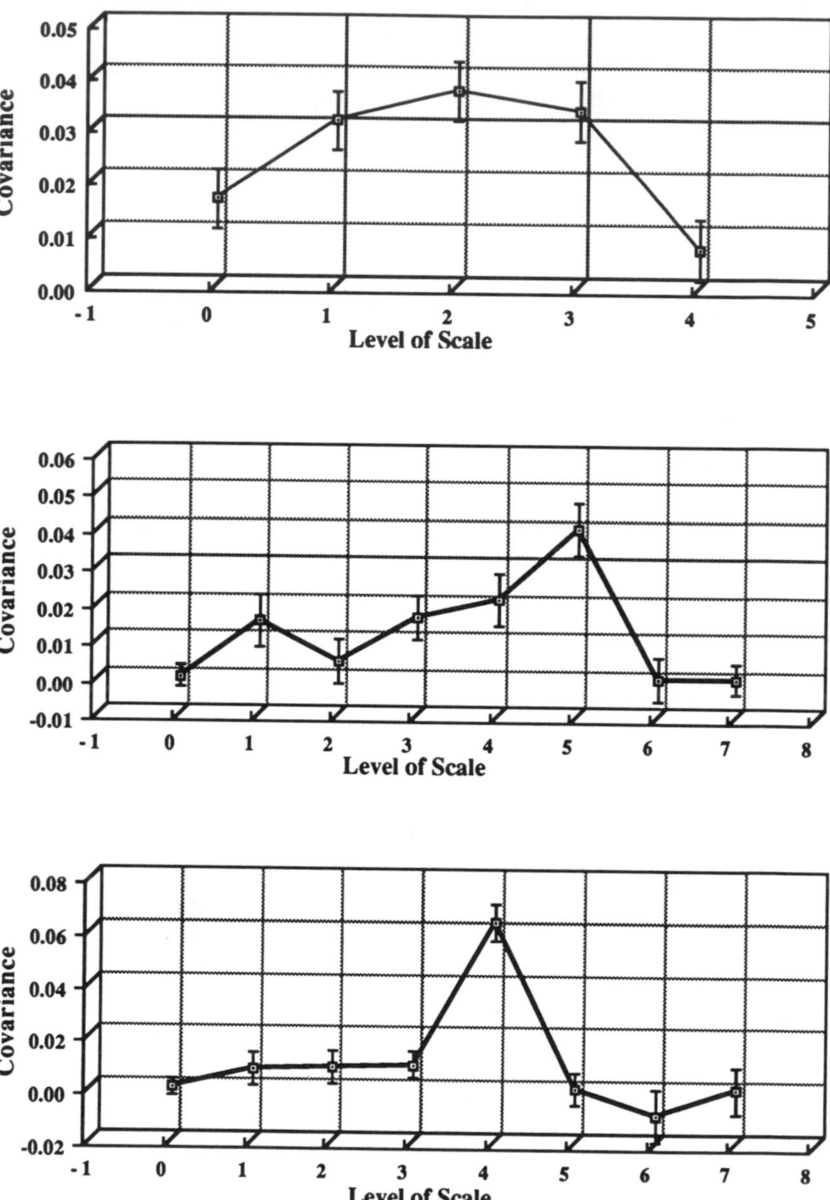

Fig. 8.1. Plots of raw (unsmoothed) mean covariance among all combinations of indicators at each level of the scale of the remaining indicators from the 1962 (upper), 1972–4 (middle), and 1986–9 (lower) analyses.

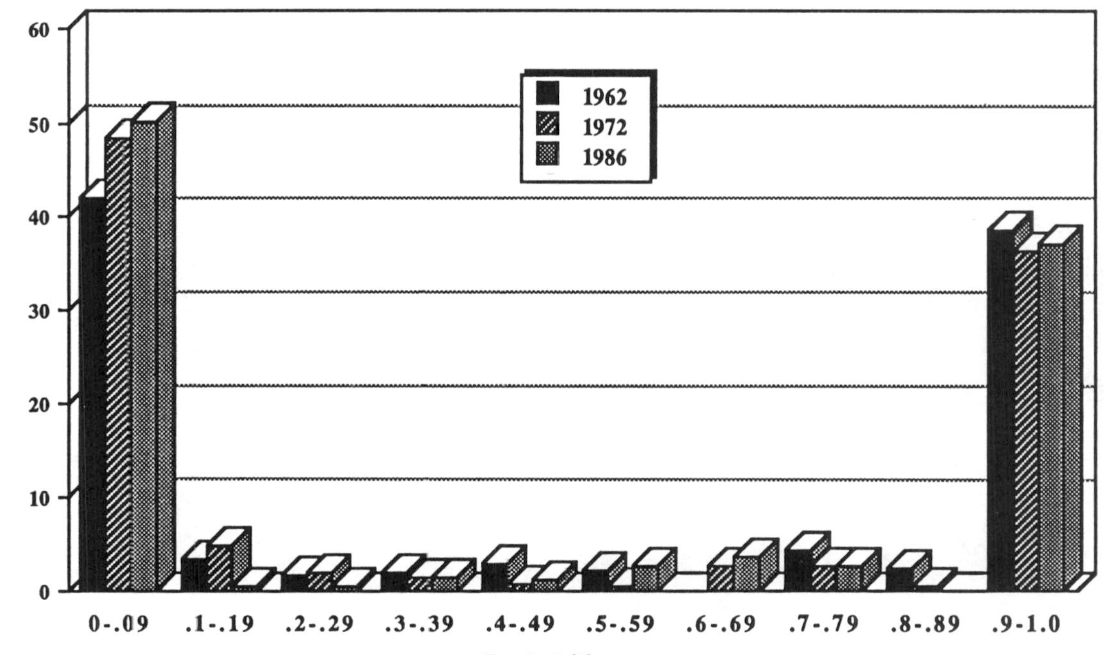

Fig. 8.2. Frequency distribution of model-based Bayesian probabilities of taxon membership from the 1962, 1972–4, and 1986–9 analyses.

1986–9 assessments. All three distributions are markedly U-shaped, and are thus consistent with a latent bimodal liability distribution.

To maximize specificity in the analyses that follow, the cutoff probability value for taxon membership was set at 0.9 for each assessment. The taxon base rates were 39%, 36%, and 37%, for the 1962, 1972–4, and 1986–9 assessments, respectively.

Taxon membership and genetic risk status

As shown in Figure 8.3, 19% of the LR, 48% of the HR, and 49% of the SHR groups were classified in the schizotypal taxon on the basis of the 1962 assessment [$\chi^2(2) = 28.98, p < .001$]. With the 1972–4 data, 21%, 43%, and 58% of the LR, HR, and SHR groups, respectively, were assigned to the taxon [$\chi^2(2) = 24.24,\ p < .001$]. The 1986–9 assessment yielded corresponding percentages of 17%, 44%, and 62% [$\chi^2(2) = 34.97, p > .001$]. The increases in the proportion of subjects classified as taxon members as a function of the number of parents with a schizophrenia-spectrum disorder in the 1972–4 and 1986–9 assessments support the genetic validity of the taxon classification. The lack of increase in the percentage of SHR compared with HR subjects in the 1962 taxon is most likely due to a relatively larger amount of measurement error associated with the indicator variables from the childhood assessment (Tyrka et al., 1995).

Taxon membership and lifetime diagnostic outcome

The percentages of subjects with lifetime DSM-III-R diagnoses of schizophrenia, spectrum personality disorders, other psychiatric disorders, and no psychiatric disorder who were classified in the taxon at each of the three assessment periods are shown in Figure 8.4. Taxon membership at each assessment significantly predicted spectrum outcome, and there was either no relationship (1962 and 1986–9) or a negative relationship (1972–4, $p < .05$, binomial distribution) between taxon membership and nonspectrum diagnoses. Thus, this classification was both highly sensitive and highly specific to spectrum disorder outcomes.

The observed rates of total spectrum disorders in the schizotypal taxon were 64%, 89%, and 92%, from the 1962, 1972–4, and 1986–9 assessments, respectively. The significance of these values can be appreciated by considering that 39%, 36%, and 37% of the spectrum outcomes would be expected to be in the schizotypal taxon by chance (i.e., based on the percent of the total number of subjects who were in the taxon at each measurement period, respectively).

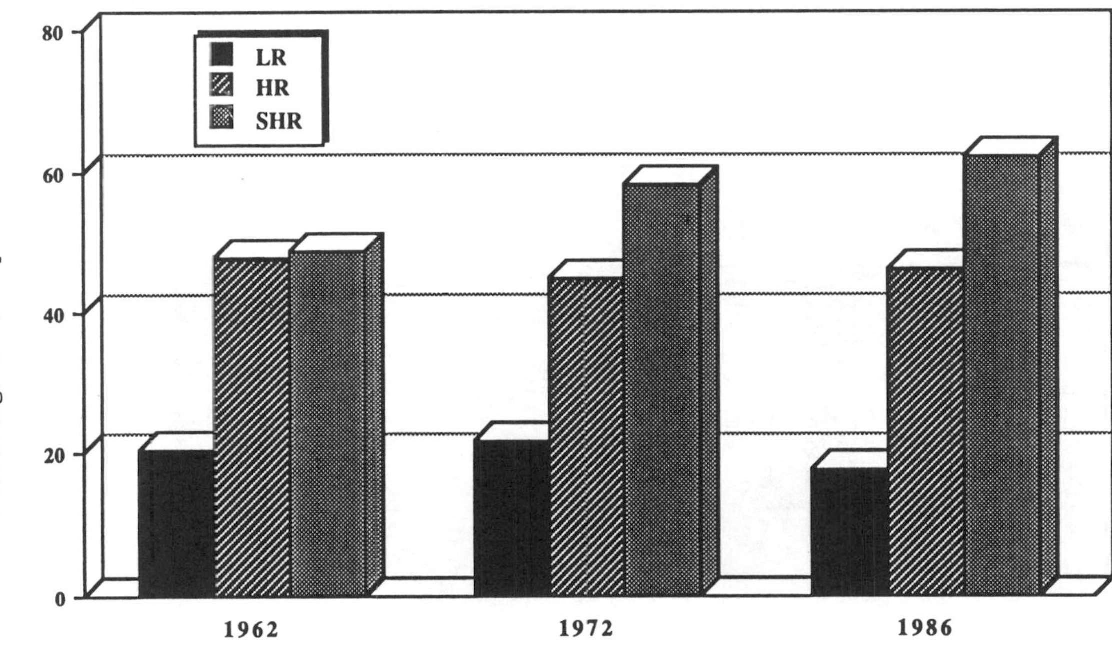

Fig. 8.3. Percentage of genetic risk groups classified in the schizotypal taxon from the 1962, 1972–4, and 1986–9 analyses.

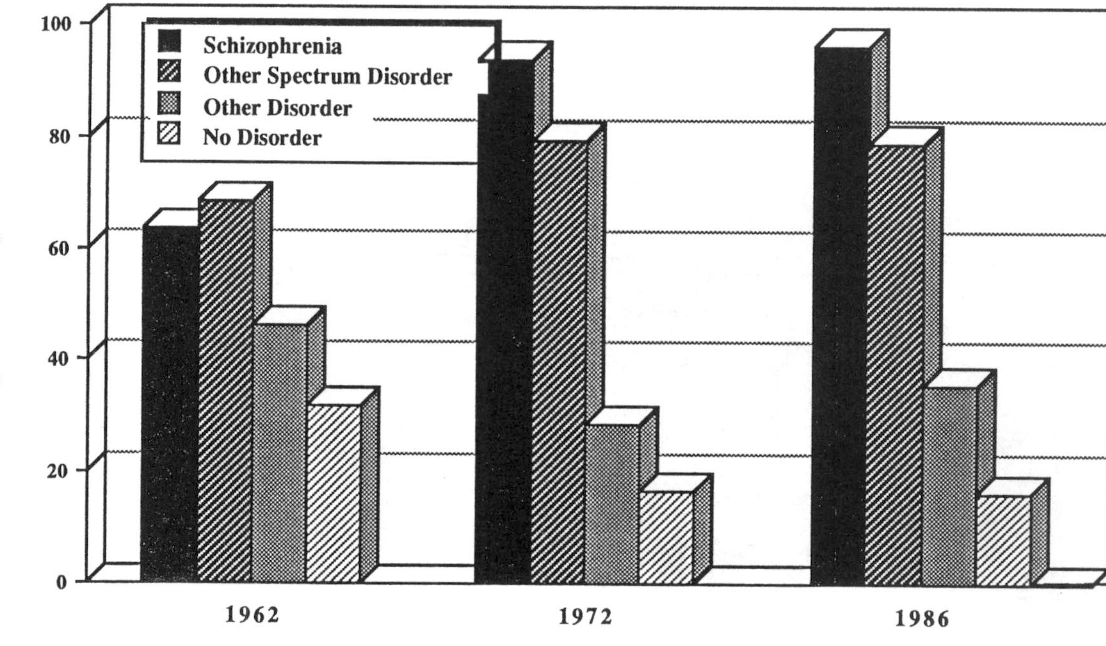

Fig. 8.4. Percentage of diagnostic outcome groups classified in the schizotypal taxon from the 1962, 1972–4, and 1986–9 analyses.

The observed proportions were all significantly larger than those expected by chance according to the binomial probability distribution (p's < .001).

Another measure of the predictive validity of the taxon classifications is the percent of taxon members who were diagnosed with spectrum disorders compared with the base rate of spectrum disorders in the total sample. Figure 8.5 shows the composition of the taxon at each assessment according to lifetime DSM-III-R diagnostic outcome. At the 1962, 1972–4, and 1986–9 assessments, respectively, 45%, 60%, and 56% of the subjects classified in the taxon were later diagnosed with schizophrenia or spectrum personality disorders. Each of these rates is significantly different from the spectrum disorder base rate in the total sample of 26% (p's < .0001). If we limit our consideration to the HR group (Figure 8.6), taxon membership at each assessment period improves the prediction of spectrum-disorder outcomes over the base rate by a factor of 1/3 to 2 (p's < .01).

It is important to note that there was not a significant difference between the percentage of subjects with schizophrenia who were classified in the taxon and the percentage of individuals with spectrum personality disorders who were classified in the taxon at any of the three assessment periods (Figure 8.4). This result indicates that schizotypal behavioral indicators were equally sensitive in predicting schizophrenia and the diagnostic categories genetically related to schizophrenia.

Longitudinal stability of latent class identification

There was substantial agreement of the taxon classifications from the three assessment periods. The overlap in taxon membership between the 1962 analysis and those for 1972–4 and 1986–9 was 68% and 64%, respectively, and the overlap between the 1972–4 and 1986–9 analyses was 74%. The average agreement was 69%. These figures indicate that taxon membership was remarkably stable from an average age of 15 years to an average age of 39 years (i.e., a 24-year period).

Conclusions

We have provided evidence that a discrete group of individuals can be identified on the basis of assessments made independently in childhood, young adulthood, and middle age, a group that (1) is characterized by deviance on sets of schizotypal signs and symptoms; (2) has an elevated level of genetic risk for schizophrenia as determined by maternal and paternal schizophrenia-spectrum diagnoses; (3) is prospectively and contemporaneously associated

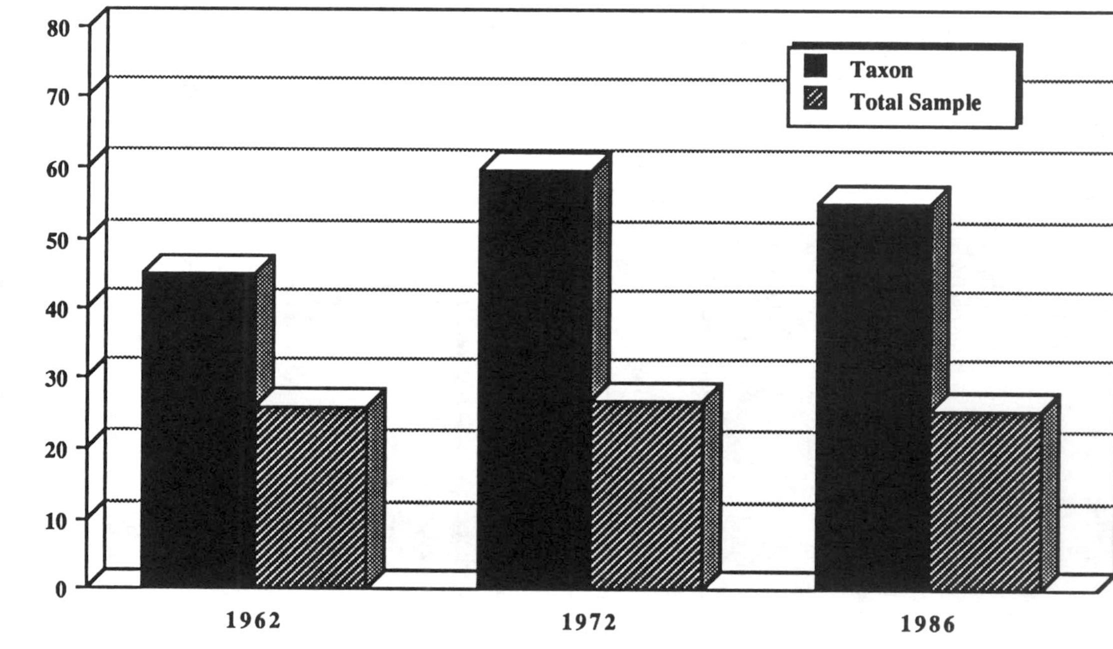

Fig. 8.5. Percentages of schizotypal taxon and total sample with spectrum-disorder outcome from the 1962, 1972–4, and 1986–9 analyses.

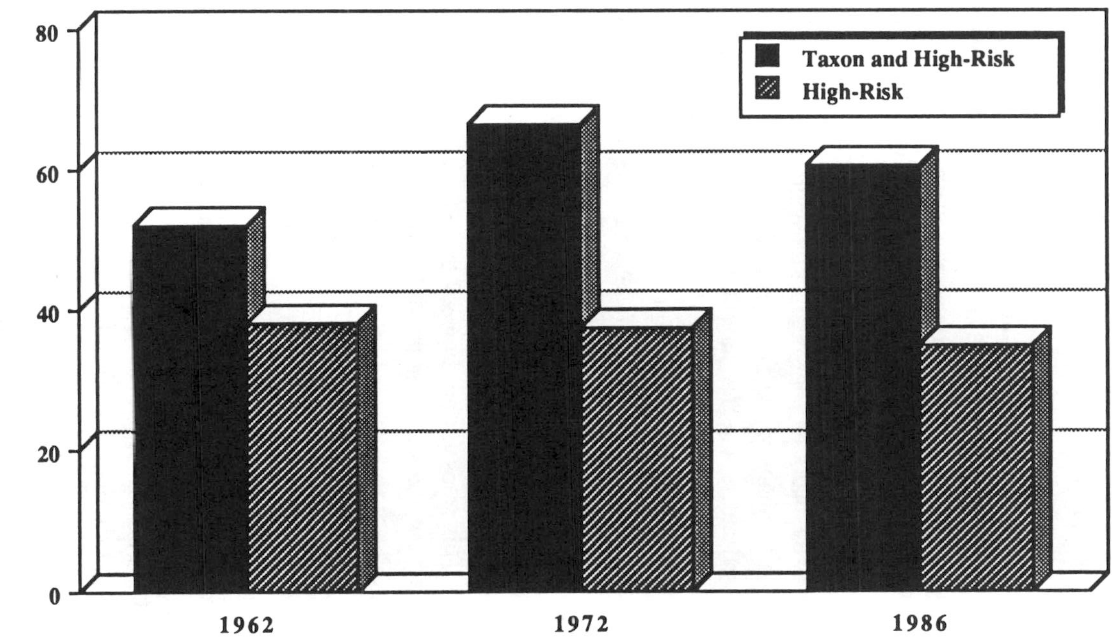

Figure 8.6. Percentages of high-risk schizotypal taxon and total high-risk group with spectrum-disorder outcome from the 1962, 1972–4, and 1986–9 analyses.

with diagnostic outcomes of schizophrenia and schizophrenia-spectrum personality disorders but not nonspectrum mental illness; and (4) is stable in terms of membership from age 15 through age 39.

The results of these analyses thus confirm several predictions of the diathesis – stress model. First, several previous studies found that schizotypy, as defined by perceptual, personality, or cognitive and neuromotor variables, is dichotomously distributed in samples of college students, nonpsychotic inpatients, and children of schizophrenic parents (Erlenmeyer-Kimling et al., 1989; Golden & Meehl, 1979; Lenzenweger & Korfine, 1992; Moldin et al., 1990). This study extends this work by showing that the aggregation of signs and symptoms analogous to many of the DSM-III-R diagnostic criteria for SPD is dichotomously distributed in at-risk subjects. Second, numerous studies have found evidence consistent with a genetic link between schizophrenia and schizotypal traits (Baron et al., 1985; Battaglia et al., 1991; Grove et al., 1991; Kendler & Gruenberg, 1984; Kety, 1987, 1988; Parnas et al., 1993; Rosenthal, 1975; Squires-Wheeler et al., 1989; Stephens et al., 1975; Thaker et al., 1993). This study extends this work by showing that schizotypal class membership varies significantly in proportion to the level of genetic risk for schizophrenia, increasing linearly as the number of affected parents increases from zero to one to two. This study further supports the genetic link between schizophrenia and schizotypal signs and symptoms by showing that an equal proportion of subjects with schizophrenia and spectrum personality disorders were classified in the schizotypal taxon at each measurement point. Third, schizophrenics have been found to show schizotypal signs and symptoms premorbidly (Mednick & Silverton, 1988). This study extends this finding by showing that premorbid schizotypal class membership is predictive of lifetime schizophrenia-spectrum disorder outcome as defined by modern operational diagnostic criteria (i.e., DSM-III-R). Finally, schizotypy and SPD have been shown to be stable from childhood to adulthood (Squires-Wheeler et al., 1992; Wolff et al., 1991). This study extends this work by demonstrating that membership in the latent schizotypal class is stable from age 15 through age 39.

A note is in order concerning the applicability of the taxometric method to Meehl's model of the mode of inheritance of schizophrenia. Meehl (1962, 1989, 1990) has proposed a mixed genetic model composed of a single major locus (SML) responsible for schizotypy, and polygenic and environmental potentiators that interact with the SML phenotype in the development of schizophrenia. He developed the taxometric method to test an assumption of this model – that is, that basic liability for schizophrenia is dichotomously distributed. It is important to emphasize, however, that this method tests only the nature of the latent liability distribution, not the mode of genetic transmission of the disorder. Evidence of a discrete schizotypal class does not necessarily reflect the influence of a single major gene; the results could also be due to a threshold effect in a polygenic situation or to genetic heterogeneity with independent genes having a common behavioral expression. Each of these models is consistent with a latent situation in which the base rate of the pathogenic gene(s) is larger than the base rate of schizophrenia but does not necessarily include all offspring of one or two schizophrenia-spectrum-disordered parents.

Since this study did not investigate a random sample from the general population, we are not able to provide an estimate of the base rate of schizotypy in the general population (in this study, the LR group was sociodemographically matched to the HR group which resulted in a lower than average SES and a higher than average incidence of institutional rearing during childhood). A representative sample is not a requirement of the taxometric method; rather, the procedure assumes only that a *mixed* sample of taxon- and complement-members is used and that the *n* of each group is large enough to minimize sampling error (Golden & Meehl, 1979). The use of a high-risk sample results in a larger taxon base rate, and therefore less sampling error, than would be found in a general population sample.

The finding that a smaller percentage of spectrum-outcome subjects were classified in the taxon from the 1962 assessment compared to the later assessments is most likely due to a larger amount of measurement error associated with the earlier indicators compared to the later indicators (Tyrka et al., 1995). The 1962 indicators were compiled from different sources (i.e., a psychiatric interview and a teacher questionnaire), whereas the 1972–4 and 1986–9 indicators were composed of symptom ratings from structured psychiatric interviews performed by the same interviewers (different interviewers were used, however, across assessments). The possibility that a systematic difference in genetic and/or environmental variables between correctly classified and "misclassified" spectrum-outcome subjects in the 1962 analysis is unlikely to account for this misclassification of spectrum-disorder outcomes for the following reasons: (1) Such a difference would most likely be expressed in the later assessment data as well as the 1962 data; and (2) there were no differences between the classified and misclassified spectrum-outcome subjects on variables such as demographic characteristics, severity or treatment of illness, comorbidity, or the indicator variables that did not meet the taxometric criteria (Tyrka et al., 1995).

Although we found statistically significant stability in schizotypal class membership from age 15 through age 39, the group membership of an average of 31% of the subjects changed across any two measurement points. This relatively small amount of instability could reflect developmental variability in gene expression, differential experiences with environmental potentiators preceding the different evaluations, episodic manifestations of the clinical features of schizotypy, or simple measurement error.

In conclusion, we have found evidence that the signs and symptoms of SPD define a class of individuals with high risk for schizophrenia-spectrum disorders that is relatively stable in composition from childhood to middle age. These findings may help to define the relevant phenotype for future molecular genetic and modeling studies, and may eventually prove useful in targeting individuals for prevention.

Acknowledgments

This research was supported by Grant No. R29 MH 48207 (to T. D. Cannon), and Research Scientist Award No. 1 K05 MH 00619 (to S. A. Mednick).

References

American Psychiatric Association. (1980). *Diagnostic and statistical manual of mental disorders* (3rd ed.). Washington, D.C.: Author.

American Psychiatric Association. (1987). *Diagnostic and statistical manual of mental disorders* (revised 3rd ed.). Washington, D.C.: Author.

Andreasen, N. C. (1983). *The Scale for the Assessment of Negative Symptoms* (SANS). Iowa City: The University of Iowa.

Andreasen, N. C. (1984). *The Scale for the Assessment of Positive Symptoms* (SAPS). Iowa City: The University of Iowa.

Asarnow, J. R. (1988). Children at risk for schizophrenia: Converging lines of evidence. *Schizophrenia Bulletin, 14,* 613–631.

Asarnow, R. F., Steffy, R. A., MacCrimmon, D. J., & Cleghorn, J. M. (1978). An attentional assessment of foster children at risk for schizophrenia. In L. C. Wynne, R. L. Cromwell, & S. Matthysse (Eds.), *The nature of schizophrenia* (pp. 339–358). New York: Wiley.

Baron, M., Gruen, R., Rainer, J. D., Kane, J., Asnis, L., & Lord, S. A. (1985). A family study of schizophrenic and normal control probands: Implications for the spectrum concept of schizophrenia. *American Journal of Psychiatry, 142,* 447–455.

Battaglia, M., Gasperini, M., Sciuto, G., Scherillo, P., & Bellodi, L. (1991). Psychiatric disorders in the families of schizotypal subjects. *Schizophrenia Bulletin, 17,* 659–668.

Cannon, T. D., & Mednick, S. A. (1993). The schizophrenia high-risk project in Copenhagen: Three decades of progress. *Acta Psychiatrica Scandinavica, 370,* 33–47.

Cannon, T. D., Mednick, S. A., & Parnas, J. (1990). Antecedents of predominantly negative and predominantly positive symptom schizophrenia in a high-risk population. *Archives of General Psychiatry, 47,* 622–632.

Cannon, T. D., Haslam, N. Tyrka, A. R., Mednick, S. A., Schulsinger, F., Schulsinger,

H., & Parnas, J. (1995). The latent structure of schizotypy: II. Detection of a longitudinally stable taxon of individuals at high risk for schizophrenia-spectrum disorders. (Manuscript in preparation).

Cornblatt, B., & Erlenmeyer-Kimling, L. (1985). Global attentional deviance in children at risk for schizophrenia: Specificity and predictive validity. *Journal of Abnormal Psychology, 94,* 470–486.

Endicott, J., & Spitzer, R. (1972). Current and past psychopathology scales (CAPPS). *Archives of General Psychiatry, 27,* 678–687.

Erlenmeyer-Kimling, L., Golden, R. R., & Cornblatt, B. A. (1989). A taxometric analysis of cognitive and neuromotor variables in children at risk for schizophrenia. *Journal of Abnormal Psychology, 98,* 203–208.

Fenton, W. S., & McGlashan, T. H. (1989). Risk of schizophrenia in character disordered patients. *American Journal of Psychiatry, 146,* 1280–1284.

Golden, R. R. (1982). A taxometric model for detection of a conjectured latent taxon. *Multivariate Behavioral Research, 17,* 389–416.

Golden, R. R., & Meehl, P. E. (1979). Detection of the schizoid taxon with MMPI indicators. *Journal of Abnormal Psychology, 88,* 212–233.

Gottesman, I. I., & Shields, J. (1982). *Schizophrenia: The epigenetic puzzle.* Cambridge: Cambridge University Press.

Grove, W. M., Lebow, B. S., Clementz, B. A., Cerri, A., Medus, C., & Iacono, W. G. (1991). Familial prevalence and coaggregation of schizotypy indicators: A multitrait family study. *Journal of Abnormal Psychology, 100,* 115–121.

Hanson, D., Gottesman, I. I., & Heston, L. L. (1976). Some possible childhood indicators of adult schizophrenia inferred from children of schizophrenics. *British Journal of Psychiatry, 129,* 142–154.

Hanson, D., Gottesman, I. I., & Meehl, P. E. (1977). Genetic theories and the validation of psychiatric diagnoses: Implications for the study of children of schizophrenics. *Journal of Abnormal Psychology, 86,* 575–588.

Hanson, D., Gottesman, I. I., & Heston, L. L. (1990). Long range schizophrenia forecasting: Many a slip twixt cup and lip. In J. Rolf, K. Nuechterlein, A. Masten, & D. Cicchetti (Eds.), *Risk and protective factors in the development of psychopathology* (pp. 424–444). Cambridge: Cambridge University Press.

Haslam, N. (1994). Categories of social relationship. *Cognition, 53,* 59–90.

Haslam, N., & Beck, A.T. (1994) Subtyping major depression: A taxometric analysis. *Journal of Abnormal Psychology, 103,* 686–692.

Kendler, K. S. (1983). Overview: A current perspective on twin studies of schizophrenia. *American Journal of Psychiatry, 140,* 1413–1425.

Kendler, K. S., & Gruenberg, A. M. (1984). An independent analysis of the Copenhagen sample of the Danish adoption study of schizophrenia VI: The relationship between psychiatric disorders as defined by DSM-III in the relatives and adoptees. *Archives of General Psychiatry, 41,* 555–564.

Kety, S. S. (1987). The significance of genetic factors in the etiology of schizophrenia: Results from the National Study of Adoptees in Denmark. *Journal of Psychiatric Research, 21,* 423–429.

Kety, S. S. (1988). Schizophrenic illness in the families of schizophrenic adoptees: Findings from the Danish National Sample. *Schizophrenia Bulletin, 14,* 217–222.

Lenzenweger, M. F., & Korfine, L. (1992). Confirming the latent structure and base rate of schizotypy: A taxometric analysis. *Journal of Abnormal Psychology, 101,* 567–571.

Lenzenweger, M. F., & Moldin, S. O. (1990). Discerning the latent structure of hypothetical psychosis proneness through admixture analysis. *Psychiatry Research, 33,* 243–257.

Loranger, A. W., Sussman, V. L., Oldham, J. M., & Russakoff, L. M. (1985).

Personality Disorder Examination: A structured interview for making diagnosis of DSM-IIIR personality disorders. White Plains, N.Y.: Cornell Medical College.

Mednick, S. A., Cannon, T. D., & Barr, C. E. (1991). Obstetrical events and adult schizophrenia. In S. A. Mednick, T. D. Cannon, C. E. Barr, & M. Lyon (Eds.), *Fetal neural development and adult schizophrenia* (pp. 115–133). Cambridge: Cambridge University Press.

Mednick, S. A., & McNeil, T. F. (1968). Current methodology in research on the etiology of schizophrenia: Serious difficulties which suggest the use of the high-risk group method. *Psychological Bulletin, 70,* 681–693.

Mednick, S. A., & Schulsinger, F. (1965). A longitudinal study of children with a high risk for schizophrenia: A preliminary report. In S. Vandenberg (Ed.), *Methods and goals in human behavior genetics* (pp. 255–296). Orlando, Fla: Academic Press.

Mednick, S. A., & Silverton, L. (1988). High-risk studies of the etiology of schizophrenia. In M. T. Tsuang & J. C. Simpson (Eds.), *Handbook of schizophrenia,* Vol 3: *Nosology, epidemiology and genetics* (pp. 543–562). Amsterdam: Elsevier.

Meehl, P. E. (1962). Schizotaxia, schizotypy, schizophrenia. *American Psychologist, 17,* 827–838.

Meehl, P. E. (1973). MAXCOV-HITMAX: A taxonomic search method for loose genetic syndromes. In P. E. Meehl (Ed.), *Psychodiagnosis: Selected papers* (pp. 200–224). Minneapolis: University of Minnesota Press.

Meehl, P. E. (1989). Schizotaxia revisited. *Archives of General Psychiatry, 46,* 935–944.

Meehl, P. E. (1990). Toward an integrated theory of schizotaxia, schizotypy, and schizophrenia. *Journal of Personality Disorders, 4,* 1–99.

Moldin, S. O., Rice, J. P., Gottesman, I. I., & Erlenmeyer-Kimling, L. (1990). Psychometric deviance in offspring at risk for schizophrenia: II. Resolving heterogeneity through admixture analysis. *Psychiatry Research, 32,* 311–322.

Nuechterlein, K. H., & Dawson, M. E. (1984). Information processing and attentional functioning in the developmental course of schizophrenic disorders. *Schizophrenia Bulletin, 10,* 160–203.

Nuechterlein, K. H., Dawson, M. E., Ventura, J., Goldstein, M. J., Snyder, K. S., Yee, C. M., & Mintz, J. (1992). Developmental processes in schizophrenic disorders: Longitudinal studies of vulnerability and stress. *Schizophrenia Bulletin, 18,* 387–421.

Parnas J. (1985). Mates of schizophrenic mothers: A study of assortative mating from the American–Danish high-risk study. *British Journal of Psychiatry, 146,* 490–497.

Parnas, J., Cannon, T. D., Jacobsen, B., Schulsinger, H., Schulsinger, F., & Mednick, S. A. (1993). Lifetime DSM-IIIR diagnostic outcomes in offspring of schizophrenic mothers: Results from the Copenhagen high-risk study. *Archives of General Psychiatry, 50,* 707–714.

Parnas, J., Schulsinger, F., Teasdale, T. W., Schulsinger, H., Feldman, P. M., & Mednick, S. A. (1982). Perinatal complications and clinical outcome within the schizophrenia spectrum. *British Journal of Psychiatry, 140,* 416–420.

Parnas, J., Teasdale, T. W., & Schulsinger, H. (1985). Institutional rearing and diagnostic outcome in children of schizophrenic mothers: A prospective high-risk study. *Archives of General Psychiatry, 42,* 762–769.

Rado, S. (1953). Dynamics and classification of disordered behavior. *American Journal of Psychiatry, 110,* 406–416.

Rosenthal, D. (1975). Discussion: The concept of subschizophrenic disorders. In R. R.

Fieve, D. Rosenthal, & H. Brill (Eds.), *Genetic research in psychiatry* (pp. 199–215). Baltimore: Johns Hopkins University Press.

Schulsinger, H. (1976). A ten year follow-up of children of schizophrenic mothers: Clinical assessment. *Acta Psychiatrica Scandinavica, 53,* 371–386.

Schulz, P. M., Schulz, S. C., Goldberg, S. C., Ettigi, P., Resnick, R. J., & Friedel, R. O. (1986). Diagnoses of the relatives of schizotypal outpatients. *Journal of Nervous and Mental Disease, 174,* 457–463.

Shields, J., Heston, L. L., & Gottesman, I. I. (1975). Schizophrenia and the schizoid: The problem for genetic analysis. In R. R. Fieve, D. Rosenthal, & H. Brill (Eds.), *Genetic research in psychiatry* (pp. 167–197). Baltimore: Johns Hopkins University Press.

Siever, L. J., Silverman, J. M., Horvath, T. B., Klar, H., Coccaro, E., Keefe, R. S. E., Pinkham, L., Rinaldi, P., Mohs, R. C., & Davis, K. L. (1990). Increased morbid risk for schizophrenia-related disorders in relatives of schizotypal personality disordered patients. *Archives of General Psychiatry, 47,* 634–640.

Spitzer, R. L., & Endicott, J. (1978). *Schedule for Affective Disorders and Schizophrenia–Lifetime Version* (3rd ed.). New York: New York Psychiatric Institute.

Squires-Wheeler, E., Skodol, A. E., Bassett, A., & Erlenmeyer-Kimling, L. (1989). DSM-IIIR schizotypal personality traits in offspring of schizophrenic disorder, affective disorder, and normal control parents. *Journal of Psychiatric Research, 23,* 229–239.

Squires-Wheeler, E., Skodol, A. E., & Erlenmeyer-Kimling, L. (1992). The assessment of schizotypal features over two points in time. *Schizophrenia Research, 6,* 75–85.

Stephens, D. A., Atkinson, M. W., Kay, D. W. K., Roth, M., & Garside, R. F. (1975). Psychiatric morbidity in parents and sibs of schizophrenics and non-schizophrenics. *British Journal of Psychiatry, 127,* 97–108.

Stone, M. H. (1977). The borderline syndrome: Evolution of the term, general aspects and prognosis. *American Journal of Psychotherapy, 31,* 345–365.

Syzmanski, S., Kane, J. M., & Lieberman, J. A. (1991). A selective review of biological markers in schizophrenia. *Schizophrenia Bulletin, 17,* 99–111.

Thaker, G., Adami, H., Moran, M., Lahti, A., & Cassady, S. (1993). Psychiatric illnesses in families of subjects with schizophrenia-spectrum personality disorders: High morbidity risks for unspecified functional psychoses and schizophrenia. *American Journal of Psychiatry, 150,* 66–71.

Trull, T. J., Widiger, T. A., & Guthrie, P. (1990). Categorical versus dimensional status of borderline personality disorder. *Journal of Abnormal Psychology, 99,* 40–48.

Tsuang, M. T., Gilbertson, M. W., & Faraone, S. V. (1991). The genetics of schizophrenia: Current knowledge and future directions. *Schizophrenia Research, 4,* 157–171.

Tyrka, A. R., Cannon, T. D., Haslam, N., Mednick, S. A., Schulsinger, F., Schulsinger, H., & Parnas, J. (1995). The latent structure of schizotypy: I Premorbid indicators of a taxon of individuals at-risk for schizophrenia spectrum disorders. *Journal of Abnormal Psychology, 104,* 173–183.

Wing, J. K., Cooper, J. E., & Sartorious, N. (1974). *The measurement and classification of psychiatric symptoms.* London: Cambridge University Press.

Wolff, S., Townshend, R., McGuire, R. J., & Weeks, D. J. (1991). 'Schizoid' personality in childhood and adult life II: Adult adjustment and the continuity with schizotypal personality disorder. *British Journal of Psychiatry, 159,* 620–629.

9

Fully and quasi-dimensional constructions of schizotypy

GORDON CLARIDGE and TONY BEECH

Two related themes run through this chapter. As the title indicates, one concerns the dimensionality inherent in our attempts to describe and understand schizotypy and schizotypal personality disorder (SPD). Although widely applied – and virtually definitive of the psychiatric notion of "borderline" – the concept of dimensionality is not entirely unambiguous, and constructions of it have varied. This is especially true where, as in the present case, attempts have been made to find a meeting point between ideas originating in the field of normal personality and other individual differences and those rooted more in psychiatry and clinical psychology. Here we explore some of the issues about dimensionality and suggest a preference for how it might best be applied to SPD; based upon our interpretation of the available evidence.

The second theme in the chapter is not unconnected to the above. It concerns attempts that are currently being made to discover experimental paradigms that can characterize the cognitive functioning of schizotypal and schizotypally disordered individuals; or, in another context, develop "markers" of a cognitive nature that might be helpful in high-risk and genetics research. Here it should be noted that the cognitive approach has no particular prerogative in either respect. Indeed it could be argued – and in our view probably is the case – that for many purposes the more promising lines of research are biological, especially neurodevelopmental. But the cognitive perspective does have significant claim on our attention, for two reasons. First, and most obviously, it allows us to probe the more purely psychological aspects of schizotypy; these are of interest in their own right, even though investigating them in the laboratory can be problematical. Second, the very difficulties of research in this area have given useful insights into how to go about choosing optimum experimental paradigms for investigating schizophrenic – and by extrapolation schizotypal – cognitive functioning. These observations, in turn, bear upon our constructions of dimensionality.

Issues of dimensionality

Although concentrating here on a particular example, it is worth noting that some questions about dimensionality are relevant to psychiatric disorder as a whole; that is to say, they arise whenever we consider possible continuities or connections between the major mental illnesses, the disorders of personality, and behavioral and psychological traits that fall within the normal, broadly healthy, domain (Claridge, 1985). But it happens that schizophrenia presents the case particularly well.

Two traditional views of dimensionality, illustrated in Figure 9.1, can be discerned. These roughly align to the psychiatric and the psychological, though to some extent they also seem to correspond (among psychologists at least) to some difference in North American and European usage. The psychiatric view of continuity is characteristically quasi-dimensional and thus confined to the upper half of Figure 9.1. Focusing on variations within the illness domain, and taking the abnormal (ill) state as its reference point, it construes dimensionality as degrees of expression of a disease process. The descriptors overtly defining this continuum, and forming the basis for measurement, are clinical signs and symptoms. Typical questions for debate include diagnostic and nosological issues, such as the relationship between full-blown psychosis and forms of personality disorder as possible *formes frustes* of disease: SPD in the case of schizophrenia. In contrast, the view of continuity referred to in the figure as "fully dimensional" takes normality or health as the starting point. It encloses the quasi-dimensional but adds another form of continuity, at the personality level. The connection between these two kinds of dimension – within illness and within personality – is that the latter supposedly describes predisposition to the former, while otherwise remaining part of normal individual variation (Claridge, 1987).

It is instructive to compare this model of dimensionality with those proposed by Meehl and by Eysenck, two other psychologists who have addressed the issue – and who have come to somewhat different conclusions, both from each other and from that shown in Figure 9.1. Meehl's (1962) theory similarly combines both quasi-dimensional and fully dimensional elements. Where it appears to differ is that for Meehl, schizotypy lies quite firmly in the illness domain – as partially expressed "schizotaxia," the very specific inherited neurointegrative defect which, according to him, underlies schizophrenia. He therefore appears to see no essential connection between schizophrenia and

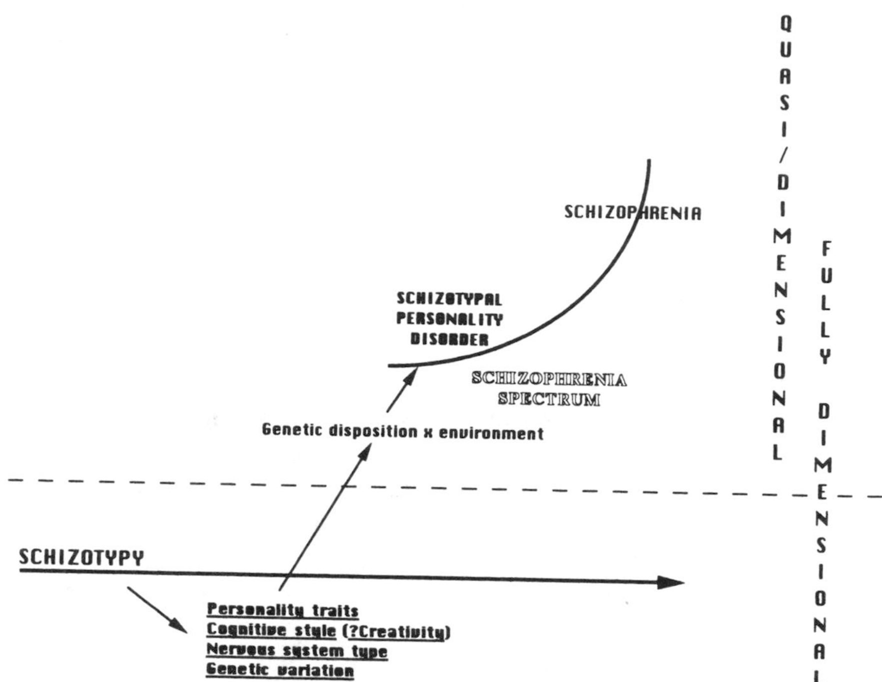

Fig. 9.1. Diagram comparing quasi-dimensional (disease based) and fully dimensional (personality-based) continuity models of schizotypy and schizophrenia.

schizotypy as a fully normal personality dimension. Where personality does enter into the equation, it does so, according to Meehl, in two respects: (1) in the form of independent polygenically determined traits that act to facilitate, or compensate for, the effects of the "schizogene"; and (2) in the form of personality aberrations that look like "true" schizophrenia but are phenocopies, genetically distinct from it (Meehl, 1990).

Eysenck's view of dimensionality is different again, and diametrically opposite, from Meehl's. According to Eysenck, mental illness is best construed entirely dimensionally, his model corresponding to what is effectively an incomplete version of Figure 9.1. Thus, he has confined his theorizing to the personality domain – below the dotted line in the figure – and takes little account of any distinctions or discontinuities that might exist between symptoms and traits. For him the psychiatric disorders, including the psychoses, merely represent the end-points of continuously variable dimensions (Eysenck, 1960; Eysenck & Eysenck, 1976). (Eysenck is also unusual, of course, in preferring what amounts to a personality version of the *Einheit-*

psychose view of psychosis; his version of Figure 9.1 would substitute "psychoticism" for "schizotypy" as the etiologically significant dimension. However, this does not materially alter the general argument here.)

Kendler (1985), albeit writing from a different perspective and with a different purpose, has also drawn out the distinction being made here: between conceptualizations of schizotypy, on the one hand, as attenuated psychotic symptoms and, on the other, as deviant personality traits. Discussing SPD (and its earlier equivalents), he notes that, historically, both approaches have been adopted to the diagnosis of these conditions. One possibility that Kendler considers is that the two types of descriptor tap vulnerabilities to quite different forms of disorder. On the other hand, it might merely be that different investigators have chosen to slant their assessments to suit their particular clinical or research end. Certainly the symptom/trait distinction per se does not seem to provide a firm basis for identifying etiologically unique features. As Kendler and his colleagues have themselves demonstrated, equivalent features of schizotypy can be measured in the same (normal) subjects evaluated, on one occasion, with a self-report questionnaire and, on another, by a clinical interview designed to assess SPD symptoms (Kendler, Och, Gorman, Hewitt, Ross, & Mirsky, 1991).

Several of the issues here are entangled with others that concern the psychometric assessment of schizotypy: what such measures are intended to tap, how they are interpreted, how they are related to one another, the reasons they were developed, and the uses to which they are put. There is now an impressive array of questionnaire scales for measuring schizotypy, psychoticism, psychosis proneness, or their other equivalents (see Table 9.1). Furthermore, the successful widespread use of these scales in nonclinical samples leaves us in no doubt that psychotic features are represented among the characteristics of the population at large. Interpretation of this fact has differed, reflecting the division of opinion about dimensionality referred to above. Thus, Meehl's emphasis on the need to develop indices that can detect membership of the so-called schizoid taxon (Golden & Meehl, 1979) has tended to define a dichotomous, categorical approach to schizotypy (Lenzenweger, 1993). This in turn has encouraged, especially among American workers, the continuing search for specific (perhaps genetically specific) questionnaire indicators that might sharply discriminate "schizotypes" from "nonschizotypes" (Lenzenweger & Loranger, 1989; Moldin, Rice, Gottesman, & Erlenmeyer-Kimling, 1990). In contrast, for workers such as ourselves, trained in the tradition of a more purely dimensional approach, this is a foreign concept. Our view would be that, although useful for certain purposes, it is entirely arbitrary to set cutoff points on scales designed to measure what are literally continuous traits. We

Table 9.1. *Psychosis-proneness scales*

Scale	Comments	References
Schizoidia	Seven-item scale derived from MMPI	Golden & Meehl (1979)
Chapman (and associates) scales	Scales measuring tendency to perceptual distortion (especially of body image), superstitious and similar belief, inability to experience pleasure, and other features of schizotypy and general psychosis-proneness	Chapman, Chapman, & Raulin (1978)
Perceptual aberration		
Magical ideation		Eckblad & Chapman (1983)
Social and physical anhedonia		Chapman, Chapman, & Raulin (1976)
Hypomanic personality		Eckblad & Chapman (1986)
Impulsive nonconformity		Chapman, Chapman, Numbers, Edell, Carpenter, & Beckfield (1984)
Intense ambivalence		Raulin (1984)
Cognitive slippage		Miers & Raulin (1985)
Social fear		Raulin & Wee (1984)
		see also Chapman, Edell, & Chapman (1980); Chapman, Chapman, & Miller (1982); Chapman & Chapman (1987)

STQ		
Schizotypal personality (STA) Borderline personality (STB)	Modeled on DSM-III criteria for SPD and BPD	Claridge & Broks (1984) *see also* Jackson & Claridge (1991)
Launay–Slade scale	Measure of "predisposition to hallucinate"	Launay & Slade (1981); Bentall & Slade (1986)
Schizophrenism	Items weighted toward attention difficulties and social anxiety	Nielsen & Petersen (1976)
Schizoid cognitions (RISC)	Designed to measure "positive" aspects of schizotypy using "nonclinical" items	Rust (1987, 1988)
Psychoticism (P-scale)	Part of four-scale Eysenck Personality Questionnaire (EPQ)	Eysenck & Eysenck (1975, 1976) Eysenck, Eysenck, & Barrett (1985)
Schizotypy	Measure of both "positive" and "negative" aspects of schizotypy	Venables, Wilkins, Mitchell, Raine, & Bailes (1990)
Schizotypal Personality Questionnaire (SPQ)	Modeled on DSM-IIIR criteria for SPD, measuring nine aspects of schizotypy	Raine (1991)

would argue that it is possible to make such distinctions only by using symptom scales – or other instruments that act in that fashion; such as the Chapman's Perceptual Aberration Scale. Notably, the latter was deliberately designed with a "strong" item content in order to maximize its discriminatory power and is the measure that has been mostly used in recent taxonometric analyses of schizotypy (see references to Lenzenweger above; and Lenzenweger & Korfine, Chapter 7, this volume).

Another strand in the debate that is now beginning to emerge concerns the multidimensional nature of schizotypy. That the latter is not a unitary concept is obvious even from casual inspection of the scales that purport to measure it; from the very beginning the prominent questionnaire constructors, such as the Chapmans, took it for granted that several instruments would be required in order to tap different facets of psychosis proneness. Recently this has been systematically examined – and validated – in a number of factor analyses of the scales shown earlier in Table 9.1. The detailed results of six such studies reported to date are collated in Table 9.2. The pattern of findings across the studies has naturally varied, reflecting the type and number of scales included for analysis. But there are striking regularities and some general conclusions can be reached (see Table 9.3 and also Claridge (1994), for further discussion).[1] Most consistent was the emergence in all six analyses of a component defined by scales measuring unusual perceptual experiences, thinking styles, and beliefs; this clearly aligns with what clinically, in relation to schizophrenia, would be labeled as "positive symptoms." Other components either seem to represent additional symptom-like features (e.g., "cognitive disorganization"), or more personality-based characteristics; among the latter the most consistently found has been a factor of "schizoid solitariness and lack of feeling," slanted toward anhedonia and perhaps roughly corresponding to negative symptomatology in the clinical domain. It is worth noting in passing that the several components necessary to define normal schizotypy map well on to those observed as symptom clusters in schizophrenia itself, where a straightforward positive/negative dichotomy is now proving oversimplistic (e.g., Liddle, 1987).

These observations raise two important, related questions. One concerns the relative status of the various components of schizotypy as measures of psychosis proneness. The other is, How clinically specific are they anyway? Some answers have emerged in the course of work using our STA scale, which we have now administered to various selected groups of subjects, some not even clinically disordered (see Table 9.4). Without exception all of these groups were typically high in STA score, equal to or even exceeding that found in diagnosed schizophrenics. Here it should be noted that the STA scale

Table 9.2. *Psychosis-proneness scales: summary of six principal components analyses*

Scales analyzed		Factors identified (with main loadings)
		Muntaner et al. (1988)
Eysenck Psychoticism (P) Extraversion (E) Neuroticism (N) Lie (L)	I	Cognitive Disturbance (STA, MgI, PAb, N)
Claridge Schizotypal Personality (STA) Borderline Personality (STB)	II	Introverted Anhedonia (SoA, E^-, PhA)
Chapman Physical Anhedonia (PhA) Social Anhedonia (SoA) Perceptual Aberration (PAb) Magical Ideation (MgI)	III	Social Nonconformity (P, L, STB)
		Raine & Allbutt (1989)[a]
Eysenck Psychoticism (P)		
Chapman Perceptual Aberration (PAb)		
Venables Schizophrenism (Sch) Social Anhedonia (SA)	I	Schizotypal Personality Disorder (STA, LSHS, Sch, STB, PAb)
Claridge Schizotypal Personality (STA) Borderline Personality (STB)		
Launay & Slade Hallucinatory Disposition (LSHS)	II	Anhedonic Psychoticism (P, SA)
		Kelley & Coursey (1992)[b]
Chapman et al. Physical Anhedonia (PhA) Perceptual Aberration (PAb) Magical Ideation (MgI) Impulsive Nonconformity (IN)	I	General Schizotypy ("positive symptoms") (all scales except PhA)
Intense Ambivalence (IA) Cognitive Slippage (CS) Social Fear (SF)	II	Anhedonia/Flat Affectivity ("negative symptoms") (PhA, MgI-, PAb-)
Nielsen & Petersen Schizophrenism (NP)		

Table 9.2. (*cont.*)

Scales analyzed	Factors identified (with main loadings)	
Golden & Meehl		
Schizoidia (MMPI 7-items)		
Schizotypy (MMPI 2-7-8)		
Claridge		
Schizotypal Personality (STA)		
	Kendler & Hewitt (1992)[c]	
Chapman		
(Shortened versions)	I	Positive Trait Schizotypy (LSHS, MgI, MgI2, PAb, PAb2, IN)
Magical Ideation (MgI)		
Perceptual Aberration (PAb)		
Impulsive Nonconformity (IN)		
Physical Anhedonia (PhA)		
Social Anhedonia (SoA)		
Claridge		
(Derived STA subscales)	II	Nonconformity (P, IN, PhA)
Perceptual Aberration (PAb2)		
Magical Ideation (MgI2)	III	Social Schizotypy (PA, SoA)
Paranoid Ideation (PI)		
Launay & Slade		
Hallucinatory Disposition (LSHS)		
Eysenck		
Psychoticism (P)		
	Bentall et al. (1989)[d]	
Eysenck		
Psychoticism (P)		
Extraversion (E)	I	"Positive symptom" (Schizotypy (HoP, MgI, P, LSHS, STA, STB, PAb)
Neuroticism (N)		
Lie (L)		
Claridge	II	Cognitive Disorganization/Anxiety (N, NP, MMPI, STA)
Schizotypal Personality (STA)		
Borderline Personality (STB)		
Chapman	III	Introverted Anhedonia (E^-, SoA, PhA)
Physical Anhedonia (PhA)		
Social Anhedonia (SoA)		
Perceptual Aberration (PAb)		
Magical Ideation (MgI)		
Hypomanic Personality (HoP)		
Nielsen & Petersen		
Schizophrenism (NP)		

Table 9.2. (*cont.*)

Scales analyzed	Factors identified (with main loadings)	
Golden & Meehl Schizoidia (MMPI)		
Launay & Slade Halluncinatory Disposition (LSHS)		
	McCreery (1993, unpublished)	
Eysenck Psychoticism (P) Extraversion (E) Neuroticism (N) Lie (L)		
Claridge		
Schizotypal Personality (STA) Borderline Personality (STB)	I	"Positive symptom" Schizotypy (MgI, LSHS, PAb, STA, HoP)
Chapman		
Physical Anhedonia (PhA) Social Anhedonia (SoA) Perceptual Aberration (PAb)	II	Cognitive Disorganization/Anxiety (NP, N, STB, E⁻, STA, MMPI)
Magical Ideation (MgI) Hypomanic Personality (HoP)	III	Asocial Schizotypy (P, L⁻, STB, HoP)
Nielsen & Petersen Schizophrenism (NP)	IV	Introverted Anhedonia (PhA, SoA, L, E⁻)
Golden & Meehl Schizoidia (MMPI)		
Launay & Slade Hallucinatory Disposition (LSHS)		

[a]Authors report more than one factor solution for data; that shown considered optimum.
[b]Only unrotated factors reported.
[c]Two other analyses included either additional personality scales or symptom measures of anxiety/depression.
[d]Also added four clinical symptom (delusions) scales to give four-factor solution: I, "Positive symptom" schizotypy; II, Cognitive disorganization/anxiety; III, Introverted anhedonia; IV, Asocial schizotypy (P, L, HoP). Compare analysis by McCreery, giving same four factors without those scales.

Table 9.3. *Summary of components of "schizotypy"*

1. Susceptibility to "positive symptoms"
   - Perceptual aberration/Magical ideation
   - Hallucinatory disposition
   - Schizotypal personality
   - Hypomanic personality
   - Delusional beliefs (Foulds scales)
2. Cognitive disorganization (social anxiety and aversiveness)
   - Schizotypal personality
   - Schizophrenism (attentional dysfunctions)
   - Neuroticism
   - Introversion
3. Schizoid solitariness with lack of feeling
   - Physical and social anhedonia
   - Introversion
   - Conforming (high "lie" score)

Note: Items under each component indicate measures referred to in Tables 9.1 and 9.2. See also endnote on page 212.

was designed as a measure of "general schizotypy," though we now know that its item content is quite weighted toward the positive-symptom component referred to above, and it does seem to be this feature in particular that is responsible for the observations made in Table 9.4.

We are faced therefore with a somewhat paradoxical situation: the aspect of schizotypy – positive symptoms – that is most generally found, even in certain nonclinical samples, is precisely that which (1) is intuitively closest to schizophrenia, (2) is expected to be psychometrically most discontinuous, and (3) emerges as the strongest and most consistent component in the analyses of schizotypy scales.

Our own interpretation of this follows. We believe that whereas the tendency to experience positive symptoms might be a necessary precondition of psychotic breakdown, it is by no means sufficient. Where present, it can predispose to a range of other clinical disorders. Or it can find expression in quite positive, rewarding psychological states – such as profound spiritual experiences (Jackson, 1991) or out-of-the-body experiences (McCreery, 1993) – and consequently be perfectly compatible with healthy adjustment. For the latter, McCreery has coined the label "happy schizotype" – in our view an extremely useful term for capturing the idea that individual features of psychosis proneness are actually neutral with respect to pathology and that it is only in certain combinations or in the presence of other factors that they con-

Table 9.4. *Samples scoring highly in "general schizotypy" (STA)*

Schizophrenics
(including in remission)
Schizophrenics' relatives
(but some paradoxically very low)
Adult dyslexics
Obsessive-compulsive disorder (OCD) patients
Eating disorder patients
Out-of-the-body experience subjects
(healthy normals)
Spiritual experience subjects
(healthy normals)

tribute to psychologically distressing experience or judged abnormal behavior.

Two other conclusions flow from what we have said. First, contrary to the simple medical – or what we have referred to here as the quasi-dimensional – model, the understanding of schizophrenia and SPD needs to proceed more from an understanding of normal schizotypy, rather than the other way around; or at least the two approaches should complement each other to a greater extent than they have hitherto. Second, given such a shift of emphasis, it is also appropriate, in seeking experimental paradigms of schizotypy, that we look for features that match its proposed status as a dimension of normal functioning rather than ones that constantly emphasize pathology or deficit. This theme is taken up in the second half of the chapter.

Cognitive paradigms of schizotypy

As noted earlier, the cognitive approach to schizotypy has a certain interest because of its emphasis on the psychological. This appeal is further enhanced by the shift proposed here toward a more broadly based construction of schizotypy, to include more reference to its normal, healthy variants in our theories about the schizophrenia spectrum: explanations that seem to be valid right along that dimension might then be very informative. Applications of cognitive psychology in schizophrenia research have a serious limitation, however. This stems from the fact that many of the research paradigms used can only predict deficit effects – for example, slower reaction time or less accurate performance. Consequently, in clinical research it is often difficult to disentangle specific from nonspecific factors and hence narrow down on unique features of schizophrenic or schizotypal functioning. The use of at-risk, rather than currently ill, subjects can overcome the problem to some extent; but even then there is a lingering feeling that nothing very interesting is being observed. The fact that researchers have been content to tolerate, or even encourage, this viewpoint on cognitive data is itself significant and reflects the predominance of the quasi-dimensional view of schizophrenia referred to earlier: disorder implies impaired functioning, conditioning us to expect evidence of defect even when extrapolating into "normal" schizotypal – that is, presumed high-risk – populations.

A new trend in cognitive research in the area has been to look for paradigms that predict performance that can in some sense be considered superior to that of other groups. In patient investigations this strategy is valuable in its own right, for obvious reasons. In studies of normal schizotypy it is interesting because it opens up the possibility of discovering features of cognitive functioning that might not in themselves be disadvantageous. Although such observations alone would not prove a fully dimensional theory, they would at least be strongly consistent with it. Here we shall consider three "superior performance" paradigms, all of which were developed in the context of schizophrenia research but also examined in relation to normal schizotypy.

Negative priming

This paradigm, which is one we ourselves have investigated extensively, was originally adopted as a test of the theory (e.g., Frith, 1979) that the positive symptoms of schizophrenia can be understood as a weakness of the mechanism that controls and limits the contents of consciousness. The aspect of cognitive psychology theory relevant to this idea is what happens to information that is processed at some level, but because of its lack of pertinence does not enter consciousness. Most recent evidence suggests that the information is not lost by passive decay, as was once thought (e.g., Broadbent, 1958); instead it is actively inhibited (Neill & Westberry, 1987; Tipper, 1985). This is demonstrated when, in a typical experiment, subjects are required to respond to a distractor they have previously ignored; here the distractor is first presented as the irrelevant part of a priming stimulus and then, in an immediately following probe phase, re-presented as a target to be named. Normally there is a delay in the latter response, due, it is argued, to a carryover of inhibition previously attached to the stimulus when being selected against at the priming stage. This "negative priming" effect is predicted to vary according to the degree of cognitive inhibition generated and to be less in schizophrenic and schizotypal individuals, leading to relatively faster response times in the probe phase.

We have tested this hypothesis in normal subjects with several negative priming procedures, using our STA scale as the measure of schizotypy. In the first of these experiments (Beech & Claridge, 1987), the task consisted of discrete priming and probe trials. Prime displays consisted of color patches (to be named) flanked by monochrome color words (to be ignored); on half the trials the latter predicted the color of a Stroop word that was then presented as a probe. The experimental measure of interest was the reaction time to probe stimuli that had been negatively primed, compared to a situation where no priming was involved. Using a median split of scores on the STA scale, we found that low schizotypal subjects showed significant negative priming, whereas high schizotypals had a tendency (though not significant) toward a facilitation effect.

We obtained identical results using a different, "list-reading," task (Beech, Baylis, Smithson, & Claridge, 1989). There subjects had to name the hue of consecutively presented color (Stroop) words, while ignoring the word itself; on 25% of occasions this ignored word predicted the hue of the next word to be named. The measure of interest here was reaction time on the "negatively primed" list compared to a control list of Stroop words when no such relation was present. A further study with the same task (Beech, Powell, McWilliam, & Claridge, 1989) examined schizophrenic patients, compared with psychiatric controls. The latter showed significant negative priming, whereas the schizophrenics did not. However, the effects were less dramatic in patients than in normal schizotypals because, it was thought, medication "normalized" the performance of schizophrenics. This would be supported by a later finding by Beech, Powell, McWilliam, and Claridge (1990) that a small dose of chlorpromazine increased the negative priming effect in normal subjects; a report by Peters (1993) that amphetamine reduces negative priming would also be consistent here.

Other observations have extended these basic comparisons. In one recent study we demonstrated a significant facilitation effect in high STA subjects when a semantic condition was included in the procedure (Beech, Baylis, Tipper, McManus, & Agar, 1991). In that case stimuli consisted of overlapping red and green words, with subjects being required to respond to one and ignore the other. (An example of a semantic relationship was naming the word CAT written in red after just ignoring the word DOG written in green.) In another experiment, we adapted the first negative priming procedure described earlier to lateralized presentation of the priming stimuli (Claridge, Clark, & Beech, 1992). Again we found significantly reduced negative priming in high schizotypals, selected on the STA. But this was the case only following primes presented to the left visual field (right hemisphere); it was also true only of males, an effect of gender regularly found in our negative priming work. These findings accord well with ongoing lines of schizophrenia and schizotypy research concerning, on the one hand, gender differences (*Schizophrenia Bulletin,* 1990) and, on the other, hemisphere functioning (Gruzelier, 1991, and Chapter 14, this volume).

Further patient studies (Laplante, Everett, & Thomas, 1992) have confirmed that negative priming is reduced in schizophrenics whereas other research, interestingly, has demonstrated that the effect is not confined to schizophrenia. Thus, Tannock, Schachar, Carr, Chajczyk, & Logan (1989) have found negative priming also to be reduced in children with attentional deficit disorder, and our own research has shown similar effects in patients suffering from obsessive-compulsive disorder (Enright & Beech, 1993). Finally (and in line with a theme introduced in the first half of this chapter), Peters, Pickering, & Hemsley (1994) used multiple measures of schizotypy in normal subjects to show that the reduction in negative priming was associated mostly with the "positive symptom" aspects of the trait. L. Williams (in press), also working with normal subjects, has similarly demonstrated this; indeed she reports that subjects with only "negative" schizotypal traits show, if anything, the reverse – namely increased negative priming.

Taken together, these results lead to conclusions that are both general and specific. On the one hand, negative priming appears to tap some common mechanism of selective attention that varies in normal subjects as a function of personality differences and is associated with vulnerability to a variety of clinical syndromes (e.g., obsessive-compulsive disorder, OCD) in addition to schizophrenia. On the other hand, negative priming seems to reflect cognitive processes that might be particularly responsible for those disorders of attention and thinking that in schizophrenia are labeled as positive symptoms.

Latent inhibition

This "superior performance" paradigm, which is currently being investigated in a number of centers, has recently been elaborated by Gray and his colleagues in a detailed neurophysiological theory of the positive symptoms of schizophrenia (Gray, Rawlins, Hemsley, & Smith, 1991). Derived from the animal learning literature, "latent inhibition" refers to the retarding effect on learning of preexposing the organism to an unreinforced stimulus to which it then has to form an association. The difficulty in learning here is due, according to Lubow (1989), to the acquisition of inhibition that interferes with subsequent excitatory conditioning. Part of the rationale for adopting latent inhibition as a paradigm for schizophrenia has been pharmacological, drawing particularly on the amphetamine/dopamine hypothesis. In this regard, it has been found that latent inhibition can be attenuated or abolished with chronic amphetamine treatment (Weiner, Lubow, & Feldon, 1984) and restored by the administration of haloperidol (Weiner & Feldon 1986). Conceptually (and, albeit over a different time scale, procedurally) similar to negative priming, latent inhibition is predicted to be weaker (and learning in the test phase therefore faster) in relation to schizophrenia.

Against this background, Baruch, Hemsley, and Gray (1988a) devised a latent inhibition task for use with schizophrenic patients. The method was such that subjects were preexposed to white noise bursts as an irrelevant distractor while performing another task. In the second phase of the experiment, the noise bursts had predictive value in terms of incrementation of a display counter (i.e., there would be a burst of white noise just before the counter moved); this constituted a rule that the subjects had to learn. The authors found that acute (though not chronic) schizophrenics did, as predicted, fail to display latent inhibition. Lubow, Weiner, Schlossberg, and Baruch (1987) failed to find this effect in schizophrenics but argued that the antipsychotic medication the subjects were receiving could have "normalized" the latent inhibition effect.

Baruch, Hemsley, and Gray (1988b) also used their same procedure in normal subjects, compared on three psychosis-proneness scales: the Eysenck P-scale, our STA, and the Launay Slade hallucinatory disposition scale (Launay & Slade, 1981). Although results for the other two scales were in the expected direction, only that for the Eysenck scale was significant: as predicted, high P scorers showed reduced latent inhibition. However, Lubow, Ingberg-Sachs, Zalstein-Orda, and Gewirtz (1992) report reduced latent inhibition for both the P and STA scales. In another recent study, Lipp and Vaitl (1992) found the more equivocal results to be obtained with the P-scale; using the STA, they observed significantly less latent inhibition in high scorers.

Given the conceptual resemblance of the latent inhibition and negative priming paradigms, some correlation between them would be expected if tested in the same subjects. As far as we are aware, there are no published data on this, though we do know of two unpublished observations (Peters, 1993; J. Williams, personal communication). Disappointingly neither demonstrated the predicted association. However, it is worth noting that, although superficially alike, the procedures for the two paradigms do differ in significant ways, and task-specific variables could easily overshadow attempts to discover whether a common process – say, of inhibition – is involved. For example, latent inhibition – unlike negative priming – does not lend itself to repeated use in the same subject; devising versions of the procedure that plausibly transfer to humans is also not easy. On the other hand, latent inhibition does have the benefit of a long history of research in the animal laboratory, helping to reveal more of its immediate physiological and pharmacological parameters than is the case with other, more strictly cognitive, paradigms.

Stimulation "below awareness"

As noted above in considering the rationale for negative priming, it can be argued that much schizophrenic cognition is ascribable to "leakage" into consciousness of semantically activated concepts that are irrelevant to ongoing thought (Frith, 1979; Maher, 1983). Cognitive psychologists would assume the mechanism of this to be preconscious, in which case the most direct way to examine it should be through the deliberate use of "below awareness" stimuli. In this way, the prediction would again be that schizotypal (and schizophrenic) subjects should, in appropriately designed experiments, be able to take advantage of their greater access to preconscious information – and hence perform better than other individuals. This theory has recently been extensively investigated in our laboratory by Evans (1992), adopting the so-called SAWCI (i.e., Semantic Activation Without Conscious Identification) paradigm (Marcel, 1983). All of her work was carried out on normal subjects evaluated for psychosis proneness with the CSTQ (Bentall, Claridge, & Slade, 1989); this is a composite questionnaire made up of many of the scales shown in Table 9.1 and the subject of two of the factor analyses referred to earlier.

Evans's prototypical experiment was a lexical decision task, based on Marcel's (1983) procedure. After assessing the subject's threshold of conscious detection, prime stimuli were then presented well below this limen, followed by probes under one of three conditions. Examples of the word pairs used are as follows:

PRIME	**PROBE**	**CONDITION**
TABLE	CHAIR	Associated
SWEET	CHAIR	Nonassociated
SWEET	UMPUL	Word/Nonword

Subjects had to respond by indicating whether the probe was a word or a nonword, reaction time (RT) being the dependent measure. All subjects were significantly faster in the associated condition than in the nonassociated condition, confirming that the prime, though not consciously reported, must have been semantically processed. Individual-differences analysis demonstrated a significant correlation (.60, $p < .02$) between STA (schizotypal personality) score and mean amount of priming (RT for nonassociated word pairs – RT for nonassociated word pairs). In other words, the higher the schizotypy the more sensitive the subjects were to the subliminal primes.

These results were confirmed and extended using a slightly different procedure, involving computer, rather than tachistoscopic, presentation of stimuli. Again significant correlations were found between amount of subliminal priming and psychosis-proneness, this time involving several scales, including Chapman's Perceptual Aberration Scale, Eysenck's P-scale, and the STB (borderline personality) scale from our STQ. These later experiments also revealed some gender variations: although both males and females showed SAWCI, the pattern of correlations with the psychosis-proneness scales differed somewhat in males and females.

Finally, Evans compared subjects performing at subliminal and at supraliminal thresholds. Under the former condition there were again the predicted significant positive correlations with schizotypy, for both Perceptual Aberration and STA. STA also correlated significantly with priming under the supraliminal condition, but now negatively so ($r = -.53$, $p < .05$). In discussing this curious reversal of the subliminal data, Evans suggests that the finding is in fact consistent with the theory behind her work. She argues that, in highly schizotypal individuals, excessive access to preconscious information might cause intrusions into consciousness which, under some rapid but supraliminal conditions of information processing, actually interferes with responding efficiently to the stimulus.

Evans has not so far attempted to validate the SAWCI paradigm in a patient sample, but a recent study by Kwapil, Hegley, Chapman, and Chapman (1990) has provided some partial confirmation of her results. They reversed the Evans procedure – using supraliminal primes and degraded targets – and found that schizophrenics performed better than both bipolar patients and normal controls on a word recognition task. They note that it is unclear whether the heightened priming they observed in schizophrenics was due to "a stronger activation or a delayed activation of associates, a greater persistence of associates, or a defect in the inhibition of associates." These questions remain to be examined, as do the relationships between the various paradigms described here. In the meantime, it does seem possible to conclude that schizotypy – or at least its positive-symptom aspects – is not necessarily associated with cognitive deficit, but rather with the opposite.

Conclusions and directions for future research

Although we regularly talk of a "schizophrenia spectrum," there are discontinuities in it that correspond – a bit too neatly perhaps – to the gaps in our understanding of it. The connection between SPD and schizophrenia seems reasonably certain, but how one jumps from the less severe personality disorder to the more severe illness is still unclear. Moving in the other direction, SPD and normal schizotypy seem more connected, but, as discussed at the beginning of this chapter, the relationship between them can at times look ambiguous. Indeed there is here an underlying dilemma about which end of the spectrum it is best to start from in order to get an understanding of the whole. If we begin with schizophrenia, then logically we are forced to admit a "defect" explanation of schizotypy as it appears in normal people: normal schizotypes are people with just a little bit of the flaw that causes schizophrenia; or they are people in whom, for some reason, the defect is not fully expressed. Either that, or we have to argue that many people who score highly on schizotypy questionnaires are not really schizotypal at all; they just look as though they are. We find this to be a nonparsimonious argument and to beg the question about what, in that case, we really mean by "schizotypy."

If we start, however, from the opposite, normal, end of the continuum and try to explain the schizophrenia spectrum from that direction, we are faced with another problem. Then we need to argue that a perfectly normal feature of personality (schizotypy) can give rise to a serious mental illness (schizophrenia) – which the currently received wisdom at least would have us believe has all the hallmarks of a neurological disease. Looked at in this way a *personality* view of schizotypy and a *disease* view of schizophrenia seem incompatible. According to either model, SPD sits awkwardly between the two extremes.

On the whole, for reasons outlined in this paper, we prefer the second – fully dimensional – approach to the problems of schizotypy, SPD, and schizophrenia. In other words, we would like to see it accepted that in the schizophrenia spectrum there are, in addition to discontinuities of function, some genuine continuities between psychotic and normal, between health and illness; with this being recognized, an important issue for research in the area would then be to find answers to the other questions that such a theory raises.

One such question is, How would we reconcile the apparent deficit state of schizophrenia with the apparent normality of schizotypy? The answer might lie in the simple notion of optimal levels of functioning. Evans's work on the SAWCI paradigm illustrates the point well. With subliminal priming, high schizotypes perform better because they have great access to below awareness data; with supraliminal priming, they perform worse because this very facility interferes with cognitive performance. Raine and Manders (1988) have offered a comparable explanation in trying to reconcile apparently similar contradictions in the enhanced performance of schizotypes and the deteriorated performance of schizophrenics on hemisphere tasks; their general point is that what may be advantageous in some circumstances may be disadvantageous in others.

Further questions then arise: What differentiates healthy schizotypy and unhealthy schizophrenia or SPD? What causes an otherwise normal mechanism to "flip" into a maladaptive state? Or, alternatively, what prevents it from doing so? One obvious factor is the natural "set point" of the mechanism itself (how schizotypal the person is in the first place); another is the presence or absence of chronic or acute stress and favorable or unfavorable life circumstances in precipitating or protecting against a dysfunctional shift in behavior. Other traits that describe the individual's personal makeup are presumably also important. An example would be high intellectual capacity; this might enable people of strongly schizotypal personality to cope better with the tendency to cognitive overload that forms part of schizotypy and which might more readily overwhelm others without the same intellectual resources. Indeed the combination of schizotypy and high intelligence might actually have a positive side, in accounting for some forms of creativity. The flexible, divergent thought style implicated in creative production could be said partly to depend upon having (to quote the SAWCI paradigm) a greatly enhanced access to preconsciously activated information. The highly intelligent, talented schizotype might be well fitted to exploit such facility, while still carrying the risk of diminished creative output if or when active psychotic illness does occur. These ideas could throw light on and clarify some ambiguities in the putative associations between schizophrenia and creativity; the crux of the argument here is that it is schizotypy, not schizophrenic disorder, that underpins the connection. (See Claridge, Pryor, & Watkins, 1990, for further discussion of this point and detailed illustration from the biographies of prominent authors who suffered periodic schizophrenic and/or schizoaffective breakdown.)

A further corollary to the above concerns possible interactions among the components of schizotypy themselves. Much of the recent emphasis has been on the latter's positive-symptom aspects; indeed all of the cognitive paradigms described here were deliberately chosen as ways of exploring those features in particular. This is understandable because in schizophrenia they seem to be the most definitive of the disorder and in schizotypy identify the strongest, most consistently observed component. It is somewhat paradoxical, then, that as questionnaire-rated traits, positive symptoms appear to be the most ubiquitous of the so-called schizophrenic features, appearing as they do in a wide range of normal and abnormal states not immediately within the schizophrenia spectrum. As noted earlier, the tendency to have positive symptom experiences would seem to be a necessary, but by no means sufficient, condition for schizophrenia. The implication here might then be that other components revealed in the recent analyses of schizotypy – for example, "cognitive disorganization," asocial, or anhedonia-related traits – are as, if not more, important in determining actual dispositions to specifically psychotic expressions of so-called positive-symptom vulnerability. We believe that this conclusion would not to be too far from that reached by Meehl and would coincide with the views of several other workers (Clementz, Grove, Iacono, & Sweeney, 1992; Siever, 1985).

In conclusion, the ideas discussed here certainly underline the need in future research to examine the questions at issue in terms of profiles of psychosis-proneness traits, rather than single constructs of schizotypy; for the latter's various components look as though they might interact to define several kinds of disposition – to schizophrenia, to other forms of psychosis, to personality disorders, even to aberrations outside the psychosis spectrum or, indeed, the illness domain altogether. Discovering the relative clinical and etiological significance of these different permutations of traits is an important priority for high-risk research and requires, among other things, a systematic dissection of their laboratory correlates. Here two, mutually compatible research strategies suggest themselves. One is to choose, on the basis of informed guesswork, what appear to be the most promising experimental paradigms for investigating each component of schizotypy. These could then be refined and elaborated in order to give them greater specificity. For example, SAWCI seems ideally suited to investigating the cognitive aspects but, like its rivals – for example, negative priming and latent inhibition – it does not yet enable us to identify which of the two components of schizotypy it is mostly tapping. In addition to this intensive research on individual paradigms, more large-scale, multivariate investigations would be worthwhile. We are thinking here of studies in which all of the currently available experimental measures of psychosis proneness could be administered to the same subjects, together with the full range of questionnaire scales. The combined data set could then be factor-analyzed, with a view to discovering how the descriptive and laboratory measures line up with one another. These two complementary research strategies would usefully extend our knowledge of the structure of schizotypy and take our understanding of its contribution to schizophrenia into a new phase.

Note

1. More recent research confirms that the four components found by McCreery (see Table 9.2) provide the most complete account of the factor structure of schizotypy (Claridge, McCreery, Mason, Bentall, Boyle, Slade, & Popplewell, in press).

References

Baruch, I., Hemsley, D. R., & Gray, A. (1988a). Differential performance of acute and chronic schizophrenics in a latent inhibition task. *Journal of Nervous and Mental Disease, 176,* 598–606.

Baruch, I., Hemsley, D. R., & Gray, A. (1988b). Latent inhibition and 'psychotic proneness' in normal subjects. *Personality and Individual Differences, 1988,* 777–783.

Beech, A., Baylis, G. C., Smithson, P., & Claridge, G. (1989a). Individual differences in schizotypy as reflected in measures of cognitive inhibition. *British Journal of Clinical Psychology, 28,* 117–129.

Beech, A. R., Baylis, G. C., Tipper, S., McManus, D., & Agar, K. J. (1991). Individual differences in cognitive processes: Towards an explanation of schizophrenic symptomatology. *British Journal of Psychology, 82,* 417–426.

Beech, A., & Claridge, G. (1987). Individual differences in negative priming: Relations with schizotypal personality traits. *British Journal of Psychology, 78,* 349–356.

Beech, A. R., Powell, T., McWilliam, J., & Claridge, G. S. (1989b). Evidence of reduced 'cognitive inhibition' in schizophrenia. *British Journal of Clinical Psychology, 28,* 109–116.

Beech, A. R., Powell, T. J., McWilliam, J., & Claridge, G. S. (1990). The effect of a small dose of chlorpromazine on a measure of 'cognitive inhibition.' *Personality and Individual Differences, 11,* 1141–1145.

Bentall, R. P., Claridge, G. S., & Slade, P. D. (1989). The multidimensional nature of schizotypal traits: A factor analytic study with normal subjects. *British Journal of Clinical Psychology, 28,* 363–375.

Bentall, R. P., & Slade, P. D. (1986). Reliability of a scale for measuring disposition towards hallucinations: A brief report. *Personality and Individual Differences, 6,* 527–529.

Broadbent, D. E. (1958). *Perception and communication.* London: Pergamon Press.

Chapman, L. J., & Chapman, J. P. (1987). The search for symptoms predictive of schizophrenia. *Schizophrenia Bulletin, 13,* 497–503.

Chapman, L. J., Chapman, J. P., & Miller, E. N. (1982). Reliabilities and intercorrelations of eight measures of proneness to psychosis. *Journal of Consulting and Clinical Psychology, 50,* 187–195.

Chapman, L. J., Chapman, J. P., & Raulin, M. L. (1976). Scales for physical and social anhedonia. *Journal of Abnormal Psychology, 85,* 374–382.

Chapman, L. J., Chapman, J. P., & Raulin, M. L. (1978). Body-image aberration in schizophrenia. *Journal of Abnormal Psychology, 87,* 399–407.

Chapman, L. J., Edell, W. S., & Chapman, J. P. (1980). Physical anhedonia, perceptual aberration, and psychosis proneness. *Schizophrenia Bulletin, 6,* 639–653.

Chapman, L. J., Chapman, J. P., Numbers, J., Edell, W. S., Carpenter, B., & Beckfield, D. L. (1984). Impulsive nonconformity as a trait contributing to the prediction of psychotic-like and schizotypal symptoms. *Journal of Nervous and Mental Disease, 172,* 681–691.

Claridge, G. S. (1985). *Origins of mental illness.* Oxford: Blackwell.

Claridge, G. (1987). 'The schizophrenias as nervous types' revisited. *British Journal of Psychiatry, 151,* 735–743.

Claridge, G. S. (1994). A single indicator of risk for schizophrenia: Probable fact or likely myth? *Schizophrenia Bulletin, 20,* 151–168.

Claridge, G. S., & Broks, P. (1984). Schizotypy and hemisphere function – I. Theoretical considerations and the measurement of schizotypy. *Personality and Individual Differences, 5,* 633–648.

Claridge, G., Clark, K. H., & Beech, A. R. (1992). Lateralization of the 'negative priming' effect: Relationships with schizotypy and with gender. *British Journal of Psychology, 83,* 13–23.

Claridge, G., McCreery, C., Mason, O., Bentall, R., Boyle, G., Slade, P., & Popplewell, D. (in press). The factor structure of 'schizotypal' traits: A large replication study. *British Journal of Clinical Psychology.*

Claridge, G., Pryor, R., & Watkins, G. (1990). *Sounds from the bell jar: Ten psychotic authors.* London: Macmillan.

Clementz, B. A., Grove, W. M., Iacono, W. G., & Sweeney, J. A. (1992). Smooth-pursuit eye movement dysfunction and liability for schizophrenia: Implications for genetic modeling. *Journal of Abnormal Psychology, 101,* 117–129.

Eckblad, M., & Chapman, L. J. (1983). Magical ideation as an indicator of schizotypy. *Journal of Consulting and Clinical Psychology, 51,* 215–225.

Eckblad, M., & Chapman, L. J. (1986). Development and validation of a scale for hypomanic personality. *Journal of Abnormal Psychology, 95,* 214–222.

Enright, S., & Beech, A R. (1993). Evidence of reduced inhibition in obsessive-compulsive disorder. *British Journal of Clinical Psychology, 32,* 67–74.

Evans, J. L. (1992). Schizotypy and preconscious processing. D. Phil. thesis, University of Oxford.

Eysenck, H. J. (1960). Classification and the problem of diagnosis. In H. J. Eysenck (Ed.), *Handbook of abnormal psychology.* London: Pitman.

Eysenck, H. J., & Eysenck, S. B. G. (1975). *Manual of the Eysenck Personality Questionnaire.* London: Hodder & Stoughton.

Eysenck, H. J., & Eysenck, S. B. G. (1976). *Psychoticism as a dimension of personality.* London: Hodder & Stoughton.

Eysenck, S. B. G., Eysenck, H. J., & Barrett, P. (1985). A revised version of the Psychoticism Scale. *Personality and Individual Differences, 6,* 21–29.

Frith, C. D. (1979). Consciousness, information processing and schizophrenia. *British Journal of Psychiatry, 134,* 225–235.

Golden, R. R., & Meehl, P. E. (1979). Detection of the schizoid taxon with MMPI indicators. *Journal of Abnormal Psychology, 88,* 217–233.

Gray, J. A., Rawlins, J. N. P., Hemsley, D. R., & Smith, A. D. (1991). The neuropsychology of schizophrenia. *Behavioral and Brain Sciences, 14,* 1–84.

Gruzelier, J. H. (1991). Hemisphere imbalance: Syndromes of schizophrenia, premorbid personality, and neurodevelopmental influences. In S. R. Steinhauer, J. H. Gruzelier, & J. Zubin, J. (Eds.), *Handbook of schizophrenia, Vol. 5: Neuropsychology, psychophysiology and information processing.* London: Elsevier.

Jackson, M. (1991). A study of the relationship between psychotic and spiritual experience. D. Phil. thesis, University of Oxford.

Jackson, M., & Claridge, G. (1991). Reliability and validity of a psychotic traits questionnaire (STQ). *British Journal of Clinical Psychology, 30,* 311–323.

Kelley, M. P., & Coursey, R. D. (1992). Factor structure of schizotypy scales. *Personality and Individual Differences, 13,* 723–731.

Kendler, K. S. (1985). Diagnostic approaches to schizotypal personality disorder. *Schizophrenia Bulletin, 11,* 538–553.

Kendler, K. S., & Hewitt, J. (1992). The structure of self-report schizotypy in twins. *Journal of Personality Disorders, 6,* 1–17.

Kendler, K. S., Och, A. L., Gorman, A. M., Hewitt, J. K., Ross, D. E., & Mirsky, A. F. (1991). The structure of schizotypy. *Psychiatry Research, 36,* 19–36.

Kwapil, T. R., Hegley, D. C., Chapman, L. J., & Chapman, J. P. (1990). Facilitation of word recognition by semantic priming in schizophrenia. *Journal of Abnormal Psychology, 99,* 215–221.

Laplante, L., Everett, J., & Thomas, J. (1992). Inhibition through negative priming with Stroop stimuli in schizophrenia. *British Journal of Clinical Psychology, 31,* 307–326.

Launay, G., & Slade, P. (1981). The measurement of hallucinatory predisposition in male and female prisoners. *Personality and Individual Differences, 2,* 221–234.

Lenzenweger, M. F. (1993). Explorations in schizotypy and the psychometric high-risk paradigm. In L. J. Chapman, J. P. Chapman, & D. C. Fowles (Eds.), *Progress in experimental personality and psychopathology research.* New York: Springer.

Lenzenweger, M. F., & Loranger, A. W. (1989). Detection of familial schizophrenia using a psychometric measure of schizotypy. *Archives of General Psychiatry, 46,* 902–907.

Liddle, P. (1987). The symptoms of chronic schizophrenia: A re-examination of the positive–negative dichotomy. *British Journal of Psychiatry, 151,* 221–234.

Lipp, O. V., & Vaitl, D. (1992). Latent inhibition in human Pavlovian differential conditioning: Effect of additional stimulation after preexposure and relation to schizotypal traits. *Personality and Individual Differences, 13,* 1003–1012.

Lubow, R. E. (1989). *Latent inhibition and conditioned attentional theory.* New York: Cambridge University Press.

Lubow, R. E., Ingberg-Sachs, Y., Zalstein-Orda, N., & Gewirtz, J. C. (1992). Latent inhibition in low and high 'psychotic-prone' normal subjects. *Personality and Individual Differences, 13,* 563–572.

Lubow, R. E., Weiner, I., Schlossberg, A., & Baruch, I. (1987). Latent inhibition and schizophrenia. *Bulletin of the Psychonomic Society, 25,* 464–467.

McCreery, C. A. S. (1993). Schizotypy and out-of-the-body-experiences. D. Phil. thesis, University of Oxford.

Maher, B. A. (1983). A tentative theory of schizophrenic utterance. In B. A. Maher & W. B. Maher (Eds.), *Progress in experimental personality research,* Vol. 12. New York: Academic Press.

Marcel, H. A. (1983). Conscious and unconscious perception: Experiments on visual masking and word recognition. *Cognitive Psychology, 15,* 197–237.

Meehl, P. E. (1962). Schizotaxia, schizotypy, and schizophrenia. *American Psychologist, 17,* 827–383.

Meehl, P. E. (1990). Toward an integrated theory of schizotaxia, schizotypy, and schizophrenia. *Journal of Personality Disorders, 4,* 1–99.

Miers, T. C., & Raulin, M. L. (1985). The development of a scale to measure cognitive slippage. Paper presented at the Eastern Psychological Association Convention, Boston.

Moldin, S. O., Rice, J. P., Gottesman, I. I., & Erlenmeyer-Kimling, L. (1990). Psychometric deviance in offspring at risk for schizophrenia: II. Resolving heterogeneity through admixture analysis. *Psychiatry Research, 32,* 311–322.

Muntaner, C., Garcia-Sevilla, L., Fernandez, A., & Torrubia, R. (1988). Personality dimensions, schizotypal and borderline personality traits and psychosis. *Personality and Individual Differences, 9,* 257–268.

Neill, W. T., & Westberry, R. L. (1987). Selective attention and the suppression of cognitive noise. *Learning, Memory and Cognition, 13,* 327–334.

Nielsen, T. C., & Petersen, N. E. (1976). Electrodermal correlates of extraversion, trait anxiety, and schizophrenism. *Scandinavian Journal of Psychology, 17,* 73–80.

Peters, E. (1993). Cognitive processes involved in the formation of positive symptomatology in schizotypal, amphetamine-treated and psychotic populations. Ph.D. thesis, University of London.

Peters, E., Pickering, A. D., & Hemsley, D. R. (1994). 'Cognitive inhibition' and positive symptomatology in schizotypy. *British Journal of Clinical Psychology, 33,* 33–48.

Raine, A. (1991). The Schizotypal Personality Questionnaire (SPQ): A scale for the assessment of schizotypal personality based on DSM-IIIR criteria. *Schizophrenia Bulletin, 17,* 555–564.

Raine, A., & Allbutt, J. (1989). Factors of schizoid personality. *British Journal of Clinical Psychology, 28,* 31–40.

Raine, A., & Manders, D. (1988). Schizoid personality, interhemispheric transfer, and left hemisphere overactivation. *British Journal of Clinical Psychology, 27,* 333–347.

Raulin, M. L. (1984). Development of a scale to measure intense ambivalence. *Journal of Consulting and Clinical Psychology, 52,* 63–72.

Raulin, M. L., & Wee, J. L. (1984). The development and initial validation of a scale of social fear. *Journal of Clinical Psychology, 40,* 780–784.

Rust, J. (1987). The Rust Inventory of Schizoid Cognitions (RISC): A psychometric measure of psychoticism in the normal population. *British Journal of Clinical Psychology, 26,* 151–152.

Rust, J. (1988). The Rust Inventory of Schizotypal Cognitions (RISC). *Schizophrenia Bulletin. 14,* 317–322.

Schizophrenia Bulletin. (1990). Issue theme: Gender and schizophrenia. *16,* 179–344.

Siever, L. J. (1985). Biological markers in schizotypal personality disorder. *Schizophrenia Bulletin, 11,* 564–575.

Tannock, R., Schachar, R. J., Carr, R. P., Chajczyk, D., & Logan, G. D. (1989). Effects of methylphenidate on inhibitory control in hyperactive children. *Journal of Abnormal Child Psychology, 17,* 473–491.

Tipper, S. P. (1985). The negative priming effect: Inhibitory priming by ignored objects. *Quarterly Journal of Experimental Psychology, 37A,* 571–590.

Venables, P. H., Wilkins, S., Mitchell, D. A., Raine, A., & Bailes, K. (1990). A scale for the measurement of schizotypy. *Personality and Individual Differences, 11,* 481–495.

Weiner, J., & Feldon, J. L. (1987). Facilitation of latent inhibition by haloperidol in rats. *Psychopharmacology, 91,* 248–253.

Weiner, I., Lubow, R. E., & Feldon, J. (1984). Abolition of the expression but not the acquisition of latent inhibition by chronic amphetamine in rats. *Psychopharmacology, 83,* 194–199.

Williams, L. M. (in press). Further evidence for a multidimensional personality disposition to schizophrenia in terms of cognitive inhibition. *British Journal of Clinical Psychology.*

PART V

Psychophysiology and psychopharmacology

10

Schizotypal personality and skin conductance orienting

ADRIAN RAINE, TODD LENCZ, and DEANA S. BENISHAY

Psychophysiological approaches to schizotypal personality are of potentially great value because psychophysiology lies at the interface between clinical science, cognitive science, and neuroscience (Dawson, 1990). Within the field of the psychophysiology of schizophrenia, one of the most widely used measures that has also produced one of the most replicated findings is the skin conductance orienting response (SCOR). As such, this chapter focuses on the growing literature on the application of SCOR to schizotypal personality and attempts to place the findings of this field into a wider neuroscience context.

The nature of SC orienting as a sensitive measure of information processing will first be outlined together with a very brief summary of key findings on SC orienting in schizophrenic patients and subjects at risk for schizophrenia. Findings from 10 previous studies of SC orienting and schizotypal personality will then be reviewed together with an initial interpretation of these findings. Three new analyses from two other studies will then be described. Interpretation of these studies will focus on the notion of increased variability of attentional processes and disinhibition in schizotypals, and the notion that prefrontal dysfunction may underlie these and other cognitive and psychophysiological deficits. Main conclusions and directions for future research will be outlined. The central idea to be put forward in this chapter is that prefrontal dysfunction represents the common mechanism that underlies not only orienting deficits but also disinhibition, eye tracking abnormalities, and working memory deficits.

Skin conductance orienting as a measure of attention

A detailed review of the electrodermal response system and SC orienting may be found in Dawson, Schell, and Filion (1990) and Roy, Boucsein, Fowles, and Gruzelier (1993). Presentation of a new (e.g., 75-dB nonsignal tone) or significant stimulus (e.g., loud tone) in most cases results in an orienting response that can be assessed by measuring changes in the electrical activity of the skin. The SCOR has been viewed by many as a sensitive measure of information processing, reflecting the extent to which the subject pays attention to and cognitively processes the orienting stimulus (Dawson & Nuechterlein, 1984; Dawsin, Filion, & Schell, 1989). Various features of the orienting response (including number of responses, amplitude, and recovery time) also have significant heritability (Venables, 1993). This demonstration of heritability is of significance in the context of SC orienting deficits as a possible genetic marker for schizophrenia.

According to one influential information processing model of SC orienting developed by Ohman (1979, 1985), orienting occurs when automatic preattentive processes make a "call" for additional controlled processing. In this model, orienting reflects a change from automatic to controlled processing as a result of initial preattentive processing of the novelty and significance of the stimulus. The call for controlled processing can be made in one of two situations. In the first, preattentive mechanisms fail to recognize the presented stimulus because it does not match with a neural model of the stimulus that has been built up in short-term memory after a prior presentation of that stimulus. Habituation, on the other hand, occurs when there is no mismatch between this neural model and the actual stimulus presented. In the second situation calling for controlled processing, the preattentive mechanisms recognize that the stimulus is significant. As such, SC orienting constitutes a fairly accurate and easily measured autonomic measure that provides a relatively sensitive measure of the allocation of attentional resources within the stimulus field.

Previous findings on SC orienting in schizophrenics

Detailed reviews of this literature may be found in Bernstein et al. (1982), Ohman (1981), and Dawson and Nuechterlein (1984). Two main findings have emerged from this extensive empirical literature. First, a sizable proportion (about 40–50%) of schizophrenics fail to give any SCORs, a much larger percentage than found in normal groups. Second, a significant minority of schizophrenics tend to be hyperresponsive and show a relative failure to habituate. These orienting abnormalities do not appear to be a secondary effect of symptomatology or medication, and reduced SC orienting in particular has been very well replicated across laboratories and patient groups.

Reviews have suggested that there may be relations between type of SC orienting abnormality and symptom type in schizophrenics, with hyporesponsivity associated with more negative symptoms and hyperresponsivity associated with more positive symptoms (Dawson et al., 1989; Zahn, 1986). Gruzelier and Manchanda (1981) have also found that asymmetries in SC orienting are related to syndromes of schizophrenia, with higher left- than right-hand responses being associated with a more active syndrome and the reverse pattern being associated with a more withdrawn or negative syndrome.

Abnormal orienting patterns have also been found in studies of the children of schizophrenics. Reviews of the literature on this high-risk population indicate that while findings are weaker for children of schizophrenics than for schizophrenic patients, there is still a tendency for the former to show greater SC responses to significant (aversive) stimuli (Dawson et al., 1989; Venables, 1993); unlike schizophrenic patients, however, they show no differences with respect to neutral orienting stimuli.

Key questions

A number of key questions can be identified which will guide our review of SC orienting in schizotypals.

1. Most fundamentally, are there orienting abnormalities in schizotypals that parallel those found in either schizophrenics or the high-risk children of schizophrenics?
2. Are response abnormalities found for orienting stimuli, significant stimuli, or both types of stimuli? Schizophrenic patients show SC differences only to neutral stimuli and not significant stimuli (Bernstein et al., 1982), whereas the reverse tends to be true for children at risk for schizophrenia.
3. Is the form of SC orienting abnormality associated with syndromes or factors of schizotypal personality? On the basis of the schizophrenia literature, it is expected that hyporesponsivity may be associated with more negative schizotypal symptoms whereas hyperresponsivity will be associated with more positive schizotypal features.
4. Are there relations between SC orienting deficits and other neuropsychological and psychophysiological deficits in schizophrenia? Specifically, orienting abnormalities may be related to frontal deficits related to a lack of inhibition.
5. More speculatively, may some patterns of orienting deficits be related to other psychopathologies that may be present in schizotypals? For example, antisocials have been found to show reduced orienting (Raine, Venables, & Williams, 1990); is the reduced orienting in schizotypals a function of concomitant antisociality in some schizotypals?

SC orienting and schizotypal personality

There have been 10 studies that have assessed relationships between aspects of schizotypal personality and SC orienting activity. Almost all of these have assessed individual differences in schizotypal personality in normal populations; only one has assessed SC orienting in clinically diagnosed schizotypals. Furthermore, 8 of the 10 studies have employed undergraduate students as subjects. As such, much of what we know about SC orienting and schizotypal personality is based on selected, biased samples. These 10 studies will be briefly reviewed below. In summary, these studies provide some limited evidence for (1) nonresponding and hyporesponding in relation to "negative" schizotypal features, (2) nonresponding and hyporesponding in relation to more "positive" schizotypal features, (3) hyperresponding in relation to "positive" schizotypal features, and (4) erratic orienting in relation to schizotypy.

"Negative" schizotypal features and nonresponding/hyporesponding

Three studies support the notion that more negative schizotypal features such as anhedonia are related to either SC nonresponding or SC hyporesponsivity to orienting stimuli. Summaries of the key findings in these studies are shown in Table 10.1.

Simons (1981)

Simons (1981) found a Group × Trials interaction indicating that anhedonics had lower SC amplitudes on the first trial than the other two groups, though by trial 2 this group effect was lost. This was partly accounted for by the fact that the physical anhedonia group showed only a small drop-off in response amplitude from trial 1 to trial 2 in contrast to the more usual steep drop in the other two groups. We shall return to this issue later. Simons (1981) also found the Physical Anhedonia group to show a greater incidence of SC nonresponding and fast habituation. The Perceptual Aberration group did not differ from the normal controls.

Bernstein and Riedel (1987)

These authors exposed subjects to 30 "signal" stimuli in which they had to give a motor response to half of the tones (those with a higher frequency). A greater incidence of SC nonresponding was found in the Physical Anhedonia group. The fact that no group differences were observed in SC responding to

Table 10.1. *Key findings on "negative" schizotypal features and SC nonresponding/hyporesponding*

Authors	Population	No. subjects/ Schizotypal measure	Key findings
Simons (1981)	Undergraduates	18/Physical Anhedonia 26/Perceptual Aberration 22/Controls	Reduced trial 1 responding in physical anhedonics
Bernstein & Riedel (1987)	Undergraduates	16/Physical Anhedonia 18/Perceptual Aberration 17/Controls	Nonresponding in physical anhedonics
Raine (1987)	Criminals	36/Schizophrenism and Anhedonia–Psychoticism indices	High schizotypal scores related to reduced orienting in those from intact homes

the signal stimuli was interpreted as consistent with data from schizophrenics. Trials were averaged across blocks of 6 trials, thus preventing examination of the drop-off from trials 1 to 2 as discussed above for Simons (1981).

Raine (1987)

Raine used indices created from several self-report schizotypy scales. The first index, "Schizophrenism," included both cognitive–perceptual and interpersonal schizotypal features. The second index, "Anhedonia–Psychoticism," largely consisted of features of psychosis proneness not generally contained in DSM-III-R criteria of schizotypal personality. Digit Span and Arithmetic subscales of the Wechsler Adult Intelligence Scale – Revised (WAIS-R) were summated to form an index of "Attention–Distraction" or verbal working memory.

High scores on both schizotypy indices were associated with reduced SC orienting ($r = -.41, -.51$) and also poorer scores on working memory ($r = -.61, -.62$) in criminals from intact homes. These relationships were not observed in criminals from broken homes, and were specific to neutral orienting tones as opposed to more significant consonant–vowel and defensive stimuli. Partialing out the effect of working memory (but not arousal as measured by SC levels) effectively abolished the schizotypy-orienting relationship. Schizotypy was unrelated to verbal or performance IQ. These results suggest that (1) schizotypy in the context of antisocial behavior is linked to SC hyporesponsivity; (2) such effects are strongest where the "social push" toward schizotypy is minimized (intact homes); (3) the orienting–schizotypy link is almost entirely mediated by deficits in working memory.

Miller (1986)

While not reporting on orienting to neutral stimuli, Miller failed to observe effects for signal stimuli. Sixteen undergraduates with high scores (two SDs above mean) on the Physical Anhedonia Scale and 16 subjects with high scores on the Perceptual Aberration Scale did not differ from 16 controls in responses to signal stimuli. It was reported, however, that group effects did not approach significance. These findings appear consistent with most studies failing to find effects for significant tone stimuli (e.g., Bernstein & Riedel, 1987).

Positive schizotypal features and nonresponding/hyporesponsivity

Four studies provide some evidence for the notion that more positive schizotypal traits such as perceptual aberration may also be related to nonresponding and hyporesponsivity. Key findings are shown in Table 10.2.

Simons, Losito, Rose, and MacMillan (1983)

Simons and colleagues took a different approach to assessing schizotypal personality–SC orienting links by first identifying a group of 24 male and 24 female subjects who were SC nonresponders as well as 24 controls, and then assessing them on several schizotypal and psychosis-proneness scales. Groups did not differ on any of three scales (Physical Anhedonia, Perceptual Aberration, Schizoidia), and no trends toward significance were observed. In a second analysis, a group of stable nonresponders (defined as subjects showing SC nonresponding on two test sessions two weeks apart; $N = 12$) were compared to unstable responders (SC nonresponders on session 1 but showing some SC responding on session 2; $N = 12$) on the psychosis-proneness scales. Stable nonresponders were now found to have higher scores on Perceptual Aberration and Schizoidia, but scores on Physical Anhedonia were nonsignificantly *lower* than those of unstable responders.

Venables (1993)

Venables reported data collected from the Mauritius longitudinal study in which SC orienting at age 3 was related to self-report schizotypal personal-

Table 10.2. *Key findings on "positive" schizotypal features and nonresponding/hyporesponding*

Authors	Population	No. subjects/ Schizotypal categories or measure	Key findings
Simons (1983)	Undergraduates	12/Stable nonresponders 12/Unstable responders	High Perceptual Aberration and Schizoidia scores in stable nonresponders
Raine (1987)	Criminals	36/Schizophrenism and Anhedonia–Psychoticism indices	High schizotypal scores related to reduced orienting in those from intact homes
Lencz et al. (1991)	Normal adults	18/STA	High STA scores in subjects showing both reduced orienting and reduced frontal lobe area
Venables (1993)	3-year-olds	1,795/Nonresponders, hyperresponders, median responders	Higher Schizophrenism scores in both nonresponders and hyperresponders defined by defensive stimuli

ity scores measured at age 16–17 years. In common with Simons et al. (1983), groups were defined on the basis of SC nonresponding, SC hyperresponding, and median responders (within 0.5 SD of the group mean). Unlike Simons et al. (1983), however, groups were defined separately using (1) orienting stimuli and (2) defensive stimuli. When these groups were defined on the basis of defensive responses, both nonresponders and hyperresponders were found to have significantly higher scores on Schizophrenism relative to controls (median responders). No significant effects were observed when group membership was based on orienting stimuli. Results on Anhedonia were less clear-cut, with the main result being that hyperresponders on orienting stimuli had *lower* Anhedonia scores relative to the nonresponders and median responders. These more mixed findings for Anhedonia may be a function of the fact that Venables's Anhedonia Scale combines both physical and social anhedonia, whereas other studies have just focused on the former.

Lencz, Raine, Sheard, and Reynolds (1991)

In this study, subjects filled out the STA and underwent MRI testing which provided measures of prefrontal area and a ventricle-to-brain ratio (VBR) of the lateral ventricles. Orienting and MRI measures were also available on 15 schizophrenics and 15 affective disordered control patients. A cluster analysis of the MRI and SC orienting measures revealed three clusters made up of (1) those with reduced SC orienting and reduced frontal area, (2) reduced SC orienting and ventricular enlargement, and (3) normal orienting and normal prefrontal and ventricular area. A significant chi-square demonstrated that normal controls were associated with normal MRI and SC measures, affective patients were associated with reduced SC orienting and ventricular enlargement, whereas schizophrenics were associated with reduced SC orienting and reduced prefrontal area (and to some extent with reduced SC orienting and ventricular enlargement). Importantly, three of the normal controls fell into the pathological group of reduced SC orienting and reduced prefrontal area. While only a small group, they were found to have significantly higher scores on the STA relative to the other groups of normal subjects. Consequently, this study shows a joint association between more positive schizotypal features (as measured by the STA) and both reduced SC orienting and reduced prefrontal area, suggesting the possibility that prefrontal deficits may underlie both SC orienting deficits and positive schizotypal features.

Raine (1987)

As outlined in the section above on negative schizotypal features, this study also observed a significant association in criminals from intact homes between high Schizophrenism scores and reduced SC orienting. That this schizotypy index was made up of Perceptual Aberration and Schizophrenism may be viewed as relating to positive schizotypal features. Again, it should be noted that working memory deficits entirely accounted for the relationship between schizotypy and SC orienting.

"Positive" schizotypal features and hyperresponsivity

Three studies find some support for a linkage between the more positive schizotypal features and increased SC orienting activity. Key findings are shown in Table 10.3.

Table 10.3. *Key findings on "positive" schizotypal features and hyperresponsivity*

Authors	Population	No. subjects/ Schizotypal measure	Key findings
Nielsen & Petersen (1976)	Undergraduates	Schizophrenism Cognitive deficits	High scores on both scales related to higher SC amplitudes
Lipp & Vaitl (1993)	Undergraduates	24/High STA 24/Low STA	Reduced latent inhibition (greater responding) in high STA scores
Venables 1993	3-year-olds	1,795/Nonresponders, hyperresponders, and median responders	Higher Schizophrenism scores in both non-responders and hyper-responders defined by defensive stimuli

Nielsen and Petersen (1976)

Nielsen and Petersen (1976) recorded SC in 34 female college students aged 19–25 years who were administered a scale of "Schizophrenism." This 14-item scale was constructed by Nielsen and Petersen to reflect characteristics thought to be typical of early schizophrenics, and included 10 items tapping social anxiety, hypersensitivity to criticism, and shyness. Four additional items reflect distractibility and make up a Cognitive subscale. High SCOR amplitude (averaged over trials) correlated significantly with high scores on both Schizophrenism (r = .30) and Cognitive Distractibility subscales (r = .35). No relationships were found with scores on Neuroticism (r = .05), indicating specificity of findings for schizophrenism as opposed to generalized anxiety. Consistent with other studies, no relationships were observed for amplitudes to defensive (105-dB) stimuli.

Lipp and Vaitl (1992)

Lipp and Vaitl (1992) do not report individual orienting trial data, but instead report on the process of latent inhibition as measured by the first interval SC response (described in Claridge & Beech, Chapter 9, this volume). Subjects were divided above and below the median on the STA scale of Claridge and Broks (1984) which measures three features of schizotypal personality. Low-scoring subjects showed the expected latent inhibition effect as indicated by retardation of the first-interval conditioned response. High STA scorers, however, showed a reliably larger first-interval response to the CS+, indicating a lack of latent inhibition. Such effects were not observed when groups were divided above and below the median on the Psychoticism Scale (Eysenck & Eysenck, 1975) or the Hallucination Scale (Launay & Slade, 1981). Although data for the habituation series were not presented, Lipp and Vaitl (1992) state that there were no overall group differences on this initial preexposure paradigm. These results for STA subjects may be interpreted as indicating a lack of inhibitory processes in these subjects and a failure to learn that a stimulus is irrelevant.

Venables (1993)

As noted above in the section on negative schizotypal features, this study observed a relationship between hyperresponsivity at age 3 and high Schizophrenism scores at ages 16–17 years, when hyperresponsivity was defined on the basis of defensive stimuli, but not when defined in terms of orienting stimuli. However, a more recent analysis of these data (Venables, Chapter 6, this volume) indicated that this effect was due largely to the "disorganized/social impairment" subfactor of Schizophrenism rather than a more "positive" schizotypal subfactor. Again, no effects were observed for SC responses to orienting stimuli.

Erratic orienting and schizotypal personality

The final study does not provide evidence for either hyporesponsivity or hyperresponsivity in relation to schizotypal personality. Instead, it suggests that schizotypal personality is associated with inconsistent and erratic orienting activity (see Table 10.4).

Wilkins (1988)

Wilkins (1988) recorded SC orienting in groups of undergraduate subjects with high scores on Schizophrenism and Physical Anhedonia scales, as well as in a group of controls. Reorienting was assessed on the fourth of nine stimuli. A significant Group × Trials interaction for SC amplitudes to the first three stimuli indicated that whereas the Schizophrenism and control groups showed normal habituation to the orienting stimuli, the Physical Anhedonia group showed an *increase* in responding from trials 1 to 2, with relatively high values for trial 3 (see Figure 10.1). Interestingly, this interaction effect was also observed for trials 4 and 5. These effects were specific to orienting

Table 10.4. *Erratic responding and schizotypal personality*

Authors	Population	No. subjects/ Schizotypal measures or categories	Key findings
Wilkins (1988)	Undergraduates	12/Physical Anhedonia	Increased responding in trials
		16/Schizophrenism	1–2 in physical anhedonics
Raine et al. (1994a)	Undergraduates	15/Controls 13/Clinical schizotypals 22/Normals	Increased responding in trials 1–3 in schizotypals

stimuli and were not observed for more defensive stimuli. In addition to this effect for the Physical Anhedonia group, Wilkins (1988) commented that the Schizophrenism group also gave what was termed an "irregular pattern of responding across trials" which appeared to be almost random in nature as compared to controls. The pattern observed by Wilkins (1988) is unusual, but, as will be indicated in the next section, it is not an isolated finding.

Interpretation of SCOR findings in schizotypal personality

Interpretation of the above-mentioned 10 studies is made difficult by the fact that studies vary widely in terms of SC recording methodology (e.g., medial versus distal phalange), subjects (e.g., undergraduates versus criminals), intensities of orienting stimuli, paradigms used (e.g., orienting, defensive, latent inhibition), types of self-report schizotypal scales (STA, Schizophrenism, differing versions of Anhedonia), use of clinical versus self-report assessments, and timing of data collection (e.g., prospective versus concurrent).

Nevertheless, one clear finding is that schizotypal personality, as variously defined, has been associated with some form of SC orienting abnormality in each of these studies. Equally consistent, group differences are almost universally specific to orienting stimuli as opposed to more defensive stimuli, a finding consistent with the literature on schizophrenia. One exception to this general finding is the study of Venables (1993), though these findings were reported as preliminary and requiring further elaboration. We shall return to this issue below.

Set against this positive general finding, it must be remembered that the

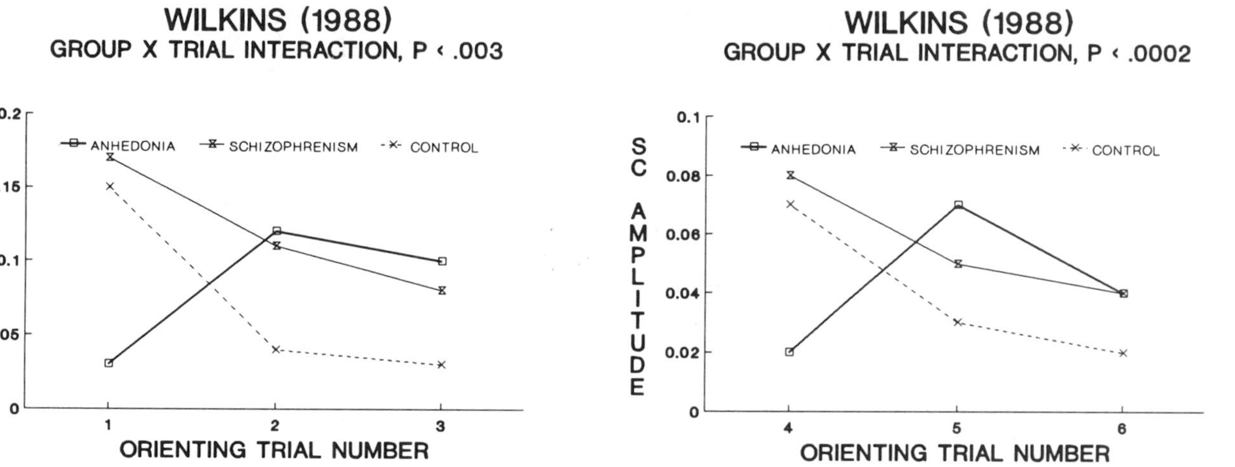

Fig. 10.1. SC orienting for schizophrenism, anhedonia, and control groups from Wilkins (1988).

form of this relationship is very variable, and, as indicated by the structure of the review, some evidence exists for all of the following: (1) negative schizotypy and hyporesponsivity, (2) positive schizotypy and hyporesponsivity, (3) positive schizotypy and hyperresponsivity, and (4) schizotypy and erratic responding. These findings, taken together, are clearly contradictory. Furthermore, many studies often measure both positive and negative schizotypy but find significant effects only for one of these measures. Effectively, therefore, studies grouped under one set of significant findings often fail to replicate findings in another group. For example, physical anhedonia is sometimes cited in the literature as being consistently related to reduced amplitude on the first trial and a greater frequency of nonresponding (Bernstein & Riedel, 1987; Simons, 1981), yet this review shows that there are several studies that do not obtain this effect (Simons et al., 1983; Venables, 1993; Wilkins, 1988).

One further potential difficulty in interpreting a link between physical anhedonia and reduced SC orienting is that such a link may merely reflect the fact that subjects scoring high on the Physical Anhedonia Scale show no interest in physical stimuli of the type used to elicit SC orienting responses. That is, physical anhedonics may not pay attention to tone stimuli (and therefore do not give SC responses) because such subjects are identified on the basis of lacking pleasure and interest in physical events. As such, nonresponding in physical anhedonics may indicate validity for the way physical anhedonia is measured, but may not reflect a factor of etiologic significance.

Another trend in the data argues against the notion that the SCOR–Physical Anhedonia data are artifactual. Wilkins found that although physical anhedonics do start off giving a lower SC response to the first orienting stimulus, they show an *increased* response to the second stimulus in contrast to other groups who show an expected decline and habituation. Such an increase cannot be explained by the notion that anhedonics merely show a lack of interest in external stimuli, but instead indicates some orienting abnormality. Some support for these findings is provided in a study by Raine, Benishay, Lencz, and Scerbo (1994) reported below.

The study of Wilkins (1988) is of interest in showing a different form of orienting deficit from that shown in other studies. Variability in SC responding has, however, been observed in the schizophrenia literature. For example, inspection of figure 2 in Gruzelier, Eves, Connolly, and Hirsch (1981) indicates that nonhabituating schizophrenics show large (more than double) increases in SC amplitudes from trials 4 to 5 to 6 in a standard orienting (75-dB) sequence, with this increase being especially exaggerated on the right hand. A similar effect was noted by Gruzelier et al. (1981) in a second series of conspicuous (90-dB) tones in which they pointed out that "perhaps the major difference between the patients and controls was the irregularity in responding across trials" (p. 201), with the nonhabituators giving particularly large responses midway through the paradigm. The irregular, random, and at times heightened pattern of SC orienting across all task conditions was interpreted as consistent with an attentional deficit that may result from a joint product of decremental inhibitory processes and incremental excitatory processes. As is outlined below, a similar interpretation may well apply to schizotypal personality.

New studies on the links between SC orienting abnormalities and schizotypal personality

Before we fully interpret the findings from the above studies, we present three new studies in order to complete the presentation of the empirical data in this review. One analysis provides confirmatory support for the findings of Wilkins (1988) indicating erratic orienting in schizotypals. A second analysis indicates that this form of orienting deficit may be specific to schizotypals with positive features. A third study suggests that an analogue of schizotypal personality in adolescence is related to SC hyporesponsivity and also to antisocial behavior. An overview of these studies is following by an interpretation of these data focusing on the finding of erratic orienting in schizotypals.

Erratic resource allocation in subjects with schizotypal personality disorder

Raine et al. (1994a) recorded SC orienting in 13 male and female undergraduates with a DSM-III-R diagnosis of schizotypal personality disorder (SPD) as assessed with the Structured Clinical Interview for DSM-III-R Personality Disorders (SCID-II), and a score above 42 on the Schizotypal Personality Questionnaire (SPQ; Raine, 1991). Controls scored in the bottom 10% of scores on the SPQ and did not receive a clinical diagnosis of SPD.

Results are shown in Figure 10.2. A significant Group × Trial interaction ($p < .05$) indicated that schizotypals showed an *increase* in SC amplitude from trial 1 to 2, and a further increase to 3, followed by normal habituation, whereas controls showed the expected decrease across trials and normal habituation. These results are similar to the earlier findings of Wilkins (1988) and indicate a disinhibitory failure in schizotypals and erratic attentional resource allocation. Furthermore, they extend the previous findings revealed earlier by showing that resource allocation abnormalities in relation to indi-

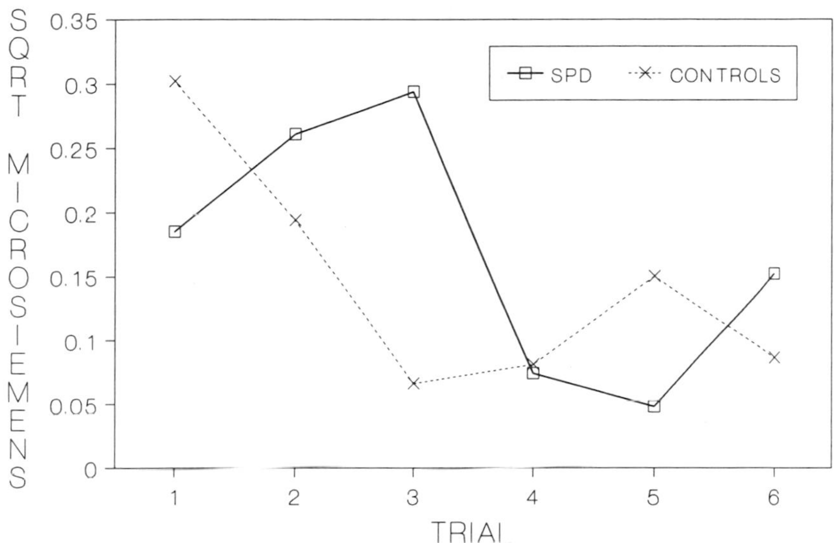

Fig. 10.2. SC orienting for diagnosed schizotypals compared to normal controls. (From Raine et al., 1994a.)

vidual differences in schizotypal personality also exist in clinically diagnosed schizotypals.

We attempted to replicate and extend the above finding of an orienting abnormality in schizotypals by taking a dimensional (as opposed to categorical) conceptualization of schizotypy using an individual difference design on a new sample of subjects. This design has the advantages of (1) assessing generalization of the previous findings from a categorical to a dimensional conceptualization of schizotypy, and (2) allowing an assessment of the links between abnormal orienting and three factors of schizotypal traits.

Subjects consisted of 30 volunteers (12 male, 18 female, mean age = 20.5 years) from a new sample of undergraduate students. All subjects were administered the SPQ, providing both a total score and subscores on three main factors of schizotypy. These subscores were derived from a confirmatory factor analysis of the nine SPQ subscales, which yielded factors labeled "Cognitive–Perceptual" (Unusual Perceptual Experiences, Magical Thinking, Ideas of Reference, and Paranoid Ideation subscales), "Interpersonal Deficits"

(Constricted Affect, No Close Friends, and Social Anxiety subscales), and "Disorganization" (Odd Speech and Odd Behavior) (see Raine, Reynolds, Lencz, Scerbo, Triphon, & Kim, 1994, for full details). All subjects received the same SC orienting paradigm as detailed above. Amplitude of the trial 1 response was subtracted from the amplitude of the trial 3 response to create an individual-difference score for each subject which would reflect the degree of abnormal orienting reported in the categorical analyses above.

Total SPQ scores were significantly correlated with the difference score (rho = .47, $p < .004$) in the expected direction of more abnormal orienting (i.e., less habituation from trial 1 to trial 3) in those with high SPQ scores. Using a Bonferroni-corrected alpha of 0.017, we observed significant correlations also for the Cognitive–Perceptual subscale (rho = .51, $p < .002$) and Interpersonal Deficits subscale (rho = .48, $p < .004$), but not for Disorganized subscale (rho = .02, $p > .45$).

Syndromes of schizotypal personality and erratic resource allocation

The above findings indicate a possible failure of inhibitory mechanisms in a group of subjects with SPD. An important conceptual question in schizotypal personality research concerns whether deficits observed in schizotypals are specific to subgroups of schizotypals delineated on the basis of syndrome type. The replication study suggests that this deficit is common for both Cognitive–Perceptual and Interpersonal Deficits. However, if erratic SC orienting reflects an attentional deficit linked to some fundamental lack of inhibitory process, it could be hypothesized that this SC orienting abnormality may be specific to a subgroup of schizotypals who fall into the more "positive" or "cognitive–perceptual deficit" syndrome characterized by faulty perceptual and cognitive processes (e.g., perceptual aberration, magical thinking). Such linkage of "faulty filtering" to cognitive and perceptual schizophrenic deficits represents a classical notion in schizophrenia research (e.g., Venables, 1964). Conversely, such linkage may be less likely to account for more behavioral/interpersonal or "negative" features such as no close friends and inappropriate/blunted affect.

To test this hypothesis, we cluster-analyzed the 13 diagnosed schizotypals, using scores on the nine schizotypal traits drawn from the SCID-II schedule (rated on a 1–3 scale) employed to derive the DSM-III-R diagnosis using a small-sample clustering procedure. Fusion coefficients indicated a two-cluster solution. ANOVAs conducted on the two groups for the nine SPQ subscales indicated that the larger cluster 2 ($N = 9$) was defined in terms of significantly higher scores on Ideas of Reference, Unusual Perceptual Experiences, and Magical Thinking scales – features that make up three of the more positive or cognitive–perceptual features of SPD. The smaller cluster 1 ($N = 4$) was defined in terms of significantly higher scores on the Social Anxiety and No Close Friends scales – features that make up two of the three main negative/interpersonal features of SPD. Group comparisons on other SPQ subscales were nonsignificant.

Data for these two schizotypal subgroups (alongside the normal control group) are shown in Figure 10.3. A MANOVA conducted on SC amplitudes to the six orienting stimuli revealed a significant Group × Trial interaction ($p < .03$). It can be seen from Figure 10.3 that whereas the Interpersonal Deficits cluster showed normal habituation to the tone series (i.e., habituation similar to that shown by the "normal" control group), the Cognitive–Perceptual group showed only a very small response to the first trial, followed by an increase in response to tone 2, and yet another increase on trial 3 which was virtually as large as the very first response given by the Interpersonal Deficit cluster. Following a decline on trial 4, the Cognitive–Perceptual group showed a further increase in responding across trials 5 and 6. As with the total group analysis described earlier, no group differences or interactions were observed for the more attention-grabbing, defensive stimuli making up trials 7–10, indicating that the effect was specific to orienting stimuli.

We have previously reported that the total group of 14 SPDs have significantly poorer smooth-pursuit eye tracking than normal controls (Lencz, Raine, Surbo, Holt, Redman, & Brodish, 1993). Poor eye tracking has been associated with a loss of inhibitory functions and consequent increased saccadic intrusions that disrupt smooth-pursuit tracking. If the SC-orienting abnormality represents one aspect of a more general lack of inhibitory functions, it would be predicted that the Cognitive–Perceptual group who show the SC attentional deficit putatively associated with a lack of inhibition should be particularly characterized by eye tracking deficits. This prediction was confirmed, with the Cognitive–Perceptual schizotypals showing significantly poorer eye tracking than the Interpersonal Deficit schizotypals ($p < .05$).

These findings must be treated as preliminary and viewed with caution since the sample sizes are small. Nevertheless, several significant findings emerged which warrant further investigation and which give rise to the following tentative conclusions:

1. At least two subclusters of SPDs can be identified, those with cognitive–perceptual features and those with interpersonal deficits. A three-cluster

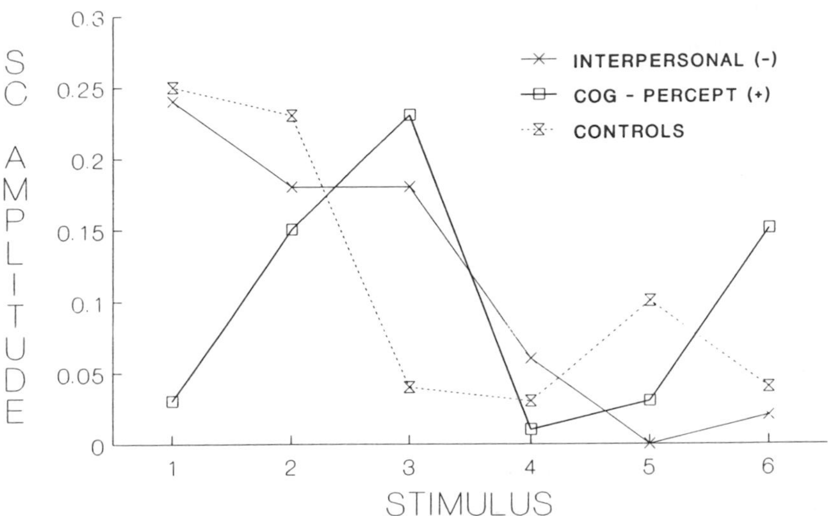

Fig. 10.3. SC orienting for two subclusters of diagnosed schizotypals and normal controls. (From Raine et al., 1994a.)

solution that had been suggested by our recent work (Raine et al., 1994b) was not confirmed with this small sample, though it is possible that a larger sample would reveal the presence of a third, "disorganized" subgroup of schizotypals.

2. Erratic attention as shown in the total group of clinical SPDs is confined to those schizotypals who cluster together on schizotypal symptomatology to form a cognitive–perceptual deficit subgroup.
3. This same group also has eye tracking deficits.
4. Taken together, these data may be taken as indicating an attentional deficit related to a lack of inhibitory processes, and suggest that such inhibitory deficits may be an important pathophysiological processes in understanding positive-symptom SPD.
5. One inconsistency with previous findings is that Wilkins (1988) observed erratic orienting to relate to anhedonia but not schizophrenism, whereas the reverse association would be expected on the basis of the results described above. A second inconsistency is that the individual-difference replication study found abnormal orienting to correlate with both cognitive–perceptual and interpersonal features of schizotypy.

Adolescent analogues to schizotypal personality

There has been very little or no research on analogue forms of schizotypal personality in adolescents and its relationship to skin conductance orienting or to other psychophysiological measures. An analysis of previously collected data was conducted in order to assess (1) whether personality analogues of schizotypal features in adolescence can be observed in a nonclinical population, (2) whether such individuals also demonstrate abnormalities in orienting and resource allocation, and (3) whether any such hyporesponsive schizotypal-like adolescents are also characterized by antisocial behavior. This last hypothesis was stimulated by the one previous study of orienting, schizotypal personality, and antisocial behavior, which showed that criminals who also have high schizotypal scores are hyporesponsive (Raine, 1987).

This analysis took advantage of a sample consisting of 101 normal 15-year-old male schoolboys (see Raine, Venables, & Williams, 1990, for more details of subject characteristics and selection). Psychophysiological testing was conducted at age 15 in which SC orienting was measured to a series of 65-dB stimuli. Subjects completed the EPQ (Eysenck & Eysenck, 1975) and other personality measures of antisocial behavior (see Raine & Venables, 1982, for further details), while teachers provided ratings of their antisocial behavior using the Unsocialized–Psychopathic subscale of the Behavior Problem Checklist (Quay & Parsons, 1970).

The three Eysenck Personality Questionnaire (EPQ) scales of Psychoticism, Neuroticism, and Extraversion provide the basis for delineating a possible analogue of schizotypal personality in this normal population. It was hypothesized that the combination of a high Psychoticism score, high neuroticism score, and low Extraversion score would delineate an analogue of schizotypal personality at this age (Eysenck & Eysenck, 1975; Gruzelier, Burgess, Stygall, Irving, & Raine, 1994; Venables, Chapter 6, this volume).

Cluster analysis was conducted on the Extraversion, Psychoticism, and Neuroticism scales. A four-group cluster revealed the presence of a small subgroup of subjects who were characterized by very high Psychoticism scores, high Neuroticism scores, and Extraversion scores that, although not particularly low, were below the mean for the group and in the direction of Introversion. Interestingly, this group made up 6% of the sample, a prevalence rate very similar to that observed for SPD in previous studies.

We then conducted ANOVAs on the four groups, using SC orienting measures as independent variables. Cluster 4 (the putatively schizotypal-like group) had significantly smaller amplitudes on the first orienting response than all three other groups ($p < .05$). No significant group differences were found, however, for frequency of SCORs, nor was there any evidence for irregular SC responding across trials. This schizotypal-like cluster also had significantly higher self-report ($p < .05$) and teacher ratings ($p < .05$) of antisocial behavior. They did not show differences in autonomic arousal, but did show approximately twice as much EEG power in the beta 2 frequency band than each of the other three groups ($p < .05$, two-tailed).

Results of this study suggest several things:

1. A small cluster with a schizotypal-like personality profile of high Psychoticism, high Neuroticism, and lower Extraversion (scores) can be identified with a similar prevalence rate (6%) as exists for schizotypal personality in adult populations.
2. This subgroup shows an SC orienting abnormality in the direction of reduced orienting, indicating reduced allocation of attentional resources to external events.
3. The failure to show the pattern of irregular SC responding shown in some other studies may be due to the fact that this cluster also has extreme antisocial behavior.
4. These findings cannot be explained by the higher rates of antisocial behavior per se within the schizotypal-like group. Antisocials have been found to have lower heart rate, skin conductance, and EEG, whereas the schizotypal-like cluster showed no difference in autonomic arousal and showed *higher,* not lower, EEG arousal.
5. The increased beta-2 resting EEG activity in the schizotypal-like subgroup is consistent with previous work showing increased beta power in children at risk for schizophrenia (e.g., Itil, Hsu, Saletu, & Mednick, 1974) and the recent finding that children at risk for schizophrenia who go on to develop schizophrenia as adults also show significantly higher beta-2 EEG activity (Gore & Mednick, under review). This provides further supporting evidence for the notion that a schizotypal-like group can be observed in a "normal" male population.

Interpretation of inconsistent responding across trials in schizotypals

Perhaps the more provocative of the new analyses reported above is the finding of inconsistent orienting in diagnosed schizotypals, particularly those characterized by more cognitive–perceptual deficits. There are several different but related ways in which this finding may be interpreted.

Increased variability in allocation of attentional resources

Inconsistent orienting may be viewed as reflecting variability in the allocation of attentional resources to external events across time. Rather than showing a failure to allocate attentional resources at all (nonresponding) or failing to gate out irrelevant stimuli (hyperresponding), schizotypals with inconsistent orienting show several fluctuations in attentional processing across time, ranging from very proficient attentional processing to very poor processing. This may represent an attentional deficit that is less severe than that shown in schizophrenics (hyperresponding or nonresponding), but is nevertheless disruptive. Paying too much attention to environmental stimuli that should normally be ignored may in part underlie schizotypal symptoms such as ideas of references and magical thinking, while variability in the allocation of attentional resources may give rise to perceptual distortions of auditory and visual stimuli, thus in part accounting for the unusual perceptual experiences of schizotypals. In this context, it is perhaps not surprising that the subcluster of schizotypals that are specifically characterized by this orienting deficit are those with ideas of reference, unusual perceptual experiences, and magical thinking.

Template mismatching

Erratic orienting shown by schizotypals may in part reflect template mismatching and a deficit in the type of comparator process that is thought to underlie orienting (Siddle, 1991). Normal habituation occurs when a new stimulus (actual stimulation) matches the "neuronal model" or template that has been built up by prior stimulation. The increment in responding shown by schizotypals on trial 2 relative to trial 1 may result from faulty perceptual processing of the second stimulus as significantly different from the first, resulting in a mismatch and a call for attentional resources.

Frontal systems, working memory, eye tracking, and SC orienting

The orienting abnormalities shown in schizotypals may reflect a deficit in working memory and a disruption to frontal brain systems involved in orienting, working memory, and eye tracking. This deduction may be drawn from a number of potentially interrelated findings. At one level, reduced SC orienting to neutral (but not significant) tones has been shown to correlate relatively highly ($r = .59$, $r = .70$) with reduced verbal working memory as indexed by the Arithmetic and Digit Span subscales of the WAIS (Raine, 1987); frontal systems are thought in part to underlie working memory processes. Reduced SC orienting also shows substantial correlations with reduced area of prefrontal cortex as measured by magnetic resonance imaging (MRI) in normal humans (Raine, Reynolds, & Sheard, 1991) and also with reduced glucose metabolism in frontal cortex in schizophrenics (Hazlett, Dawson, Buchsbaum, & Nuechterlein, 1993). As such, reduced SC orienting, reduced working memory, and prefrontal structure/function may represent interrelated deficits.

At a second level, Park, Holzman, and Levy (1991) have shown that schizophrenics have working memory deficits and, furthermore, that schizophrenics with bad eye tracking perform more poorly on delayed response tasks that rely on working memory and that may index prefrontal pathology (see Holzman et al., Chapter 15, this volume). The study reported above similarly finds that schizotypals with predominantly positive symptoms show both poor eye tracking and SC orienting deficits that may reflect deficits in the working memory process of template matching. This is consistent with the notion that deficits to prefrontal regions may underlie both SC orienting abnormalities and eye tracking deficits in this subgroup.

One piece of evidence against the notion that erratic orienting in positive-symptom schizotypals reflects a working memory, frontally related deficit is that the undergraduate schizotypals were not characterized by cognitive deficits (see Lencz, Raine, Benishay, Mills, & Bird, Chapter 13, this volume). It is possible, however, that because undergraduates are selected for proficient cognitive ability (but not for proficient psychophysiological characteristics), the nature of the sample is biased against finding effects on cognitive measures. Future studies assessing SC orienting, working memory, and frontal functioning in nonselected SPD subjects are needed to test this prefrontal hypothesis of SPD more clearly.

That frontal deficits may be specific to more positive schizotypal symptoms is suggested by the fact that structural prefrontal deficits have been related to positive-symptom scales like the STA, but not to anhedonia (Raine, Sheard, Reynolds, & Lencz, 1993). Furthermore, inspection of table 1 of Lencz et al. (Chapter 13, this volume) indicates that it is the more positive rather than negative features of schizotypy that relate more clearly to neuropsychological measures of frontolimbic functioning.

Inhibitory deficits

A more general approach to the wider body of findings on SC orienting is to suggest that schizotypal personality is associated with a lack of inhibitory processes, and at times heightened SC orienting. This interpretation is suggested by findings that link an increase in SC orienting to schizotypal personality. Studies that at least in part support this view include Nielsen and Petersen (1976), Wilkins (1988), Lipp and Vaitl (1992), Raine et al. (1993), and Venables (1993).

The lack of latent inhibition observed by Lipp and Vaitl (1992) in high STA scorers is also consistent with a lack of inhibitory processes in schizotypals, suggesting that schizotypals overrespond to stimuli that should normally be interpreted as having no signal value. Such lack of latent inhibition as indicated by SC is also consistent with studies showing a lack of negative priming in high STA subjects (see Claridge & Beech, Chapter 9, this volume), indicating a reduction in the operation of active inhibitory processes in schizotypals.

Two important associated issues are whether this inhibitory deficit is relatively specific to positive-symptom schizotypy, and whether such deficits are closely related to the prefrontal deficit outlined above. A review by Levin, Yergulun-Todd, and Craft (1989) of neuropsychological deficits in schizophrenia concluded that positive-symptom schizophrenics tend to be characterized by more intrusions on attentional tasks, and the linkage of a lack of inhibition to positive-symptom schizophrenia would be consistent with the view here that erratic orienting is specific to positive-symptom schizotypal personality. However, Wilkins's (1988) findings of a link between erratic orienting and anhedonia makes clear conclusions on this issue unwarranted at the present time.

An important inconsistency that needs to be addressed concerns the fact that some studies find evidence for hyporesponsivity and consequently an *excess* of inhibitory processes. How can such conflicting data be reconciled with the view of an inhibitory deficit? The new study reported above by Raine et al. (1994a) offers some clues. Out of 13 diagnosed schizotypals, 6 were found to show some form of abnormal increment in orienting across trials 1 to 2 to 3. Of the remaining 7, one subject was found to show a normal profile of habituation, while the other 6 were all SC nonresponders. Consequently, almost half of the subjects in this sample were nonresponders, and because those who showed inconsistent orienting were characterized by cognitive–perceptual deficits, it seems likely that the nonresponders were more negative-symptom schizotypals.

It seems therefore that there may be subgroups of schizotypals, some of whom are characterized by a lack of inhibitory processes as indicated by erratic orienting, and others who are characterized by excessive inhibition and SC nonresponding. A key deficit in schizotypal personality may therefore be a disruption to the balance between excitatory and inhibitory processes, with the direction of this imbalance giving rise to either positive- or negative-symptom schizotypy. Furthermore, it is quite possible that there are elements of both dysfunctions in the same group of schizotypals. For example, the cognitive–perceptual schizotypal group in Figure 10.3 who show increments in SC orienting across early trials start off at a lower orienting level on trial 1 relative to other groups and, consequently, may in relative terms show an initial lack of attention allocation. Again, this specific study is more suggestive of variability in excitatory and inhibitory processes rather than one extreme or another.

Attentional proficiency

Although these interpretations focus on erratic orienting as a deficit, it is important to bear in mind that at times, schizotypals may show better stimulus processing than controls. This better stimulus processing may give some clues as to the superior performance and creativity sometimes shown in such individuals (Claridge & Beech, Chapter 9, this volume).

Hyporesponding in antisocial schizotypals?

The finding that adolescents who score low on Extraversion, high on Psychoticism, and high on Neuroticism are both SC hyporesponders and antisocial is consistent with one previous study of antisocial populations (Raine, 1987) and suggests the possibility that hyporesponding is a particular characteristic of schizotypals who are also antisocial. Similarly, Blackburn (1979) found that secondary psychopaths with schizotypal personality profiles showed reduced SC orienting. The four diagnosed schizotypals referred to above, all of whom were SC nonresponders, were found to have a prominent family history of antisocial and criminal behavior, although such behavior was not formally assessed in the subjects themselves to confirm this link.

The linkage of schizotypal personality with antisocial behavior has been made since Heston's (1966) innovative study showing that the offspring of schizophrenics tended to be criminal as well as schizophrenic. More recently, adoption studies have suggested that the link between schizophrenia and crime is not due to assortative mating but is instead mediated by a common genetic link (Silverton, 1988), and it has been argued that frontal dysfunction may represent one common link between crime and schizophrenia-spectrum disorders (Raine & Venables, 1992). Meehl (1989) has suggested that either the majority or a large minority of psychopaths are schizotaxic. High rates of

SPD have been found in juvenile delinquents (e.g., McManus, Alessi, Grapentine, & Brickman, 1984), and a surprising proportion of patients with SPD (19.2%) have been reported to be also comorbid for antisocial personality disorder (Siever et al., 1990).

If it is true that there is a nonartifactual link between schizotypal personality and antisocial behavior, then concurrent assessment of factors such as antisocial personality may well be required in order to obtain a clearer understanding of SPD. It may well be the case that schizotypals with conjoint antisocial or psychopathic tendencies may show a psychophysiological profile very different from that of schizotypals without such antisociality. Findings to date support this notion, in that when schizotypal personality coexists with antisocial behavior, the orienting abnormality consists of reduced resource allocation (SC hyporesponsivity) as opposed to either irregular or excessive resource allocation (SC hyperresponsivity).

Implications and directives for future research

A number of directives for future research are envisaged as follows:

1. Neuropsychological and psychophysiological studies might usefully look further than overall group means in data analysis of schizotypal personality. Variability like erratic SC orienting may be missed in many data analyses that plot habituation curves across subjects and consequently "smooth" out these variations. Alternatively, such variability in responding may be interpreted by researchers as noise and, as such, ignored.
2. Linear extrapolation from research findings in schizophrenia may be erroneous. Erratic orienting is an unexpected finding in schizotypal personality in that it has not been a prominent finding in the schizophrenia literature. It may nevertheless be consistent with the evolution in the disease process from schizotypal personality to clinical manifestations of schizophrenia, which could result in an evolution in the manifestation of the vulnerability factor for schizophrenia (e.g., changing from erratic orienting in positive schizotypals to hyperresponding in positive schizophrenics). For instance, the implication is that researchers in the field of schizotypal personality may be advised not to discard automatically any unusual or unpredicted findings.
3. More studies are needed on clinically diagnosed schizotypals to ascertain whether the findings that are emerging on individual differences in the normal population are also found in clinical populations, or alternatively whether a different pattern of deficits hold for more severe manifestations

of schizotypal personality. No studies to date on SC orienting have been conducted on diagnosed schizotypals drawn from the community. Future studies need to focus on less selected, nonundergraduate populations.

4. Longitudinal studies are needed to help clarify cause–effect relationships and determine the relationship of orienting deficits to breakdown. Do orienting deficits precede the onset of positive schizotypal symptoms? Are those schizotypals who become schizophrenic the ones who are characterized by orienting abnormalities such as erratic responding or nonresponding?
5. More control groups need to be included in order to assess the specificity of orienting deficits to schizotypal personality. Are such deficits also observed in subjects with depression or antisocial personality? For example, nonresponding may also be found in depression, but erratic orienting may be specific to schizotypal personality.
6. Clinical artifacts and possible mediators need to be more thoroughly explored. Are orienting deficits in schizotypals a function of concomitant alcohol abuse? Are they specific to schizotypals with a family history of schizophrenia-spectrum disorders? Are orienting deficits relatively specific to schizotypals who are also antisocial?
7. A more formal analysis of the relationship between schizotypal syndromes and orienting is required in order to assess whether erratic orienting and hyperresponding is related to positive schizotypal features, with hyporesponding and nonresponding related to more negative features. What relationship exists between orienting deficits and the disorganized aspect of schizotypal personality?
8. Bilateral recording of SC orienting would be valuable in order to assess links between lateral asymmetries and schizotypal symptomatology. Gruzelier and Manchanda (1981) have argued that greater left- than right-hand responses characterized the more active syndrome of schizophrenia, with the reverse pattern characterizing the more withdrawn syndrome. Can this pattern of activity be extended to schizotypal symptomatology?
9. None of the studies reviewed above have analyzed for sex differences owing to the relatively small sample sizes involved. Given symptom differences between male and female schizophrenics and schizotypals (Raine, 1992), it would be of value to pursue the hypothesis that male schizotypals (possibly characterized by more negative symptoms) are more likely to be hyporesponsive, whereas females may be more hyperresponsive.
10. SC orienting deficits need to be related to other putative psychophysiological risk factors in order to shed more light on the nature of the orient-

ing deficit. If erratic SC orienting reflects a relative lack of inhibitory processes, do schizotypals with this deficit also show the startle eye-blink deficits that may also reflect a lack of protective inhibition (see Dawson, Schell, Hazlett, Filion, & Nuechterlein, Chapter 11, this volume).

11. Finally, one of the most important directives for future research lies in brain imaging studies. These are greatly required for two reasons: the first reason is that we need to understand more about the neural networks that play an *inhibitory* role with respect to SC orienting. To date we have some knowledge about excitatory centers from PET and MRI studies, but none regarding possible inhibitory centers. Such research is essential to gain a better understanding of a possible lack of such inhibition in schizotypals. The second reason is that such studies can help test hypotheses concerning the dysfunctional brain mechanisms that provide a common basis to interrelated cognitive and psychophysiological deficits, such as prefrontal dysfunction.

Almost inevitably this review has provided only a partial answer to the original questions raised, while raising a considerable number of other questions. Research along the lines above would nevertheless provide some answers to these questions, and in turn provide greater insights into a disorder that we are only now beginning to define, let alone understand.

Summary

This chapter reviews findings from 10 previous studies which have related SC orienting to individual differences in schizotypal personality in normals. While all studies find significant effects, findings are very diverse, and all of the following receive some support: (1) negative schizotypy and hyporesponding, (2) positive schizotypy and hyporesponding, (3) positive schizotypy and hyperresponding, and (4) schizotypy and erratic responding. Three analyses from two new studies are presented. Clinically diagnosed schizotypals are characterized by erratic orienting (increased responding from the first to third orienting stimulus). Cluster analysis of these schizotypals reveals cognitive–perceptual and interpersonal-deficit subgroups. Erratic orienting was found to be specific to schizotypals with cognitive–perceptual symptoms, and this same subgroup also showed eye tracking abnormalities. A cluster analysis of the EPQ in 15-year-old normal males revealed a small cluster characterized by low Extraversion, high Psychoticism, and high Neuroticism scores with a similar base rate to SPD (6%). This possible adolescent analogue to schizotypal personality was characterized by SC hyporesponsivity, antisocial behavior, and excessive EEG beta activity that has been previously observed in children of schizophrenics. It is hypothesized that (1) positive-symptom schizotypals may be characterized by SC orienting deficits (erratic orienting or hyperresponsivity) that reflect a lack of inhibition and working memory deficits underpinned by prefrontal dysfunction; and (2) hyporesponsivity may be specific to schizotypals who are also antisocial. Brain imaging and longitudinal studies of SC orienting in schizotypal personality are viewed as two of the most important directions for future research.

Acknowledgments

Research described in this chapter was supported by an NIMH Shared Instrumentation Grant and by BRSG S07 RR07012-21 awarded by the Biomedical Research Support Grant Program, Division of Research Resources, the National Institutes of Health.

The authors are grateful to Mike Dawson, Ted Zahn, Peter Venables, and John Gruzelier for the helpful comments provided.

References

Bernstein, A. S., Frith, C. D., Gruzelier, J. H., Patterson, T., Straube, E., Venables, P. H., & Zahn, T. P. (1982). An analysis of the skin conductance orienting response in samples of American, British, and German schizophrenics. *Biological Psychology, 14,* 155–211.

Bernstein, A. S., & Riedel, J. A. (1987). Psychophysiological response patterns in college students with high physical anhedonia: Scores appear to reflect schizotypy rather than depression. *Biological Psychiatry, 22,* 829–847.

Blackburn, R. (1979). Cortical and autonomic response arousal in primary and secondary psychopaths. *Psychophysiology, 16,* 143–150.

Claridge, G., & Broks, P. (1984). Schizotypy and hemisphere function I: Theoretical considerations and the measurement of schizotypy. *Personality and Individual Differences, 5,* 633–648.

Dawson, M. E. (1990). Psychophysiology at the interface of clinical science, cognitive science, and neuroscience: Presidential Address, 1989. *Psychophysiology, 27,* 243–255.

Dawson, M. E., Filion, D. L., & Schell, A. M. (1989). Its elicitation of the autonomic orienting response associated with allocation of processing resources? *Psychophysiology, 26,* 560–572.

Dawson, M. E., & Nuechterlein, K. H. (1984). Psychophysiological dysfunction in the developmental course of schizophrenic disorders. *Schizophrenia Bulletin, 10,* 204–232.

Dawson, M. E., Schell, A. M., & Filion, D. L. (1990). The electrodermal system. In J. T. Cacioppo & L. G. Tassinary (Eds.), *Principles of psychophysiology* (pp. 295–324). Cambridge: Cambridge University Press.

Eysenck, H. J., & Eysenck, S. G. B. (1975). *Manual of the Eysenck Personality Questionnaire.* London: Hodder & Stoughton.

Gore, L. R., & Mednick, S. A. (1994). *Computer-analyzed EEG findings predictive of schizophrenia.* Manuscript under review.

Gruzelier, J., Eves, F., Connolly, J., & Hirsch, S. (1981). Orienting, habituation, sensitization, and dishabituation in the electrodermal system of consecutive, drug free, admissions for schizophrenia. *Biological Psychology, 12,* 187–209.

Gruzelier, J. H., & Manchanda, R. (1981). The syndromes of schizophrenia: Relations between electrodermal response lateral asymmetries and clinical ratings. *Biological Psychology, 12,* 187–209.

Hazlett, E., Dawson, M., Buchsbaum, M. S., & Nuechterlein, K. (1993). Reduced regional brain glucose metabolism asessed by PET in electrodermal nonresponder schizophrenics: A pilot study. *Journal of Abnormal Psychology, 102,* 39–46.

Heston, L. L. (1966). Psychiatric disorders in foster-home reared children of schizophrenic mothers. *British Journal of Psychiatry, 112,* 819–825.

Itil, T. M., Hsu, W., Saletu, B., & Mednick, S. A. (1974). Computer EEG and auditory evoked potential investigations in children at high risk for schizophrenia. *American Journal of Psychiatry, 131,* 892–900.

Launay, G., & Slade, P. (1981). The measurement of hallucinatory predisposition in male and female prisoners. *Personality and Individual Differences, 2,* 221–234.

Lencz, T., Raine, A., Scerbo, A., Holt, L., Redmon, M., Brodish, S., & Bird, L. (1993). Impaired eye tracking in undergraduates with schizotypal personality disorder. *American Journal of Psychiatry, 150,* 152–154.

Lencz, T., Raine, A., Sheard, C., & Reynolds, G. (1991). Two neural bases of electrodermal hypo-responding in schizophrenia. *Psychophysiology, 28,* 37.

Levin, S., Yurgelun-Todd, D., & Craft, S. (1989). Contributions of clinical neuropsychology to the study of schizophrenia. *Journal of Abnormal Psychology, 98,* 341–356.

Lipp, O. V., & Vaitl, D. (1992). Latent inhibition in human Pavlovian conditioning: Effect of additional stimulation after preexposure and relation to schizotypal traits. *Personality and Individual Differences, 13,* 1003–1012.

McManus, M., Alessi, N. E., Grapentine, W. L., & Brickman, A. (1984). Psychiatric disturbance in serious delinquents. *Journal of the American Academy of Child Psychiatry, 23,* 602–615.

Meehl, P. E. (1989). Schizotaxia revisited. *Archives of General Psychiatry, 46,* 935–944.

Miller, G. A. (1986). Information processing deficits in anhedonia and perceptual aberration: A psychophysiological analysis. *Biological Psychiatry, 21,* 100–115.

Nielsen, T. C., & Petersen, K. E. (1976). Electrodermal correlates of extraversion, trait anxiety, and schizophrenism. *Scandinavian Journal of Psychology, 17,* 73–80.

Ohman, A. (1979). The orienting response, attention, and learning: An information processing perspective. In H. D. Kimmel, E. H. van Olst, & J. F. Orlebeke (Eds.), *The orienting reflex in humans* (pp. 443–471). Hillsdale, N.J.: Lawrence Erlbaum.

Ohman, A. (1981). Electrodermal activity and vulnerability in schizophrenia: A review. *Biological Psychology, 12,* 87–145.

Ohman, A. (1985). Face the beats and fear the face: Animal and social fears as prototypes for evolutionary analyses of emotion. *Psychophysiology, 23,* 123–145.

Park, S., Holzman, P. S., & Levy, D. L. (1991). Spatial working memory deficit in the relatives of schizophrenic patients is associated with their smooth pursuit eye tracking performance. *Schizophrenia Research, 9,* 185.

Quay, H. C., & Parsons, L. B. (1970). *The differential classification of the juvenile offender.* Washington, D.C.: Bureau of Prisons.

Raine, A. (1987). Effect of early environment on electrodermal and cognitive correlates of schizotypy and psychopathy in criminals. *International Journal of Psychophysiology, 4,* 277–287.

Raine, A. (1991). The Schizotypal Personality Questionnaire (SPQ): A scale for the assessment of schizotypal personality based on DSM-III-R criteria. *Schizophrenia Bulletin, 17,* 555–564.

Raine, A. (1992). Sex differences in schizotypal personality in a non-clinical population. *Journal of Abnormal Psychology, 101,* 361–364.

Raine, A., Benishay, D. S., Lencz, T., & Scerbo, A. (1994a). *Abnormal electrodermal orienting in schizotypal personality disorder.* Manuscript under review.

Raine, A., Reynolds, C., Lencz, T., Scerbo, A., Triphon, N., & Kim, D. (1994b). Cognitive/perceptual, interpersonal and disorganized features of schizotypal personality. *Schizophrenia Bulletin, 20,* 191–201.

Raine, A., Reynolds, G. P., & Sheard, C. (1991). Neuroanatomical correlates of skin conductance orienting in normal humans: A magnetic resonance imaging study. *Psychophysiology, 28,* 548–557.

Raine, A., Sheard, S., Reynolds, G. P., & Lencz, T. (1993). Evidence for pre-frontal structural and functional deficits associated with schizotypal personality: A magnetic resonance imaging study. *Schizophrenia Research, 7,* 237–247.

Raine, A., & Venables, P. H. (1982). Locus of control and socialization. *Journal of Research in Personality, 16,* 147–156.

Raine, A., & Venables, P. H. (1992). Antisocial behavior: Evolution, genetics, neuropsychology, and psychophysiology. In A. Gale & M. Eysenck (Eds.), *Handbook of Individual Differences: Biological Perspectives* (pp. 287–321). Chichester: Wiley.

Raine, A., Venables, P. H., & Williams, M. (1990). Orienting and criminality: A prospective study. *American Journal of Psychiatry, 147,* 933–937.

Roy, J. C., Boucsein, W., Fowles, D. C., & Gruzelier, J. (1993). *Progress in electrodermal research.* New York: Plenum.

Siddle, D. A. T. (1991). Orienting, habituation, and resource allocation: An associative analysis. Presidential Address, 1990. *Psychophysiology 28,* 245–260.

Siever, L. J., Keefe, R., Bernstein, D. P., Coccaro, E. F., Klar, H. M., Zemishlany, Z., Peterson, A. E., Davidson, M., Mahon, T., Horvath, T., & Mohs, R. (1990). Eye tracking impairment in clinically identified patients with schizotypal personality disorder. *American Journal of Psychiatry, 147,* 740–745.

Silverton, L. (1988). The genetic relationship between antisocial behavior and schizophrenia: A review of the literature. In W. Buikuisen (Ed.), *Explaining crime.* Leiden: Brill.

Simons, R. F. (1981). Electrodermal and cardiac orienting in psychometrically defined high-risk subjects. *Psychiatry Research, 4,* 347–356.

Simons, R. F., Losito, B. D., Rose, S. C., & MacMillan, F. W. (1983). Electrodermal nonresponding among college undergraduates: Temporal stability, situational specificity, and relationship to heart rate change. *Psychophysiology, 20,* 498–506.

Venables, P. H. (1964). Input dysfunction in schizophrenia. In B. Maher (Ed.), *Progress in experimental personality research* (pp. 1–41). New York: Academic Press.

Venables, P. H. (1993). Electrodermal indices as markers for the development of schizophrenia. In J. C. Roy, W. Boucsein, D. C. Fowles, & J. Gruzelier (Eds.), *Progress in electrodermal research.* New York: Plenum.

Wilkins, S. (1988). *Behavioral and psychophysiological aspects of information processing in schizotypics.* Ph.D. dissertation, University of York, U.K.
Zahn, T. P. (1986). Psychophysiological approaches to psychopathology. In M. G. H. Coles, E. Donchin, & S. W. Porges (Eds.), *Psychophysiology: Systems, processes, and applications* (pp. 508–610). New York: Guilford.

11

Attention, startle eye-blink modification, and psychosis proneness

MICHAEL E. DAWSON, ANNE M. SCHELL, ERIN A. HAZLETT, DIANE L. FILION, and KEITH H. NUECHTERLEIN

Attentional and information processing dysfunctions have long been considered to be core deficits of schizophrenia (Bleuler, 1911/1950; Kraepelin, 1919). According to this view, many of the characteristic symptoms of schizophrenia are consequences of underlying attentional and information processing dysfunctions. Despite the apparent consensus concerning the importance of these dysfunctions, close examination of the literature reveals considerable disagreement about their specific nature. Some investigators have suggested that schizophrenic patients suffer from primary deficits in controlled attentional processes (e.g., Callaway & Naghdi, 1982; Gjerde, 1983; Nuechterlein & Dawson, 1984b). Others have hypothesized primary deficits in the automatic, preattentive stages of information processing (e.g., Braff & Geyer, 1990; Frith, 1979; Venables, 1984). The possibility that primary deficits in automatic processing might lead to dysfunctions in controlled processing in some situations has also been considered (e.g., Nuechterlein & Dawson, 1984b).

The distinction between automatic and controlled cognitive processes has been prominent in cognitive psychology since the 1970s (Posner & Snyder, 1975; Shiffren & Schneider, 1977). Although there is not perfect agreement about all characteristics that distinguish automatic and controlled processes, there is nevertheless fundamental agreement about the key distinctions (Schneider, Dumais, & Shiffrin, 1984). Automatic cognitive processes occur rapidly, in parallel, demand little or no conscious attention and effort, and are difficult if not impossible to suppress voluntarily. Controlled cognitive processes, in contrast, occur slowly, in series, demand allocation of attentional resources and effort, and are under voluntary control. Most cognitive psychologists agree that automatic and controlled processes may occur in rapid sequence following presentation of salient stimuli. The first "automatic" or "preattentive" process serves to detect the stimulus and perform preliminary evaluation. Following this rapid preattentive processing, "controlled" or "attentive" processes may be engaged if the stimulus is considered either novel or important (Öhman, 1979).

A variety of empirical evidence has been cited that the primary cognitive deficit in schizophrenia involves controlled processing dysfunctions. For example, Callaway and Naghdi (1982) cited findings of speeded EEG alpha blocking to a visual stimulus (a hypothesized automatic process) coupled with slowed behavioral reaction time (a hypothesized controlled process) as evidence that schizophrenic patients do not have a deficiency in automatic cognitive processes but do have a deficiency in controlled processes. In fact, these authors suggested that schizophrenics may have supernormal automatic processes. Nuechterlein and Dawson (1984b) concluded that tasks with high processing demands were more likely to reveal deficiencies than tasks with low processing demands, suggesting that schizophrenic patients and persons at risk for schizophrenia have a reduced amount of controlled processing capacity available for task-relevant cognitive operations. Although emphasizing deficits in controlled processing, Nuechterlein and Dawson (1984b) did not rule out the possibility that there may be an impairment in automatic processes in some schizophrenic patients.

Many theorists who argue that automatic or preattentive deficits are central to schizophrenia emphasize evidence of impaired sensory filtering of irrelevant stimuli, because sensory filtering is considered an automatic process (Braff & Geyer, 1990; Frith, 1979; McGhie & Chapman, 1961; Venables, 1984). One line of evidence relevant to the notion of an impaired sensory filter comes from the empirical and theoretical work of Braff, Geyer, and their colleagues. The operational definition of impaired sensorimotor gating emphasized by these investigators involved dysfunctions in the modification of the startle eye-blink reflex. Because modification of the startle eye-blink reflex is the primary measure reported in this chapter, we now turn to a review of this topic in (1) normal subjects, (2) schizophrenic patients, and (3) schizotypal patients and putatively psychosis-prone subjects. Following this introductory material, we present results obtained with a new paradigm that permits assessment of both automatic and controlled modulation of the startle eye-blink reflex, first in schizophrenic patients and then in putatively psychosis-prone subjects.

Startle eye-blink modification in normal subjects

The startle reflex is elicited in a variety of species by any abrupt or unexpected stimulus change of sufficient intensity. In humans, the startle reflex consists of a rapid sequence of muscle movements completed within approximately 300 ms. Landis and Hunt (1939) captured this pattern of responding with high-speed motion pictures of human subjects startled by the noise of pistol shots. These investigators noted that the fastest and most reliable component of the startle pattern to a loud noise was the eye-blink response.

What has captured the interest and imagination of the contemporary research community is not the startle eye-blink reflex per se, but rather its plasticity in the context of a startle eye-blink modification (SEM) paradigm. In the SEM paradigm, the size and/or latency of the eye-blink component of the human startle reflex to a startling stimulus (e.g., sudden loud noise) is altered by innocuous stimuli that immediately precede the startling stimulus. The amplitude of the startle reflex can be either inhibited or facilitated depending upon the stimulus conditions, particularly the lead-interval between onset of the first stimulus (prestimulus) and onset of the startle stimulus. When the lead-interval is short (i.e., between approximately 30 and 500 ms), there is a reduction in startle eye-blink amplitude compared to the response elicited in the absence of a prestimulus, with the maximum inhibition occurring at approximately 100 ms. We refer to this phenomenon, sometimes also called "prepulse inhibition," as "short lead-interval SEM."

Short lead-interval SEM is unlearned (i.e., it occurs on the first trial), requires only midbrain and lower brain structures in rats (Leitner & Cohen, 1985), and is evident in human adults even while asleep (Silverstein, Graham, & Calloway, 1980). For these reasons, coupled with its speed of occurrence, this SEM inhibition effect has been hypothesized to reflect an automatic sensorimotor gating mechanism initiated by the prestimulus to allow the early, preattentive stages of information processing of the prestimulus to proceed relatively undisturbed by other stimulus events (Braff & Geyer, 1990; Graham, 1975, 1980). Thus, the degree of inhibition of startle in a short lead-interval SEM paradigm may be a useful index of the protective aspects of the automatic processing of the prestimulus.

In contrast to the short lead-interval SEM inhibition effect, the amplitude of the startle blink is enhanced when a sustained prestimulus in the same modality as the startle stimulus is employed with a relatively long lead-interval (e.g., greater than 1000 ms). The long lead-interval facilitation effect is hypothesized to reflect, at least partially, sensory enhancement associated with orienting and modality-specific selective attention (Bohlin & Graham,

1977). In support of a selective attention model of long lead-interval SEM, blink amplitude is facilitated if attention is directed to the modality of the startle stimulus, whereas blink amplitude is inhibited if attention is directed to a modality different from that of the startle stimulus (see reviews by Anthony, 1985; Putnam, 1990). Thus, the degree and direction of modification of the startle response in a long lead-interval SEM paradigm may be a useful index of the degree and direction of allocation of controlled attentional resources.

Evidence is accumulating that the short lead-interval SEM effect also can be modulated by selective attention, suggesting that it is not an entirely automatic process in all situations. These studies demonstrated that short lead-interval blink inhibition is enhanced by instructions to attend to the prestimulus (DelPezzo & Hoffman, 1980; Filion, Dawson, & Schell, 1993; Hackley & Graham, 1987; Hackley, Woldorff, & Hillyard, 1987).

Filion et al. (1993), for example, employed a selective attention paradigm in which to-be-attended and to-be-ignored tones served as prestimuli for the startle-eliciting noise. They found greater short lead-interval SEM inhibition at a 120-ms lead-interval (but not at a 60-ms lead-interval), and greater facilitation of the blink reflex at a long lead-interval (2000 ms), following the to-be-attended prestimulus than following the to-be-ignored prestimulus. These results clearly demonstrate that the degree of both short lead-interval and long lead interval SEM can be modulated by attention in normal college students.

In summary, the measurement of SEM and its attentional modulation may provide a sensitive nonverbal, nonvoluntary metric of either automatic or controlled attentional processes, depending upon the task demands and lead-interval. In a passive attention paradigm without demands to actively engage attentional mechanisms, SEM at short lead-intervals may index automatic preattentive processing of the prestimulus. In an active attention paradigm, in addition to automatic processing, SEM may index both a controlled attentional process at short lead-intervals (e.g., 120 ms), and a later sustained controlled attentional process at long lead-intervals (e.g., 2000 ms). The fact that attentional modulation of short lead-interval SEM is apparent with a 120-ms lead-interval but not with a 60-ms lead-interval suggests that automatic processes are predominant at 60 ms even in an active attention paradigm, whereas controlled processes become engaged by 120 ms. Thus, SEM is a potentially useful tool for understanding the automatic and controlled nature of the cognitive dysfunctions in schizophrenia.

SEM in schizophrenic patients

Three SEM studies employing the passive attention paradigm with schizophrenic patients have been published to date. Braff and colleagues (Braff,

Stone, Callaway, Geyer, Glick, & Bali, 1978; Braff, Grillon, & Geyer, 1992; Grillon, Ameli, Charney, Krystal, & Braff, 1992) measured SEM in heterogeneous groups of hospitalized chronic and acute medicated schizophrenic patients with no instructions to attend to any of the stimuli. In each study, schizophrenic patients exhibited significantly less short lead-interval blink inhibition than did normal control subjects. The findings were interpreted as reflecting an impairment in automatic, preattentive central nervous system inhibition (sensorimotor gating) (Braff & Geyer, 1990; Geyer & Braff, 1987). The deficiency in sensorimotor gating was suggested to be a "trait-linked longitudinal deficit in central inhibition and gating mechanisms" (Braff & Geyer, 1990, p. 187) which increases the vulnerability to cognitive fragmentation and disorganization in schizophrenia.

SEM in schizotypal patients and putatively at-risk subjects

The inference that the deficit in short lead-interval SEM inhibition is trait-related, as suggested by Braff and Geyer (1990), would be strengthened if one could find similar impairments in subjects who were hypothesized to be in the schizophrenic spectrum of psychopathology but were not suffering from psychotic symptoms. One approach to this issue is to study patients with schizotypal personality disorder (SPD). Cadenhead, Geyer, and Braff (1993) measured short lead-interval blink inhibition with the passive attention paradigm in patients diagnosed with SPD according to DSM-III-R (American Psychiatric Association, 1987) criteria, most of whom were unmedicated. They found impaired eye-blink inhibition in the SPD patients compared to normal controls across three short lead-intervals (30, 60, 120 ms). Thus, SPD patients appear to exhibit deficits in passive sensorimotor gating similar to those shown by schizophrenic patients.

Still another approach to the basic issue is to study subgroups of the normal population that are psychometrically identified to be putatively at risk for psychosis, and/or are hypothesized to have some of the same underlying psychobiological dysfunctions as schizophrenic patients. This approach has the advantage of identifying subjects before patient status has been reached, although it is not without disadvantages as well (Nuechterlein, 1990). The Chapmans have developed a number of widely used self-report questionnaires that are hypothesized to identify psychosis-prone samples (Chapman & Chapman, 1987). Simons and Giardina (1992) studied SEM with an uninstructed passive attention paradigm using both short (60 and 120 ms) and long (2,000 ms) lead-intervals in college students deemed to be psychosis-prone on the basis of high scores on either the Perceptual Aberration Scale (Chapman, Chapman, &

Raulin, 1978) or the Physical Anhedonia Scale (Chapman, Chapman, & Raulin, 1976). "Perceptual aberrators" showed significantly less blink inhibition at the 120-ms lead-interval than did the controls, whereas the "anhedonics" fell between the other two groups and did not differ from the controls at the 120 ms lead-interval. All three groups exhibited moderate facilitation at 2,000 ms, but there were no group differences at the long lead-interval. The finding of reduced short lead-interval blink inhibition in perceptual-aberrator college students is consistent with previous findings with schizophrenic patients reviewed above. Simons and Giardina (1992) interpreted these results as suggesting that nonpatient subjects with perceptual aberrations may share with schizophrenic patients an underdeveloped preattentive mechanism that functions to protect sensory information from interference by subsequent stimuli.

The SEM studies described above with schizophrenic patients, SPD patients, and putatively at-risk subjects have employed only the uninstructed passive attention paradigm. As emphasized earlier, there is strong evidence that instructions to attend to the prestimuli can enhance both the short lead-interval blink inhibition, and the long lead-interval blink facilitation in normal subjects. We describe below two studies recently completed in our laboratory using our selective attention paradigm. The first study tested relatively remitted, recent-onset schizophrenic patients (Dawson, Hazlett, Filion, Nuechterlein, & Schell, 1993), whereas the second study tested college students putatively at risk based on high scores on scales measuring Physical Anhedonia, Perceptual Aberration, or Magical Thinking (Schell, Dawson, Hazlett, & Filion, 1995). All subjects in both studies were instructed to attend to one tone pitch (prestimulus) and to ignore another tone pitch. Thus, there were intermixed presentations of a task-relevant, to-be-attended prestimulus, and a task-irrelevant, to-be-ignored prestimulus. Short lead-interval SEM to the to-be-ignored prestimulus was expected to provide an estimate of predominantly automatic cognitive processes, whereas SEM to the to-be-attended prestimulus was expected to provide an estimate of automatic-plus-controlled attentional processes. Therefore, differential SEM to the to-be-ignored and the to-be-attended prestimuli at the 120-ms and 2000-ms lead-intervals should reflect the effect of controlled processing above and beyond the automatic processing of the to-be-ignored prestimuli.

The following studies constitute the first tests of attentional modulation of SEM in schizophrenic patients and putatively psychosis-prone college students. The overall goals of the studies were to determine whether the relatively remitted patients and putatively at-risk students exhibit similar SEM deficits, and to determine whether these deficits qualify as impairments in automatic or controlled cognitive processes, or both.

Attentional modulation of SEM in schizophrenic patients

The subjects in our initial study were 15 schizophrenic patients and 14 matched normal controls (Dawson et al., 1993). The schizophrenic subjects were outpatients at the UCLA Aftercare Clinic and were or had been participants in a longitudinal study of the early phases of schizophrenia (Nuechterlein et al., 1992). The first psychotic episode began not longer than two years before entry into the main longitudinal project and occurred an average of 2.9 years (SD = 2.6 years) before testing in the present project. Thus, at the time of assessment, the patients were still in the relatively early phases of schizophrenia and were without a long history of medication and institutionalization. The patients also were either on a standardized low-to-moderate dose of injectable fluphenazine (Prolixin) decanoate or off all psychoactive medication at the time of the SEM test session. It is important to note that the patients were relatively asymptomatic at the time of their testing, as assessed by independent ratings on the Brief Psychiatric Rating Scale (BPRS). Thus, any observed SEM impairments are not likely to be secondary effects of concurrent symptoms.

The matched normal controls also were drawn from participants in the longitudinal research project. These normal controls were matched to the schizophrenic outpatients on age, sex, race, and educational level.

All subjects were instructed to listen to a series of high and low pitch tones presented through headphones, to count silently the number of "longer than usual" (7 vs. 5 s) tones of one pitch, and simply to ignore the tones of the other pitch. Subjects also were told that a brief loud noise burst would be presented occasionally throughout the tone-counting task, but that it was unrelated to the task and could be ignored.

A total of 48 tone trials was presented during the task, 24 high (1,200 Hz) and 24 low (800 Hz) pitch tones with intertone intervals ranging between 25 and 35 s. Of the 24 tones of each pitch, 16 included the startle-eliciting white noise (102 dB). Of these 16 trials, there were 4 presentations of the startle-eliciting noise at each of four lead-intervals: 60, 120, 240, and 2000 ms. In effect, then, there was a to-be-attended prestimulus and a to-be-ignored prestimulus each presented with the startling noise at three short lead-intervals (60, 120, and 240 ms) and one long lead-interval (2,000 ms).

In addition to the startle-noise presentations at critical lead-intervals, startle stimuli also were presented at preselected times during the intertone intervals in order to provide a baseline measure of startle amplitude. Startle eye-blink modification (SEM) scores were then computed as differences between the baseline intertone interval blink amplitude and the during-tone blink amplitudes, expressed as percent changes. A positive SEM score indicated startle facilitation relative to baseline, whereas a negative SEM score indicated startle inhibition relative to baseline.

Figure 11.1 presents the mean SEM scores of the schizophrenic patients and the matched controls at each of the four lead-intervals following the to-be-attended prestimulus and the to-be-ignored prestimulus. As described earlier, it was anticipated that SEM to the to-be-ignored prestimulus would provide an estimate of predominantly automatic cognitive processes. Therefore, the SEM scores at the short lead-intervals following the to-be-ignored prestimulus were submitted to a 2 (Group) × 3 (Lead-interval: 60, 120, 240 ms) analysis of variance (ANOVA). This analysis revealed neither a group main effect nor an interaction effect, indicating that the patients did not differ from normal subjects in short lead-interval blink inhibition following the to-be-ignored prestimulus. Similarly, no difference between the groups was found in blink facilitation at the 2,000-ms long lead-interval following the to-be-ignored prestimulus.

As indicated previously, differences in SEM between the to-be-attended and to-be-ignored prestimuli are expected to provide an estimate of predominantly controlled attentional modulation of startle eye-blink. In order to evaluate statistically these effects at the short lead-interval, a 2 (Group) × 2 (Prestimulus) × 3 (Lead-interval) ANOVA was performed on the SEM scores obtained at the three short lead-intervals (the 60-, 120-, and 240-ms points in Figure 11.1). This analysis revealed a significant Group × Prestimulus × Lead-interval interaction effect. Simple effects tests confirmed that the matched normal controls showed significantly greater blink inhibition following the to-be-attended prestimulus than following the to-be-ignored prestimulus at 120 ms, consistent with our previous findings with normal college students (Filion et al., 1993). However, as can be seen in Figure 11.1, the patients failed to show differential inhibition at any short lead-interval. Thus, the normal controls demonstrate attentional modulation of short lead-interval SEM inhibition, whereas the patients show a lack of attentional modulation of SEM inhibition. This short lead-interval finding suggests that patients fail to engage the normally enhanced protective inhibition following the to-be-attended prestimulus.

We next performed a 2 (Group) × 2 (Prestimulus) ANOVA on the SEM scores at the long lead-interval (the 2,000-ms point in Figure 11.1). The Group × Prestimulus interaction was significant, indicating that the groups differed in their differential blink modification to the to-be-attended and to-be-ignored prestimuli. Simple effects tests confirmed that the normal controls exhibited significantly greater SEM facilitation at 2,000 ms following the to-

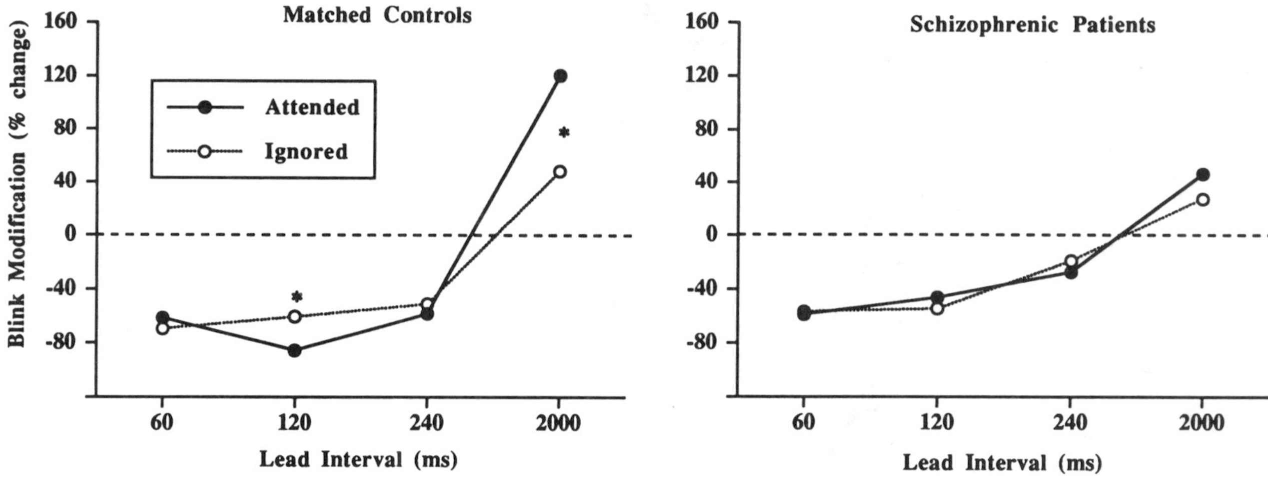

Fig. 11.1. Mean startle eye-blink modification scores as a function of prestimulus type and lead-interval for the matched control subjects and the schizophrenic patients. Asterisks indicate significant differences between attended and ignored prestimuli.

be-attended prestimulus than the to-be-ignored prestimulus, again consistent with past findings in normal college students, whereas the schizophrenic patients failed to respond differentially. Thus, as in the short lead-interval findings, only the normal control group exhibited significant attentional modulation of the startle blink at the long lead-interval. This long lead-interval finding suggests that the patients fail to maintain a strong selective attention focus during the to-be-attended prestimulus, at least at 2,000 ms following onset of the to-be-attended prestimulus.

Analyses of individual subject data, as opposed to group means, were conducted in order to examine the consistency of the group effects across individuals. In order to assess the attentional modulation effect at the individual case level, differences were computed between the SEM scores for the to-be-attended and the to-be-ignored prestimuli at the 120-ms and the 2,000-ms lead-intervals for each individual subject. Negative-difference scores indicate more inhibition following the to-be-attended prestimulus, whereas positive-difference scores indicate more facilitation following the to-be-attended prestimulus. The difference scores for individual subjects at the 120-ms lead-interval are shown in panel A of Figure 11.2. As can be seen, 13 of 14 normal controls exhibited greater inhibition following the to-be-attended prestimulus; the one exception was a subject who showed 100% inhibition to both the to-be-attended and to-be-ignored prestimuli and hence had a zero difference score. In contrast, 9 of the 15 patients showed this direction of difference, and as can be seen, most of their difference scores hovered near zero.

Panel B of Figure 11.2 shows the SEM difference scores for individual subjects at the 2,000-ms lead-interval for normal controls and schizophrenic patients. As can be seen, 13 of the 14 normal controls exhibited greater startle-blink facilitation following the to-be-attended prestimulus than the to-be-ignored prestimulus. Ten of the 15 schizophrenic patients responded in this direction, and most of these were small differences.

All in all, the results demonstrate that recent-onset, relatively asymptomatic schizophrenic patients have impaired attentional modulation of SEM at both short lead-intervals and long lead-intervals. However, the patients did not differ from normal in SEM following the to-be-ignored prestimulus; instead the impairment was specific to the attended prestimulus at the 120-ms and 2,000-ms lead-intervals. These results suggest that controlled attentional modulation of SEM is impaired in schizophrenia in the active attention paradigm. Moreover, this impairment may represent a traitlike vulnerability factor because it is present in relatively asymptomatic outpatients.

If the impaired attentional modulation of SEM is related to underlying vulnerability to schizophrenia, then we would expect to find similar impairments

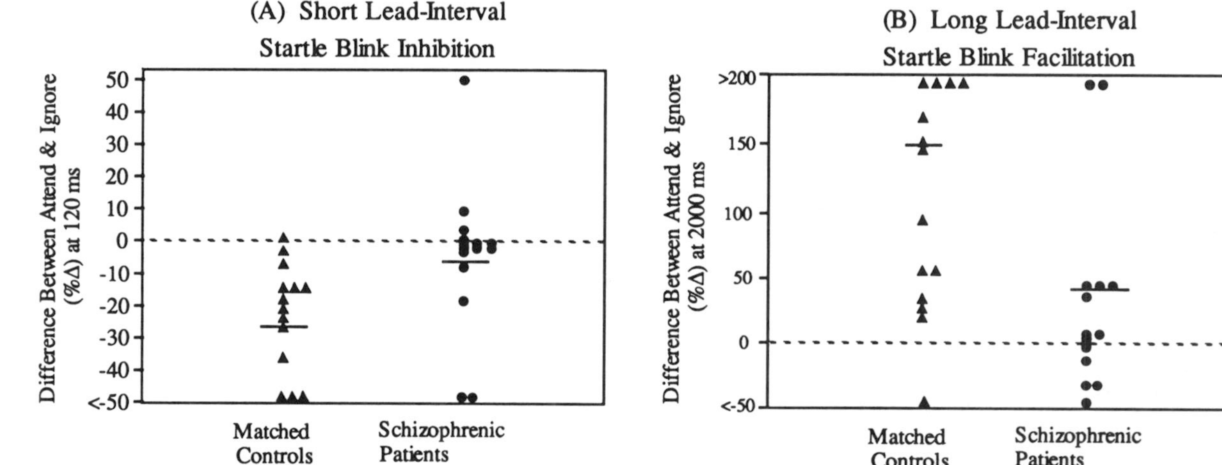

Fig. 11.2. Difference scores between attended and ignored prestimuli for each individual subject in the matched control group and the schizophrenic group at the 120-ms short lead-interval (panel A) and the 2000-ms long lead-interval (panel B). A negative score indicates greater startle inhibition following the attended prestimulus, whereas a positive score indicates greater facilitation following the attended prestimulus. Horizontal bars indicate group means.

in subjects at-risk for schizophrenia. Therefore, we turn next to an examination of SEM impairments in college students putatively at-risk for psychosis based on selected Chapman Psychosis Proneness Scales.

Attentional modulation of SEM in putatively at-risk subjects

A total of 984 students from Introduction to Psychology classes at the University of Southern California were administered questionnaires containing items of the Physical Anhedonia Scale (Chapman et al., 1976), Perceptual Aberration Scale (Chapman et al., 1978), and the Magical Ideation Scale (Eckblad & Chapman, 1983). More details regarding these scales can be found in Chapman, Chapman, and Kwapil (Chapter 5, this volume). Students who scored two or more standard deviations above the same sex means on the Physical Anhedonia, Perceptual Aberration, or Magical Ideation scales were identified and recruited for participation in the present study. Because scores on the Perceptual Aberration and Magical Ideation scales tend to be highly correlated, students who scored high on either scale were combined into a single "Per-Mag" group, following the practice of Chapman and Chapman (1987). In addition, control subjects were recruited if they had scores no greater than .5 standard deviation above or below the same sex means of any of the three psychosis-proneness scales. The number of subjects who participated in the SEM paradigm and yielded usable SEM data included 17 anhedonics, 25 Per-Mags, and 27 controls. These three groups of college students were administered the same paradigm described previously, involving selective attention to prestimuli.

Figure 11.3 shows the mean SEM scores at each of the four lead intervals following the to-be-attended and to-be-ignored prestimuli for all three groups of college students. As described earlier, SEM following the to-be-ignored prestimulus is expected to provide an estimate of automatic cognitive processing. Therefore, we performed a 3 (Group) × 3 (Lead-interval) × 2 (Trial block) ANOVA on the SEM scores recorded at the three short lead-intervals following the to-be-ignored prestimulus, and a separate 3 (Group) × 2 (Trial block) ANOVA on the SEM scores at the 2,000-ms long lead-interval following the to-be-ignored prestimulus. In neither of these analyses was the main effect of group or any of its interactions significant. Thus, as in results described previously for the schizophrenic patients, there was no evidence of impaired automatic SEM following the to-be-ignored prestimuli in the at-risk groups.

We next analyzed data for deficits in attentional modulation of SEM by

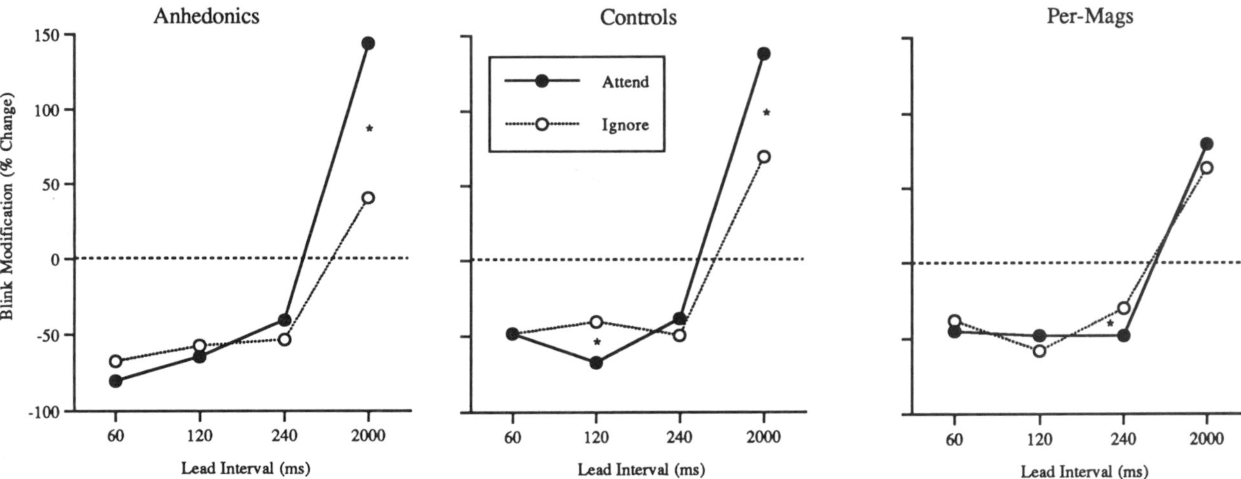

Fig. 11.3. Mean startle eye-blink modification scores as a function of prestimulus type and lead-interval for three groups of college student subjects (anhedonics, controls, and Per-Mags). Asterisks indicate significant differences between attended and ignored prestimuli.

examining differential SEM following to-be-attended and to-be-ignored prestimuli. In order to evaluate these effects at the short lead-intervals, we conducted a 3 (Group) × 2 (Prestimulus) × 3 (Lead-interval) × 2 (Trial block) ANOVA on the SEM scores at the 60-, 120-, and 240-ms lead-intervals. There was a highly significant effect of trial block, owing to less inhibition during the second half of the trials than during the first. There was also a significant Group × Prestimulus × Lead-interval interaction, reflecting group differences in differential inhibition following the to-be-attended and to-be-ignored prestimuli across the short lead-intervals. As can be seen in Figure 11.3, the control group exhibited significantly greater inhibition after the to-be-attended prestimulus than after the to-be-ignored prestimulus at the 120-ms lead-interval. This finding replicates our previous findings with normal college students (Filion et al., 1993) and with normal control subjects demographically matched with schizophrenic patients (Dawson et al., 1993). In contrast, both of the putatively at-risk groups failed to exhibit significant differential inhibition at the 120-ms lead-interval. The lack of attentional modulation of short lead-interval SEM inhibition in the anhedonic and Per-Mag college students at 120 ms is consistent with a similar failure in the relatively asymptomatic schizophrenic patients. The anhedonics failed to show differential inhibition at all of the short lead-intervals. The Per-Mags, however, showed significant differential attentional effects at the 240-ms lead-interval, unlike the other two groups. This finding suggests that attentional modulation develops more slowly in the Per-Mag group.

Attentional modulation of long lead-interval SEM was tested by performing a 3 (Group) × 2 (Prestimulus) × 2 (Trial block) ANOVA on SEM scores at the 2,000-ms lead-interval. This ANOVA revealed a significant Group × Prestimulus × Trial block interaction. The interaction effect reflects the fact that differential SEM facilitation shows a different pattern across the two trial blocks for the three groups. Differential SEM facilitation was more pronounced in the control group than in either at-risk group in the first block of trials, owing to heightened facilitation following the to-be-attended prestimulus, but the control group showed a decline in differential facilitation during the second trial block. In fact, differential facilitation in the control group was significant only during the first trial block. The Per-Mag group also showed a decline in differential facilitation across trial blocks; however, for this group differential facilitation was not significant during both early and late trial blocks. On the other hand, the anhedonic group showed an increase in differential facilitation over trials, with significant facilitation only on the second block of trials. The increased long lead-interval SEM facilitation of the anhedonic group in the second half of the task suggests that this group tended to "normalize" selective allocation of attention as the task progressed.

The individual subject data for the three groups of college students were examined at the 120-ms and 2,000-ms lead-intervals, as had been done with the schizophrenic patients and their controls. Because the groups differed with respect to long lead-interval facilitation primarily during the early trial block, the individual data for the 2,000-ms lead-interval are presented only for the first trial block.

Panel A of Figure 11.4 shows the individual SEM difference scores between the to-be-attended and to-be-ignored prestimuli at the 120-ms lead-interval. As can be seen, 20 of the 27 control subjects exhibited greater short lead-interval SEM inhibition following the to-be-attended prestimulus than following the to-be-ignored prestimulus. In contrast, 11 of the 17 anhedonics exhibited greater inhibition following the to-be-attended prestimulus, and 6 showed equal or reversed inhibition. Even more striking, 11 of the 25 Per-Mags showed greater inhibition following the to-be-attended prestimulus, and 14 showed reversed inhibition.

Panel B of Figure 11.4 shows the individual SEM difference scores at the long lead-interval for the first trial block for all three groups. Of the 27 controls, 26 exhibited greater SEM facilitation following the to-be-attended pre-stimulus than following the to-be-ignored prestimulus, and only one showed reversed differential facilitation. Of the 17 anhedonics, 7 exhibited greater facilitation following the to-be-attended prestimulus, and 10 showed equal or reversed differential facilitation. Of the 25 Per-Mags, 14 exhibited greater facilitation following the to-be-attached prestimulus than the to-be-ignored prestimulus, and 11 showed reversed differential facilitation.

In summary, impairments in attentional modulation of SEM found in Per-Mag college students are similar to those found in relatively asymptomatic schizophrenic outpatients. In fact, the impairments appear somewhat more frequent and severe in the Per Mag subjects than the schizophrenic outpatients (compare Figure 11.2, depicting the schizophrenia results, with Figure 11.4, depicting the Per-Mag results at the short lead-intervals). This may be because impaired attentional modulation of SEM is associated specifically with perceptual aberrations (and/or magical thinking), and the Per-Mag subjects are relatively homogeneous in this regard, whereas only some of the patients have these specific symptoms. The anhedonic college students, on the other hand, showed less consistent impairments in short lead-interval SEM inhibition. At the long lead-interval, however, a substantial subgroup of anhedonics (10/17 or 59%; see Figure 11.4) exhibited distinct impairments in attentional modulation of SEM on the first half of the trials.

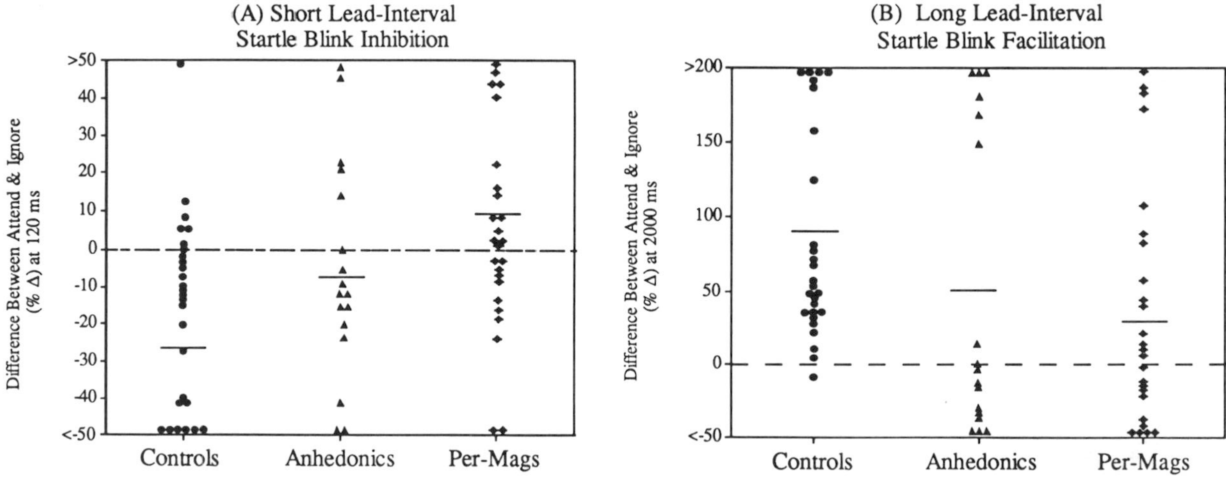

Fig. 11.4. Difference scores between attended and ignored prestimuli for each individual subject in the control group, the anhedonia group, and the Per-Mag group at the 120-ms short lead-interval (panel A) and the 2000-ms long lead-interval (panel B). A negative score indicates greater startle inhibition following the attended prestimulus, whereas a positive score indicates greater facilitation following the attended prestimulus. Horizontal bars indicate group means.

Conclusions and directions for future research

The primary conclusion suggested by the findings reported here is that both relatively asymptomatic young schizophrenic outpatients and Per-Mag college students exhibit deficits in controlled attentional modulation of SEM, but not in automatic components of SEM, when tested with a paradigm involving differential attention to prestimuli. This conclusion is based on our hypotheses that SEM following the to-be-ignored prestimulus, and SEM at the very short lead-interval (60 ms) following the to-be-attended prestimulus, both reflect primarily automatic information processing, whereas differential SEM at the 120-ms and 2,000-ms lead-intervals represents primarily controlled modulation of SEM (Dawson et al., 1993). However, processing of the to-be-ignored prestimulus may not be entirely an automatic process because subjects must discriminate to-be-attended and to-be-ignored pre-stimuli, and therefore likely allocate sufficient attention to the to-be-ignored prestimulus to identify it as the task-irrelevant stimulus.

Although the present results suggest impairments in controlled processes and not automatic processes in an active attention paradigm, other investigators have found SEM impairments in an uninstructed passive attention paradigm in schizophrenic patients (Braff et al., 1978, 1992; Grillon et al., 1992), in schizotypal patients (Cadenhead et al., 1993), and in putatively at-risk college students (Simons & Giardina, 1992). The latter findings suggest impairments in automatic components of SEM. Clearly, one important direction of future research is to measure SEM from the same subjects in both active and passive attentional paradigms. This will serve to test whether deficits in automatic processes revealed by the passive attention paradigm, and deficits in controlled processing revealed by the active attention paradigm, occur in the same subjects or different subgroups of subjects.

The finding of SEM impairments in relatively asymptomatic schizophrenic outpatients and putatively psychosis-prone college students suggests that the impairments are not merely secondary correlates of psychotic symptoms. SEM impairments may provide nonverbal, reflexive, state-independent markers of vulnerability to schizophrenia. Although our findings indicate that impaired attentional modulation of SEM is not secondary to current psychotic symptoms, it is still necessary to test the same patients during a psychotic state and again during a remitted state to determine if state effects exist. Vulnerability indicators should show abnormalities during a remitted state, but some vulnerability indicators may show increased deviance during a psychotic phase (Nuechterlein & Dawson, 1984a).

The striking similarity of SEM impairments in schizophrenics and Per-

Mags suggests that the two groups share a common dysfunction in controlled modulation of incoming stimuli. These findings are consistent with the hypothesis that perceptual aberration and magical thinking are indicators of processes that are related to the vulnerability to psychosis (Chapman & Chapman, 1987). Of course, the present data do not demonstrate that Per-Mags have an increased risk of later psychosis, but the finding of parallel SEM impairments in schizophrenic outpatients and Per-Mag college students is consistent with a basic commonality of underlying processes across the groups.

What relevance do the present results have for schizotypal personality disorder (SPD)? If we are correct that impaired attentional modulation of SEM is related to an aspect of vulnerability to schizophrenia, and if SPD is part of a continuum of schizophrenia-related disorders, then impaired attentional modulation of SEM should be detectable in at least a subgroup of SPD patients. This specific hypothesis has yet to be tested. However, as reviewed earlier, impaired short lead-interval blink inhibition has been found in SPD patients when tested with the passive attention paradigm (Cadenhead et al., 1993). This SEM impairment is presumed to reflect a deficit in automatic processing because subjects were not instructed to attend to the prestimuli. Given our current results, we consider it important in future research to determine whether SPD patients exhibit impaired controlled modulation of SEM when instructed to attend to the prestimuli.

How general or specific are the findings of impaired SEM? Other patient groups that are neither psychotic nor schizophrenic have been reported to exhibit short lead-interval SEM impairments when tested with the passive attention paradigm, such as individuals with obsessive-compulsive disorders (Swerdlow, Benbow, Zisook, Geyer, & Braff, 1993) or Huntington's disease (Swerdlow, Caine, Braff, & Geyer, 1992), and children with nocturnal enuresis (Ornitz, Hanna, & de Traversay, 1992). In addition, children with posttraumatic stress disorder have been found to exhibit a trend toward impaired short lead-interval SEM inhibition coupled with significantly enhanced long lead-interval SEM facilitation (Ornitz & Pynoos, 1989). Therefore, another important direction for future research involves differentiation of automatic and controlled SEM deficits in other patient groups. It is theoretically important to determine which groups have impairments in automatic components of SEM, which in controlled components of SEM, and which in both components. As suggested by Cadenhead et al. (1993), SEM impairments may be found in disorders characterized clinically by deficient gating of intrusive, irrelevant sensory, cognitive, and motor information. It will be fruitful to determine the extent of SEM impairments not only in patient groups but also in subjects who share the genetic vulnerability to schizophrenia but who do not have the symptoms (e.g., first-degree relatives of schizophrenics or, better yet, asymptomatic identical twins of schizophrenics).

Thus far, for convenience we have spoken of schizophrenia (and schizotypal personality disorder) as a single disorder; however, many investigators suggest that it is very likely a heterogeneous disorder. Therefore, future research should determine what is unique about those schizophrenic patients (as well as schizotypal subjects and putatively at-risk subjects) who exhibit the most profound SEM deficits versus those who exhibit mild or no SEM impairments. Are the SEM impairments related to specific disorders of perception or thought? The relationships will likely differ for impairments in short and long lead-intervals, and for impairments in automatic and controlled processes. The meaning of the SEM impairments will be better understood by relating them to behavioral and phenomenological symptoms, as well as other laboratory measures. Progress is now beginning to be made in this large and important task. For example, poor short lead-interval blink inhibition measured in a passive attention paradigm was related to an index of ego impairment by Perry, Viglione, and Braff (1992), and to increased perseveration errors on the Wisconsin Card Sorting Test by Butler, Jenkins, Geyer, and Braff (1991). Filion et al. (1993) found that weak attentional modulation of both short lead-interval inhibition and long lead-interval facilitation obtained in the active attention paradigm with normal college students were correlated with small skin conductance orienting responses to the prestimuli. These are interesting pieces of the puzzle, but much remains to be done in order to understand the behavioral, clinical, and psychophysiological significance of SEM and its impairments.

One of the attractive features of SEM methodology is that the neural circuits and neurotransmitters mediating SEM can be studied in lower animals. This line of research suggests that short lead-interval startle inhibition is mediated at the midbrain level (Leitner & Cohen, 1985), but that it can be modulated by a cortico-striato-pallidal-thalamic circuit (Geyer, Swerdlow, Mansbach, & Braff, 1990; Swerdlow & Koob, 1987). Therefore, future research may profit from the application of brain imaging techniques (e.g., positron emission tomography, PET; and functional magnetic resonance imaging, MRI) in human subjects to differentiate the central processes responsible for the impairments of automatic and controlled components of SEM.

In conclusion, SEM provides a potentially powerful methodology for examining automatic and controlled cognitive processing deficits that appear to be related to underlying vulnerability factors for schizophrenia. Perhaps most notable in the long term, SEM is a measure that has considerable potential for building meaningful bridges among cognitive science, neuroscience, and clinical science (Dawson, 1990) approaches to understanding schizophrenia and related personality disorders.

Acknowledgments

Research reported in this chapter was supported by research grants MH46433 (to M. E. Dawson), MH37705 (to K. H. Nuechterlein), and a Mental Health Clinical Research Center grant MH30911 (to R. B. Liberman) from the National Institute of Mental Health, and by a grant from the Scottish Rite Schizophrenia Research Program, N.M.J., U.S.A. (to M. E. Dawson). This chapter was prepared while the first author (M. E. Dawson) was supported by a Research Scientist Development Award (1 KO2 MH01086) from the National Institute of Mental Health.

References

American Psychiatric Association. (1987). *Diagnostic and statistical manual of mental disorders, third edition – revised.* Washington, D.C.: Author.

Anthony, B. J. (1985). In the blink of an eye: Implications of reflex modification for information processing. In P. K. Ackles, J. R. Jennings, & M. G. H. Coles (Eds.). *Advances in psychophysiology* (Vol. 1, pp. 167–218). Greenwich, Conn.: JAI Press.

Bleuler, E. (1950). *Dementia praecox or the group of schizophrenias* (J. Zinkin, trans.). New York: International Press. (Original work published 1911).

Bohlin, G., & Graham, F. K. (1977). Cardiac deceleration and reflex blink facilitation. *Psychophysiology, 14,* 423–430.

Braff, D. L., & Geyer, M. A. (1990). Sensorimotor gating and schizophrenia: Human and animal model studies. *Archives of General Psychiatry, 47,* 181–188.

Braff, D. L., Grillon, C., & Geyer, M. A. (1992). Gating and habituation of the startle reflex in schizophrenic patients. *Archives of General Psychiatry, 49,* 206–215.

Braff, D. L., Stone, C., Callaway, E., Geyer, M., Glick, I., & Bali, L. (1978). Prestimulus effects on human startle reflex in normals and schizophrenics. *Psychophysiology, 15,* 339–343.

Butler, R. W., Jenkins, M., Geyer, M. A., & Braff, D. L. (1991). Wisconsin Card Sorting deficits and diminished sensorimotor gating in a discrete subgroup of schizophrenic patients. In C. A. Tamminga & S. C. Schulz (Eds.), *Advances in neuropsychiatry and psychopharmacology: Schizophrenia research* (Vol. 1, pp. 163–168). New York: Raven Press.

Cadenhead, K. S., Geyer, M. A., & Braff, D. L. (1993). Impaired startle prepulse inhibition and habituation in schizotypal patients. *American Journal of Psychiatry, 150,* 1862–1867.

Callaway, E., & Naghdi, S. (1982). An information processing model for schizophrenia. *Archives of General Psychiatry, 39,* 339–347.

Chapman, L. J., & Chapman, J. P. (1987). The search for symptoms predictive of schizophrenia. *Schizophrenia Bulletin, 13,* 497–503.

Chapman, L. J., Chapman, J. P., & Raulin, M. L. (1976). Scales for physical and social anhedonia. *Journal of Abnormal Psychology, 85,* 374–382.

Chapman, L. J., Chapman, J. P., & Raulin, M. L. (1978). Body-image aberration in schizophrenia. *Journal of Abnormal Psychology, 87,* 399–407.

Dawson, M. (1990). Psychophysiology at the interface of clinical science, cognitive science, and neuroscience. *Psychophysiology, 27,* 243–255.

Dawson, M. E., Hazlett, E. A., Filion, D. L., Nuechterlein, K. H., & Schell, A. M. (1993). Attention and schizophrenia: Impaired modulation of the startle reflex. *Journal of Abnormal Psychology, 102,* 633–641.

DelPezzo, E. M., & Hoffman, H. S. (1980). Attentional factors in the inhibition of a reflex by a visual prestimulus. *Science, 210,* 673–674.

Eckblad, M., & Chapman, L. J. (1983). Magical ideation as an indicator of schizotypy. *Journal of Consulting and Clinical Psychology, 51,* 215–225.

Filion, D. L., Dawson, M. E., & Schell, A. M. (1993). Modification of the acoustic startle-reflex eyeblink: A tool for investigating early and late attentional processes. *Biological Psychology, 35,* 185–200.

Frith, C. D. (1979). Consciousness, information processing and schizophrenia. *British Journal of Psychiatry, 134,* 225–235.

Geyer, M. A., & Braff, D. L. (1987). Startle habituation and sensorimotor gating in schizophrenia and related animal models. *Schizophrenia Bulletin, 13,* 643–668.

Geyer, M. A., Swerdlow, N. R., Mansbach, R. S., & Braff, D. L. (1990). Startle response models of sensorimotor gating and habituation deficits in schizophrenia. *Brain Research Bulletin, 25,* 485–498.

Gjerde, P. F. (1983). Attentional capacity dysfunction and arousal in schizophrenia. *Psychological Bulletin, 93,* 57–72.

Graham, F. K. (1975). The more or less startling effects of weak prestimulation. *Psychophysiology, 12,* 238–248.

Graham, F. K. (1980). Control of reflex blink excitability. In R. F. Thompson, L. H. Hicks, & V. B. Shryrkov (Eds.), *Neural mechanisms of goal directed behavior and learning* (pp. 511–519). New York: Academic Press.

Grillon, C., Ameli, R., Charney, D. S., Krystal, J., & Braff, D. L. (1992). Startle gating deficits occur across prepulse intensities in schizophrenic patients. *Biological Psychiatry, 32,* 939–943.

Hackley, S. A., & Graham, F. K. (1987). Effects of attending selectively to the spatial position of reflex-eliciting and reflex-modulating stimuli. *Journal of Experimental Psychology: Human Perception and Performance, 13,* 411–424.

Hackley, S. A., Woldorff, M., & Hillyard, S. A. (1987). Combined use of microreflexes and event-related brain potentials as measures of auditory selective attention. *Psychophysiology, 24,* 632–647.

Kraepelin, E. (1919). *Dementia praecox and paraphrenia* (R. M. Barclay, trans.). Edinburgh: E. & S. Livingston. (Original work published 1913).

Landis, C., & Hunt, W. A. (1939). *The startle pattern.* New York: Farrar & Rinehart.

Leitner, D. S., & Cohen, M. E. (1985). Role of the inferior colliculus in the inhibition of acoustic startle in the rat. *Physiology and Behavior, 34,* 65–70.

McGhie, A., & Chapman, J. (1961). Disorders of attention and perception in early schizophrenia. *British Journal of Medical Psychology, 34,* 103–116.

Nuechterlein, K. H. (1990). Methodological considerations in the search for indicators of vulnerability to severe psychopathology. In J. W. Rohrbaugh, R. Parasuraman, & R. Johnson, Jr. (Eds.), *Event-related brain potentials: Basic issues and applications* (pp. 364–373). Oxford: Oxford University Press.

Nuechterlein, K. H., & Dawson, M. E. (1984a). A heuristic vulnerability/stress model of schizophrenic episodes. *Schizophrenia Bulletin, 10,* 300–312.

Nuechterlein, K. H., & Dawson, M. E. (1984b). Information processing and attentional functioning in the developmental course of schizophrenic disorders. *Schizophrenic Bulletin, 10,* 160–203.

Nuechterlein, K. H., Dawson, M. E., Gitlin, M., Ventura, J., Goldstein, M. J., Snyder, K. S., Yee, C. M., & Mintz, J. (1992). Developmental processes in schizophrenic disorders: Longitudinal studies of vulnerability and stress. *Schizophrenia Bulletin, 18,* 387–425.

Öhman, A. (1979). The orienting response, attention, and learning: An information processing perspective. In H. D. Kimmel, E. H. van Olst, & J. F. Orlebeke (Eds.), *The orienting reflex in humans* (pp. 443–471). Hillsdale, N.J.: Lawrence Erlbaum.

Ornitz, E. M., Hanna, G. L., & de Traversay, J. (1992). Prestimulation-induced startle modulation in attention-deficit hyperactivity disorder and nocturnal enuresis. *Psychophysiology, 29,* 437–451.

Ornitz, E. M., & Pynoos, R. S. (1989). Startle modulation in children with posttraumatic stress disorder. *American Journal of Psychiatry, 146,* 866–870.

Perry, W., Viglione, D., & Braff, D. L. (1992). The Ego Impairment Index and schizophrenia: A validation study. *Journal of Personality Assessment, 59,* 165–175.

Posner, M. I., & Snyder, C. R. R. (1975). Facilitation and inhibition in the processing of signals. In P. M. A. Rabbitt & S. Dornic (Eds.), *Attention and performance* (pp. 669–682). New York: Academic Press.

Putnam, L. E. (1990). Great expectations: Anticipatory responses of the heart and brain. In J. W. Rohrbaugh, R. Parasuraman, & R. Johnson, Jr. (Eds.), *Event-related brain potentials: Basic issues and applications* (pp. 109–129). Oxford: Oxford University Press.

Schell, A. M., Dawson, M. E., Hazlett, E. A., & Filion, D. L. (1995). Attentional modulation of startle in psychosis-prone college students, *Psychophysiology, 32,* 266–273.

Schneider, W., Dumais, S. T., & Shiffrin, R. M. (1984). Automatic and controlled processing and attention. In R. Parasuraman, & J. Davies (Eds.), *Varieties of attention* (pp. 1–27). Orlando, Fla.: Academic Press.

Shiffrin, R. M., & Schneider, W. (1977). Controlled and automatic human information processing: II. Perceptual learning, automatic attending, and a general theory. *Psychological Review, 84,* 127–190.

Silverstein, L. D., Graham, F. K., & Calloway, J. M. (1980). Preconditioning and excitability of the human orbicularis oculi reflex as a function of state. *Electroencephalography and Clinical Neurophysiology, 48,* 406–417.

Simons, R. F., & Giardina, B. D. (1992). Reflex modification in psychosis-prone young adults. *Psychophysiology, 29,* 8–16.

Swerdlow, N. R., Benbow, C. H., Zisook, S., Geyer, M. A., & Braff, D. L. (1993). A preliminary assessment of sensorimotor gating in patients with obsessive compulsive disorder. *Biological Psychiatry, 33,* 298–301.

Swerdlow, N. R., Caine, S. B., Braff, D. L., & Geyer, M. A. (1992). The neural substrates of sensorimotor gating of the startle reflex: A review of recent findings and their implications. *Journal of Psychopharmacology, 2,* 132–146.

Swerdlow, N. R., & Koob, G. F. (1987). Dopamine, schizophrenia, mania, and depression: Toward a unified hypothesis of cortico-striato-pallido-thalamic function. *Behavioral and Brain Sciences, 10,* 197–245.

Venables, P. H. (1984). Cerebral mechanisms, autonomic responsiveness, and attention in schizophrenia. In W. D. Spaulding & J. K. Cole (Eds.), *Theories of schizophrenia & psychosis: Nebraska symposium of motivation 1983* (pp. 47–91). Lincoln: University of Nebraska Press.

12

Brain and th schizo

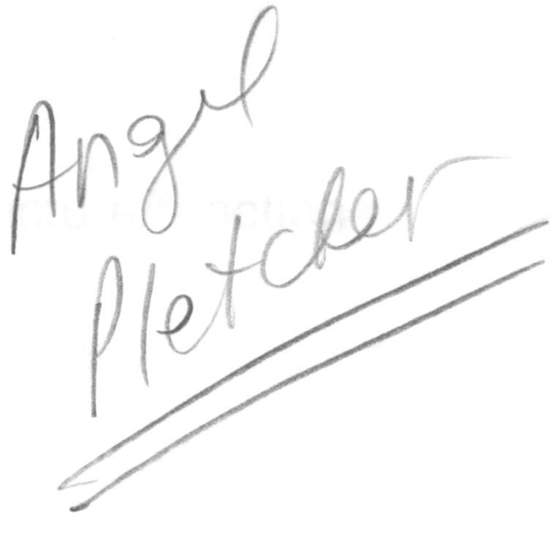

LARRY J

As the increasing complexity and multifactorial interaction of pathophysiological processes in schizophrenia are more apparent, the advantages of studying the full range of schizophrenic-spectrum disorders becomes more compelling. The milder schizophrenia-related disorders, of which schizotypal personality disorder (SPD) is the prototype, offer a unique opportunity to relatively disentangle and isolate the contingent pathophysiological processes involved in the schizophrenic disorders. Furthermore, such patients are much likelier to be free of potentially confounding artifacts such as long-term neuroleptic treatment, institutionalization, or chronic psychosis. Finally, since the genetic diathesis to schizophrenia is much more likely to be manifest as SPD or even schizotypal traits than as chronic schizophrenia, the study of SPD, especially among relatives of schizophrenic patients, may lead to a better understanding of the biology and genetics of schizophrenia and point to the appropriate selection of the affected phenotype in linkage studies currently underway.

Dopamine is implicated in the pathophysiology of schizophrenia by the antipsychotic effects of neuroleptic medications as well as by studies of plasma homovanillic acid and postmortem studies. Imaging studies suggest alterations in brain structure, whereas psychophysiological and neuropsychological tests point to abnormalities in brain function.

In this chapter, current work from our laboratory investigating the biology of SPDs is presented in the context of a model of the interaction of altered brain structure/function and the dopamine system in SPD and schizophrenia.

A model of positive and negative schizotypy

Both schizophrenic and schizotypal patients evince symptoms that are related to psychosis as well as to social deficits. The psychotic symptoms of schizophrenia include hallucinations, delusions, and evidence of gross thought disorder. The psychotic-like or "positive" symptoms of SPD include ideas of reference, magical thinking, perceptual distortions, and possibly suspiciousness. Whereas schizophrenic patients show profound impairments in social function with flat affect and social withdrawal, schizotypal patients are often characterized by deficit-like symptoms including social isolation and constricted affect (Siever, 1992). In schizophrenia, psychotic symptoms have been hypothesized to be related to abnormal dopamine activity, whereas the deficit symptoms have been hypothesized to be related to structural alterations of the brain (Crowe, 1980).

Although only limited support has been found for this dichotomy, more recent reformulations of the role of dopamine in brain structural alterations in schizophrenia emphasize decrements in cortical – particularly frontal cortical – function, associated with structural alterations in the brain and deficit symptoms, with secondary upregulation of limbic dopamine systems related to psychotic symptoms (Siever & Davis, 1991; Weinberger, 1987). Alterations in cortical circuits in frontal and related areas, related to either deficits in ascending dopaminergic tracks or descending glutaminergic tracks, could result in reduced inhibition of subcortical dopaminergic activity. The resultant hyperactivation of these circuits might account for the cognitive stereotypy and altered perceptions associated with schizophrenia. Individual differences in the sensitivity to subcortical dopaminergic upregulation secondary to cortical deafferentation might contribute to the variability in psychotic symptoms along the schizophrenic spectrum from predominantly deficit-symptom schizotypes without psychotic-like symptoms to severely psychotic chronic schizophrenic patients.

A number of lines of evidence are at least consistent with these formulations. For example, plasma homovanillic acid (HVA) concentrations are correlated with psychotic symptoms in schizophrenic patients, even though mean levels may actually be decreased (Davidson & Davis, 1988; Davis et al., 1985; Pickar et al., 1984). The Wisconsin Card Sort Task (WCST) is a neuropsychological test sensitive to frontal dysfunction. Performance of the WCST may be impaired in schizophrenic patients, and activation of dorsolateral prefrontal cortex (DLPFC) as indexed by blood flow imaging is reduced during the performance of the WCST (Weinberger, Berman, & Chase, 1986).

In one study, the decrements in performance on the WCST were correlated with the measures of decreased blood flow (Weinberger, Berman, & Zec, 1986). In a later study, the decreased blood flow during WCST performance was correlated with reductions in cerebrospinal fluid (CSF) HVA concentrations in schizophrenic patients (Weinberger, Berman, & Illowsky, 1988). The administration of apomorphine (Daniel, Berman, & Weinberger, 1989) and amphetamine to schizophrenic patients (Daniel et al., 1990) was associated with improved WCST performance and modestly increased frontal blood flow. Alterations of blood flow during the WCST has also been associated with structural damage to the hippocampus as indicated by magnetic resonance imaging (MRI) in a study of twins discordant for schizophrenia (Suddath, Casanova, Goldberg, Daniel, Kelso, & Weinberger, 1989).

Alterations in frontal, temporal, and enterorhinal cortex would be expected to impede the development of normal executive function and goal directed activity. In fact, dopaminergic activity at D_1 receptors may be important to the maintenance of working memory, a function necessary for social engagement as well as other executive functions (Sawaguchi & Goldman-Rakic, 1991). Along these lines, reduced concentrations of CSF HVA have been associated with poor outcome (Bowers, 1974; Bowers, Swigar, Jatlow, & Goicoechea, 1984) as well as social impairment (Lindstrom, 1985). The deficit symptoms of schizophrenia find a partial analogy in the motivational and cognitive deficits of Parkinson's disease, also characterized by dopaminergic deficits. In contrast to Parkinson's disease, however, hypodopaminergia in cortical areas may be associated with subcortical hyperdopaminergia in schizophrenia. However, because of these complex regional interactions, it has proved difficult to clarify the nature of these alterations in brain structure and function in relation to alterations in the dopamine system in schizophrenia.

The study of schizophrenia-spectrum personality disorders, particularly SPD, offers a relatively unique opportunity to disentangle and clarify these pathophysiological processes that may interact in chronic schizophrenia. Both "positive" and "negative" schizotypy have been found to be independently heritable and to have a differential pattern of psychophysiological correlates in studies of monozygotic twins (Kendler et al., 1989). "Positive" schizotypy includes psychotic-like symptoms of ideas of reference, magical thinking, and perceptual illusions or distortions, whereas the social deficit, or "negative," symptoms include social isolation, constricted affect, and odd comprise behavior. Neuropsychological and psychophysiological correlates like poor smooth-pursuit eye movements and poor attentional performance on the Continuous Performance Task (CPT) were particularly associated with "negative" schizotypy.

The independent heritability of these two dimensions supports the possibility that these two symptom clusters in SPD may have distinct antecedents, which may converge in chronic schizophrenia. A model of these partially distinct pathophysiological processes, which may be dissociable in SPD but converge in schizophrenia, suggests that the primary process from a genetic point of view is a neurodevelopmentally based lesion with clinical correlates of deficit-like symptoms (Siever et al., 1993b; Figures 12.1 and 12.2).

The neurodevelopmental pathophysiological process is unknown but has been hypothesized by some, for example, to represent a disorder of neuronal cell migration (Akbarian et al., 1993; Altsulter, Conrad, Kovelman, & Scheibel, 1987) that has an underlying genetic basis and that may be markedly influenced in its expression by early developmental events such as fetal hypoxia or viral infection (Murray, O'Callaghan, Castle, & Lewis, 1992). The genetic susceptibility to altered cortical development would then be reflected in malfunction of cortical processing and could be detected in information processing tasks. Deficient information processing appears to contribute to the deficit-like symptoms of SPD (Siever, Kalus, & Keefe, 1993). A neurodevelopment abnormality is thus hypothesized to be associated with the deficit-like symptoms of schizotypy, consistent with evidence suggesting that relatives of schizophrenic patients are more likely to evidence deficit-like than psychotic-like symptoms (Lenzenweger & Dworkin, 1984; Lyons, Merla, Young, & Kremen, 1991).

Structural alterations in cortical morphology reflecting a developmental impairment could be detected in histopathological studies or even more gross structural imaging. For example, cortical sulcal enlargement has been reported to be related to a genetic loading for schizophrenia-related disorders (Cannon, Mednick, & Parnas, 1989; Cannon, 1993), whereas increased ventricular size has been related to early obstetrical complications (Cannon et al., 1989, 1993). Performance on tasks sensitive to cortical (particularly prefrontal cortical) dysfunction might be hypothesized to be impaired in individuals with this developmental lesion. Other psychophysiological tasks that involve information processing and attention and require optimal cortical function would also be expected to be impaired and correlate with deficit-like symptoms including impaired eye tracking performance, poor performance on the CPT, impaired visual information processing on the backward masking test, and alterations in evoked potentials. Finally, these impairments would be hypothesized to be associated with hypofunction of the dopamine system, perhaps secondary to the neurodevelopmental structural alterations.

In contrast, the "positive" domain of schizotypal symptoms or psychotic-like symptoms would be expected to be associated with hyperdopaminergic function, particularly in subcortical areas. Increased dopaminergic activity,

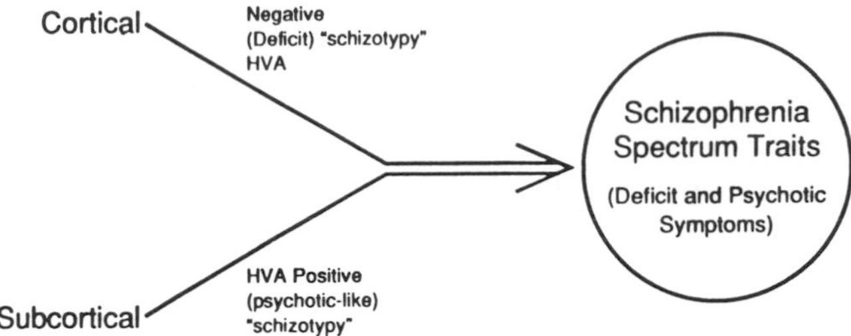

Fig. 12.1. Cortical and subcortical determinants of SPD symptoms/traits.

for example, as observed after high doses of amphetamine, might result in stereotyped cognition and even psychotic-like symptoms. Indeed, increased dopaminergic function might be associated with increased attentional performance and hypervigilance. Heightened susceptibility to increased dopaminergic activity or upregulation of subcortical dopamine systems in relation to stress or reduced cortical inhibition of subcortic might also be genetically mediated, although less specifically related to schizophrenia itself. When the second pathophysiological process occurs in isolation, that is, in the absence of prominent neurodevelopmental impairment, the result might be modest psychotic-like symptoms without the chronic psychosis of schizophrenia or its related deficit symptoms.

According to this model, individuals with mild to moderately severe neurodevelopmental impairment of cortical function might develop the deficit-like symptoms of SPD without prominent psychotic features. Such individuals would be hypothesized to be relatively less vulnerable to subcortical upregulation of dopaminergic circuits by virtue of cortical deaffrontation due to a cortical neurodevelopmental lesion. Thus, unlike chronic schizophrenic patients, "negative" schizotypes with prominent deficit-like symptoms would not go on to develop the chronic psychotic symptoms of schizophrenia. In contrast, schizophrenic individuals may be excessively vulnerable, possibly for distinct genetic reasons, to upregulation of subcortical dopaminergic systems and thus might respond to a neurodevelopmental lesion and cortical deaffrontation with pronounced increases in subcortical dopaminergic activity. This model builds on current hypotheses of the pathophysiology of schizophrenia, but incorporates the unique role of the schizophrenia-spectrum disorders where these two processes may be dissociated. Although hypotheses of regional differences or specific neurodevelopmental hypotheses relating to these two pathophysiological dimensions remain highly speculative, the presence of two relatively dissociable dimensions in schizotypy and their psy-

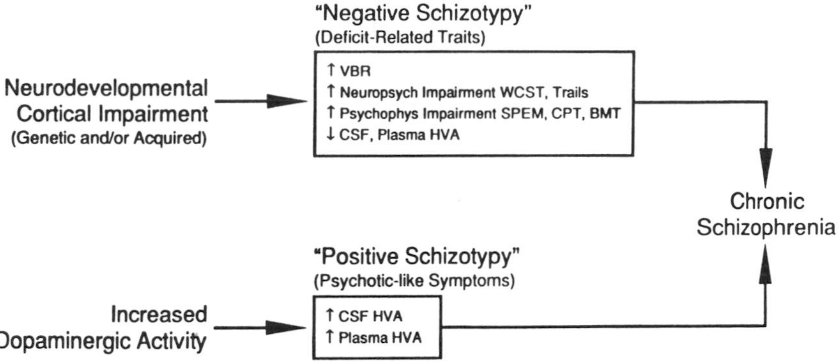

Fig. 12.2. Biological correlates of positive and negative schizotypy.

chobiologic correlates can be subjected to empirical scrutiny. In the next section, we examine available evidence from ongoing studies from our laboratory, as well as other laboratories that bear on the possibility of two pathophysiological processes in schizotypy.

"Deficit or negative" schizotypy

Structural imaging correlations

Increased ventricular size has been reported in two studies of clinically selected schizotypal patients (Cazzulo, Vita, Giobbio, Dieci, & Sacchetti, 1991; Rotter et al., 1991; Siever et al., 1993b, Siever, Rotter, Trestman, Coccaro, Losonczy, & Davis, 1993). In both studies, the lateral ventricles were enlarged. While these increases were associated with decreased psychotic-like symptoms in interim analyses of these studies from our laboratory (Rotter et al., 1991; Siever et al., 1993b), there were no symptomatic correlates in a larger extended series (Siever et al., 1993b). In the study from our laboratory, the left/right frontal horn ratio of the frontal horns was enlarged in SPD patients compared to other personality-disordered patients (Siever et al., 1993b); these findings were similar to those observed in Kraepelinian or chronic, unremitting schizophrenics (Keefe, Silverman, Siever, & Cornblatt, 1991). The left lateral ventricle was specifically enlarged in the schizotypal patients. Frontal horn size was correlated with impairment on neuropsychological tests sensitive to frontal dysfunction (e.g., the WCST and Trails B) but not with other neuropsychological tasks (Siever et al., 1993b).

Studies of relatives of schizophrenic patients have also suggested increased frontal horn size or ventricular size in some (Silverman et al., 1992) but not all studies (Olson, Nasrallah, & Lynn, 1993). In one study of offspring of schizophrenic patients, a genetic loading for schizophrenia was associated with increased cortical sulcal markings, whereas increased ventricular size was associated with obstetrical complications (Cannon et al., 1989, 1993).

Neuropsychological function

Abnormalities of performance on the WCST have been found in schizotypal volunteers selected by advertisement (Lyons et al., 1991), schizotypal volunteers selected by virtue of altered MMPI profiles (Spaulding, Garbin, & Dras, 1989), and SPD patients (DeVegvar et al., 1993; Siever et al., 1993b). In the study from our laboratory, the schizotypal patients showed impairment on the WCST as well as Trails B, but not on tests assessing more generalized cortical function, including the WAIS-R vocabulary and block design test. The SPD patients made more perseverative errors and completed fewer categories than other personality-disordered patients. Poor performance on the WCST and Trails B were correlated with deficit-related criteria for SPD as well as with increased ventricular brain ratio in frontal horn areas. Furthermore, perseverative errors on the WCST and Trails B were correlated or tended to be correlated with reduced concentrations of plasma HVA (DeVegvar et al., 1993; Wainberg, Trestman, Keefe, Cornblatt, DeVegvar, & Siever, 1993). Furthermore, abnormalities on the WCST were correlated with abnormalities on the Continuous Performance Test (CPT). In summary, schizotypal patients showed impairment on neuropsychological tests sensitive to prefrontal dysfunction; this impairment was significantly correlated with deficit-like symptoms, enlargement of frontal horn size, and tended to be correlated with reduced concentration of plasma HVA, consonant with the proposed model.

Psychophysiological/information processing tasks

A number of tests of information processing or attentional function that can be assessed psychophysiologically suggest impaired cortical information processing in SPD patients. For example, the smooth-pursuit system is recruited to enable the eye to follow a slowly moving target. Impairment has been demonstrated in schizophrenic patients and some schizotypal volunteers performing a variety of eye movement tasks including smooth pursuit tasks and antisaccade tasks (Holzman et al., Chapter 15, this volume). Impairment of eye movements on the smooth-pursuit task has been seen in 60–80% of schizophrenic patients and approximately half of their relatives (Holzman,

Solomon, Levin, & Waternaux, 1974, 1984), whereas eye movement impairment, although present in psychotic affective disorders, is not prevalent in the relatives of bipolar patients (Holzman et al., 1984) and may reflect a gene(s) underlying both eye tracking impairment and schizophrenia-related symptoms (Holzman et al., 1988). Eye movement impairment has also been found in schizotypal volunteers (Simons & Katkin, 1985) and patients with SPD (Siever et al., 1991, 1993b). Furthermore, increased prevalence of SPD and schizotypal traits was found in individuals selected from a college student population by virtue of their low tracking accuracy (Siever, Coursey, Alterman, Buchsbaum, & Murphy, 1984; Siever et al., 1989). Eye tracking impairment was correlated particularly with the deficit-like symptoms of SPDs in a number of studies (Siever et al., 1984, 1989, 1990, 1993b; Simons & Katkin, 1985; Van den Bosch, 1984). In one study of schizophrenic patients (Weinberger & Wyatt, 1982), eye tracking impairment was associated with ventricular enlargement in schizophrenic patients, but this has not been observed in other studies of schizophrenia (Siever et al., 1984) or SPD (Siever et al., 1993b).

The Continuous Performance Task (CPT) is a test of sustained attention that is rather consistently impaired in schizophrenic patients as well as schizotypal volunteers, schizophrenic offspring of schizophrenic patients, and SPD patients (see Siever et al., 1993b). In a recent study in our laboratory, errors of omission and commission did not distinguish SPD patients from other personality-disordered patients or normal controls, although very preliminary results using an identical pairs version of the CPT (Cornblatt & Erlenmeyer-Kimling, 1985) raised the possibility that this more difficult task may differentiate the SPD patients from comparison groups (Wainberg et al., 1993). In this study, CPT abnormalities were associated with impairment on the WCST as well as eye movement impairment and tended to correlate with deficit-like symptoms (Wainberg et al., 1993). In relatives of schizotypal patients, errors on the CPT were correlated with schizotypal symptoms (Moskowitz, Keefe, Harvey, Silverman, Siever, & Mohs, unpublished data). Studies of offspring of schizophrenic patients suggest that impairment of the CPT is associated particularly with deficit symptoms (Cornblatt, Lenzenweger, Dworkin, & Erlenmeyer-Kimling, 1992; Mirsky, 1988).

Other attentional tasks such as the backward masking task have been shown to be abnormal in unmedicated schizotypal patients (Braff, 1981) and schizotypal volunteers and associated with deficit symptoms in schizophrenia (Saccuzzo & Schulbert, 1981; see review by Siever, Silverman, & Bernstein, 1991). More recently, defects in sensory gating have been reported in schizotypal patients (Cadenhead et al., 1993). Evoked potential abnormalities have been found in some (Kutcher et al., 1989) but not all (e.g., Kalus et al., 1991) studies of SPD.

In summary, impairment has been found in a variety of attentional, information processing, psychophysiological tasks in schizotypal patients, or volunteers, or relatives of schizophrenic patients, and these have often, but not always consistently, been associated with the deficit-like symptoms of SPD. These tests have been less consistently evaluated in relation to measures of cortical activity and brain structure.

Functional imaging

In a variety of studies, schizophrenic patients demonstrate reduced or altered patterns of activation of prefrontal and other cortical areas during cognitive tasks (Rubin et al., 1991; Weinberger et al., 1986). In particular, reductions and activation of prefrontal areas during the WCST have been reported (Rubin et al., 1991; Weinberger et al., 1986). Functional imaging studies have not yet been reported in schizotypal patients, although preliminary studies in our laboratory raise the possibility that schizotypal patients show increased activation both of prefrontal areas and of other cortical nonfrontal areas, but relatively reduced subcortical activation, compared to normal controls. These very preliminary results hint at the possibility that schizotypal patients may overactivate frontal areas as well as utilize other cortical areas not normally recruited for the WCST to compensate for frontal inefficiency.

Dopaminergic activity and deficit-like symptoms

Reduced indices of dopaminergic activity are hypothesized to be related to deficit-like symptoms. In relatives of schizophrenic patients, primarily characterized by deficit-like symptoms in our and other laboratories (Lenzenweger & Dworkin, 1984; Lyons et al., 1991), plasma HVA concentrations are lower in relatives with SPD than in those without SPD (Amin et al., 1993). Furthermore, the reductions have been correlated with the deficit-like criteria of SPD (Amin et al., 1993), consistent with the predominance of deficit-like symptoms in relatives of schizophrenic patients (Lenzenweger & Dworkin, 1984; Lyons et al., 1991). In clinically selected schizotypal patients, there is a trend for reductions of plasma HVA to be correlated with deficit-like symptoms (Siever et al., unpublished data). However, plasma HVA concentrations in schizotypal patients are driven primarily by those with the "positive," psychotic-like symptoms.

In a preliminary study of SPD (Wainberg et al., 1993), amphetamine, which releases dopamine and blocks its reuptake thus making it more available in the synapse, appeared to improve neuropsychological performance on the WCST. Indeed, as neuropsychological performance improved, there was no worsening of clinical symptomatology. Plasma HVA concentrations tended to be reduced after amphetamine (Siever et al., unpublished data). Although further studies are required, these interim results of ongoing studies suggest that hypodopaminergia may be associated with cognitive impairment and deficit-like symptoms in SPD patients and hint at the possibility that dopamine-enhancing agents may improve the deficit-like symptoms. Those agents that enhance dopamine activation at postsynaptic D_1 receptors in the frontal cortex might be particularly valuable in this regard.

"Positive" or psychotic-like symptoms of schizotypy

In clinically selected samples of schizotypal and other personality-disordered patients, CSF and plasma HVA were found to be elevated in the schizotypal patients as compared to the other personality-disordered and/or normal control comparison groups (Siever et al., 1991, 1993a). In both cases, the increases in plasma HVA correlated positively with the psychotic-like symptoms, but not with the deficit-like symptoms, of SPD. Indeed, group differences were accounted for by those schizotypal individuals with prominent psychotic-like symptoms so that covariation for these symptoms abolished the group differences.

Neuroleptic medications have led to improvements in psychotic-like symptoms of SPD as well as positive symptoms of anxiety and obsessionality (Goldberg, Schulz, & Schulz, 1986; Hymowitz, Frances, Jacobsberg, Sickles, & Hoyt, 1986; Schulz, Cornelius, Schulz, & Soloff, 1988). These results suggest that dopamine antagonists may improve the psychotic-like symptoms of SPD, perhaps by blocking dopaminergic activation, particularly in patients with increased indices of dopaminergic activity as in schizophrenic patients (Bowers et al., 1984).

Implications of a bidimensional model for schizophrenia research

Clearly, the patterns of findings to date are based on interim results of ongoing studies, many of which are only preliminary. Although results to date conform in a number of respects with the model proposed, they can offer no definitive confirmation or disconfirmation of such a model at this time. However, such a model does have heuristic value in organizing future research on the pathophysiology and the genetics of schizophrenia. A multidimensional model calls for consideration of more complex inheritance patterns in linkage studies of schizophrenia, with the underlying genotype being more likely to be manifested as more subtle deficit-like clinical and cognitive symptomatology than is evidenced in chronic schizophrenia or even SPD. Modifying factors that may impact on dopaminergic activity may be related to amplifying this vulnerability in the direction of chronic psychosis. Both factors may need to be taken into account ultimately to define the genetics of the schizophrenia spectrum disorders.

More specific regional hypotheses of alteration in structure and dopamine activity will clearly require more specific imaging techniques to target dopaminergic activity in specific cortical regions. The specific labeling of D_1 and D_2 receptors in particular brain regions may be helpful as may be studies of fluorinated DOPA which may provide an index of presynaptic dopamine release. Basal studies of brain metabolic activity assessed by region in relation to psychotic-like and deficit-like symptoms may also be helpful. Although such studies may be complicated to interpret in schizophrenic patients, the models proposed suggest that in schizotypal patients, these advanced methodologies may be useful for effective dissociation of the psychotic-like and deficit-like aspects of the clinical picture.

Studies using pharmacological probes that enhance dopaminergic activity directly by releasing dopamine or by acting directly at D_1 receptors may be helpful in evaluating the relationship among dopamine activity, cognitive performance, and clinical symptomatology. Simultaneous imaging of functional activity before and after pharmacological challenge during a task performance may be particularly useful. Thus, for example, dopaminergic enhancement by amphetamine of the performance of WCST might be assessed by functional imaging during the WCST on and off the dopaminergic challenge. Similar strategies might be applied to the assessment of verbal learning and temporal lobe function. In these ways, the study of schizophrenia-spectrum disorders may uniquely contribute to our understanding of the pathophysiology of schizophrenia.

References

Akbarian, S., Bunney, W. E., Jr., Potkin, S. G., Wigal, S. B., Hagman, J., Sandman, C. A., & Jones, E. G. (1993). Altered distribution of nicotinamide-adenine dinucleotide phosphate-diaphorase in frontal lobe of schizophrenics implies disturbances of cortical development. *Archives of General Psychiatry, 50,* 169–177.

Altsulter, L. L., Conrad, A., Kovelman, J. A., & Scheibel, A. (1987). Hippocampal pyramidal cell orientation in schizophrenia. *Archives of General Psychiatry, 44,* 1904–1908.

Amin, F., Silverman, J. M., Dumont, L., Zaccario, M., Kahn, R. S., Schwarz, M., Davidson, M., & Siever, L. J. (1993). Plasma HVA in non-psychotic first-degree relatives of schizophrenic probands. American Psychiatric Association, *New Research Abstracts,* NR221.

Bowers, M. B. (1974). Central dopamine turnover in schizophrenic syndromes. *Archives of General Psychiatry, 31,* 50–54.

Bowers, M., Swigar, M., Jatlow, P., & Goicoechea, N. (1984). Plasma catecholamine metabolism and early response to haloperidol. *Journal of Clinical Psychiatry, 45,* 248–251.

Braff, D. L. (1981). Impaired speed of information processing in nonmedicated schizotypal patients. *Schizophrenia Bulletin, 7,* 499–508.

Cadenhead, K. S., Geyer, M. A., & Braff, D. L. (1993). Information processing at the boundaries of schizophrenia. *48th Annual Meeting of Biological Psychiatry, 33*(6A), 89.

Cannon, T. D., Mednick, S. A., & Parnas, J. (1989). Genetic and perinatal determinants of structural brain deficits in schizophrenia. *Archives of General Psychiatry, 46,* 883–889.

Cannon, T. D., et al. (1993). Developmental brain abnormalities in the offspring of schizophrenic mothers. *Archives of General Psychiatry, 50,* 551–564.

Cazzullo, C., Vita, A., Giobbio, G., Dieci, M., & Sacchetti, E. (1991). Cerebral structural abnormalities In schizophreniform disorder and in schizophrenia spectrum personality disorders. In C. A. Tamminga & S. C. Schulz (Eds.), *Advances in neuropsychiatry and psychopharmacology, Vol. 1: Schizophrenia research* (pp. 209–217). New York: Raven Press.

Cornblatt, B., & Erlenmeyer-Kimling, L. (1985). Global attentional deviance as a marker of risk for schizophrenia: Specificity and predictive validity. *Journal of Abnormal Psychology, 94,* 470–486.

Cornblatt, B. A., Lenzenweger, M. F., Dworkin, R. H., & Erlenmeyer-Kimling, L. (1992). Childhood attentional dysfunctions predict social deficits in unaffected adults at risk for schizophrenia. *British Journal of Psychology, 161* (Suppl. 18), 59–64.

Crowe, T. J. (1980). Molecular pathology of schizophrenia: More than one disease process? *British Medical Journal, 280,* 66–68.

Daniel, D. G., Berman, K. F., & Weinberger, D. R. (1989). The effect of apomorphine on regional cerebral blood flow in schizophrenia. *Journal of Neuropsychiatry, 1,* 377–384.

Daniel, D. G., Breslin, N., Clardy, J., Goldberg, T., Gold, J., Kleinman, J., & Weinberger, D. (1990). The effect of L-dopa on negative symptoms: Cognitive performance and regional cerebral blood flow in schizophrenia. *Biological Psychiatry, 27,* Abstract No. 174.

Davidson, M., & Davis, K. L. (1988). A comparison of plasma homovanillic acid concentrations in schizophrenics and normal controls. *Archives of General Psychiatry, 45,* 561–563.

Davis, K. L., Davidson, M., Mohs, R. C., Kendler, K., Davis, B., Johns, C., DeNigris, Y., & Horvath, T. (1985). Plasma homovanillic acid concentration and the severity of schizophrenic illness. *Science, 227,* 1601–1602.

DeVegvar, M., Keefe, R. S. E., Moskowitz, J., Lees, S., Knott, P., Trestman, R. L., & Siever, I. J. (1993). Frontal lobe dysfunction and schizotypal personality disorder. Washington, D.C.: American Psychiatric Association, *New Research Abstracts,* NR502.

Goldberg, S. C., Schulz, S. C., & Schulz, P. M. (1986). Borderline and schizotypal personality disorders treated with low-dose thiothixene vs placebo. *Archives of General Psychiatry, 43,* 680–686.

Holzman, P. S., Kringlen, E., Matthysse, S., Flanagan, S., Lipton, R. B., Cramer, G.,

Levin, S., Lange, K., & Levy, D. L. (1988). A single dominant gene can account for eye tracking dysfunctions and schizophrenia in offspring of discordant twins. *Archives of General Psychiatry, 45,* 641–647.

Holzman, P. S., Solomon, C. M., Levin, S., & Waternaux, C. S. (1974). Eye-tracking dysfunctions in schizophrenic patients and their relatives. *Archives of General Psychiatry, 41,* 136–139.

Holzman, P. S., Solomon, C. M., Levin, S., & Waternaux, C. S. (1984). Pursuit eye movement dysfunctions in schizophrenia; family evidence for specificity. *Archives of General Psychiatry, 41,* 136–139.

Hymowitz, P., Frances, A., Jacobsberg, L. B., Sickles, M., & Hoyt, R. (1986). Neuroleptic treatment of schizotypal personality disorders. *Comprehensive Psychiatry, 27,* 267–271.

Kalus, O., Horvath, T. B., Peterson, A., Coccaro, E. F., Mitropoulou, V., Davidson, M., Davis, K. L., & Siever, L. J. (1991). Event related potentials in schizotypal personality disorder and schizophrenia. *Biological Psychiatry, 29,* 43a–185a.

Keefe, R. S. E., Silverman, J. M., Siever, L. J., & Cornblatt, B. A. (1991). Refining phenotype characterization in genetic linkage studies of schizophrenia. *Social Biology, 38,* 197–218.

Kendler, K., Walsh, D., Su, Y., McGuire, M., Spellman, M., Lytle, C., McCormick, O., O'Neill, A., Shinkwin, R., Nuallain, N., O'Hare, A., Kidd, K., MacLean, C., & Diehl, S. (1989). The Roscommon family and linkage study of schizophrenia: Preliminary report. Abstracts presented at the 28th Annual Meeting of the American College of Neuropsychopharmacology, p. 56.

Kety, S. S., Wender, P. H., Jacobsen, B., Ingraham, L. J., Jansson, L., Faber, B., & Kinney, D. K. (1994). Mental illness in the biological and adoptive relatives of schizophrenic adoptees: Replication of the Copenhagen study in the rest of Denmark. *Archives of General Psychiatry, 51,* 442–455.

Kutcher, S. P., Blackwood, D. H. R., Gaskell, D. F., Muir, W. J., & St. Clair, D. M. (1989). Auditory P300 does not differentiate borderline personality disorder from schizotypal personality disorder. *Biological Psychiatry, 26,* 766–774.

Lenzenweger, M. F., & Dworkin, R. H. (1984). Symptoms and the genetics of schizophrenia: Implication for diagnosis. *American Journal of Psychiatry, 141,* 1541–1546.

Lindstrom, L. H. (1985). Low HVA and normal 5-HIAA CSF in drug-free schizophrenic patients compared to healthy volunteers: Correlations to symptomatology and family history. *Psychiatric Research, 14,* 265–273.

Lyons, M. J., Merla, M. E., Young, L., & Kremen, W. S. (1991). Impaired neuropsychological functioning in symptomatic volunteers with schizotypy: Preliminary findings. *Biological Psychiatry, 30,* 424–426.

Mirsky, A. (1988). Research on schizophrenia in the NIMH Laboratory of Psychology and Psychopathology. *Schizophrenia Bulletin, 14,* 151–156.

Murray, R. M., O'Callaghan, E., Castle, D., & Lewis, S. (1992). A Neurodevelopmental approach to the classification of schizophrenia. *Schizophrenia Bulletin, 18,* 319–333.

Olson, S. C., Nasrallah, H. A., & Lynn, M. B. (1993). Brain morphology in schizophrenics and their siblings. American Psychiatric Association, *New Research Abstracts,* NR221.

Pickar, D., Labarca, R., Linnoila, M., Roy, A., Hommer, D., Everett, D., & Paul, S. (1984). Neuroleptic induced decrease in plasma homovanillic acid and antipsychotic activity in schizophrenic patients. *Science, 225,* 954–956.

Rotter, M., Kalus, O., Losonczy, M., Guo, L., Trestman, R. L., Coccaro, E., Davidson, M., Davis, K. L., & Siever, L.J. (1991). Lateral ventricle enlargement in schizotypal personality disorder. *Biological Psychiatry, 29,* 43a–185a.

Rubin, P., Holm, S., Friberg, L., Videbech, P., Steen-Andersen, H., Bjerg-Bendsen, B., Stromso, N., Knud-Larsen, J., Lassen, N., & Hemmingsen, R. (1991). Altered modulation of prefrontal and subcortical brain activity in newly diagnosed schizophrenia and schizophreniform disorder: A regional cerebral blood flow study. *Archives of General Psychiatry, 48,* 987–996.

Saccuzzo, D. P., & Schubert, D. L. (1981). Backward masking as a measure of slow processing in schizophrenia spectrum disorders. *Journal of Abnormal Psychology, 90,* 305–312.

Sawaguchi, T., & Golman-Rakic, P. S. (1991). D_1 dopamine receptors in prefrontal cortex: Involvement in working memory. *Science, 251,* 947–950.

Schulz, S. C., Cornelius, J., Schulz, P. M., Soloff, P. H. (1988). The amphetamine challenge test in patients with borderline disorder. *American Journal of Psychiatry, 145,* 809–814.

Siever, L. J. (1991). The biology of the boundaries of schizophrenia. In C. A. Tamminga & S. C. Schulz (Eds.), *Advances in neuropsychiatry and psychopharmacology, Vol. 1: Schizophrenia research* (pp. 181–191). New York: Raven Press.

Siever, L. J. (1992). The schizophrenic spectrum personality disorders. In A. Tasman (Ed.), *Annual Review of Psychiatry* (pp. 25–42). Washington, D.C.: APA.

Siever, L. J., Amin, F., Coccaro, E. F., Trestman, R. L., Silverman, J. M., Horvath, T. B., Mahon, T. R., Knott, P., Davidson, M., & Davis, K. L. (1993a). Cerebrospinal fluid homovanillic acid in schizotypal personality disorder. *American Journal of Psychiatry, 150,* 149–151.

Siever, L. J., Amin, F., Coccaro, E. F., Bernstein, D., Kavoussi, R. J., Kalus, O., Horvath, T. B., Warner, P., Davidson, M., & Davis, K. (1991). Plasma homovanillic acid in schizotypal personality disorder patients and controls. *American Journal of Psychiatry, 148,* 1246–1248.

Siever, L. J., Coursey, R. D., Alterman, I. S., Buchsbaum, M. S., & Murphy, D. L. (1984). Impaired smooth-pursuit eye movement: Vulnerability marker for schizotypal personality disorder in a normal volunteer population. *American Journal of Psychiatry, 141,* 1560–1566.

Siever, L. J., Coursey, R. D., Alterman, I. S., Zahn, T., Brody, L., Bernad, P., Buchsbaum, M. S., Lake, C. R., & Murphy, D. L. (1989). Clinical, psychophysiologic, and neurologic characteristics of volunteers with impaired smooth pursuit eye movements. *Biological Psychiatry, 26,* 35–51.

Siever, L. J., & Davis, K. L. (1991). A psychobiological perspective on the personality disorders. *American Journal of Psychiatry, 148,* 1647–1658.

Siever, L. J., Kalus, O., & Keefe, R. S. E. (1993b). The boundaries of schizophrenia. *Psychiatric Clinics of North America, 16,* 217–244.

Siever, L. J., Coccaro, E. F., Klar, H. M., Zemishland, Z., Peterson, A., Davidson, M., Mahon, T., Horvath, T., & Mohs, R. (1990). Eye tracking impairment in clinically identified schizotypal personality disorder patients. *American Journal of Psychiatry, 147,* 740–745.

Siever, L. J., Rotter, M., Trestman, R. L., Coccaro, E. F., Losonczy, M., & Davis, K. L. (1993c). Increased ventricular brain ratio in schizotypal personality disorder. American Psychiatric Association, 146th Annual Meeting. *New Research Abstracts,* NR335.

Siever, L. J., Silverman, J. M., & Bernstein, D. (1991). Schizotypal personality disorder: A review of its current status. *Journal of Personality Disorders, 5,* 178–193.

Silverman, J. M., Keefe, R. S. E., Losonczy, M. F., Li, G., O'Brian, V., Mohs, R. C., & Siever, L. J. (1992). Schizotypal and neuro-imaging factors in relatives of schizophrenic probands. *Society of Biological Psychiatry Annual Meeting, 31* (April), 70a.

Simons, R. F., & Katkin, W. (1985). Smooth pursuit eye movements in subjects reporting physical anhedonia and perceptual aberrations. *Psychiatry Research, 14,* 275–289.

Spaulding, W., Garbin, C. P., & Dras, S. R. (1989). Cognitive abnormalities in schizophrenic patients and schizotypal college students. *Journal of Nervous and Mental Diseases, 177,* 717–728.

Suddath, R. L., Casanova, M. F., Goldberg, T. E., Daniel, D. G., Kelsoe, J. R., Jr., & Weinberger, D. R. (1989). Temporal lobe pathology in schizophrenia; a quantitative magnetic resonance imaging study. *American Journal of Psychiatry, 146,* 464–472.

Van den Bosch, R. J. (1984). Eye tracking impairment: Attentional and psychometric correlates in psychiatric patients. *Psychiatry Research, 18,* 277, 286.

Wainberg, M. L., Trestman, R. L., Keefe, R. S. E., Cornblatt, B., DeVegvar, M. L., & Siever, L. J. (1993). Continuous Performance Test in schizotypal personality disorder. 146th Annual Meeting of the American Psychiatric Association.

Weinberger, D. R. (1987). Implications of normal brain development for the pathogenesis of schizophrenia. *Archives of General Psychiatry, 44,* 660–669.

Weinberger, D. R., Berman, K. F., & Chase, T. N. (1986). Prefrontal cortex physiological activation in Parkinson's disease: Effect of L-dopa. *Neurology, 36* (Suppl.), 170.

Weinberger, D. R., Berman, K. F., & Illowsky, B. P. (1988). Physiological dysfunction of dorsolateral prefrontal cortex in schizophrenia. III. A new cohort and evidence for a monoaminergic mechanism. *Archives of General Psychiatry, 45*(7), 609–615.

Weinberger, D. R., Berman, K. F., & Zec, R. F. (1986). Physiologic dysfunction of dorsolateral prefrontal cortex in schizophrenia. I. Regional cerebral blood flow evidence. *Archives of General Psychiatry, 43,* 114–124.

Weinberger, D. R., & Wyatt, R. J. (1982). Cerebral ventricular size: A biological marker for subtyping chronic schizophrenia. In Usdin, E., & Hamin, I. (Eds.), *Biological markers in psychiatry and neurology* (pp. 505–512). New York: Pergamon Press.

PART VI

Neuropsychology

13

Neuropsychological abnormalities associated with schizotypal personality

TODD LENCZ, ADRIAN RAINE, DEANA S. BENISHAY, SHARI MILLS, and LAURA BIRD

As more and more evidence has accumulated to support the hypothesis of a genetic basis to schizophrenia (Fowles, 1992; Meehl, 1990), research has turned increasingly toward examining biological mechanisms that may underlie the disorder. Researchers have attempted to isolate neuroanatomical, psychophysiological, cognitive, and neuropsychological impairments in schizophrenics that may be expressions of what Meehl (1990) termed the "integrative neural defect." This defect is the phenotypic manifestation of the schizogene(s) and is theorized to set the stage for the emergence of psychotic symptomatology. Since such research is etiological in nature, the goal is to identify stable traits that are not merely the by-products of the disease or state-dependent indices of current symptomatology but rather are present irrespective of the waxing and waning of symptoms.

However, basic research into such biological mechanisms in schizophrenic subjects faces a number of potential confounds and obstacles. These include the difficulties of maintaining and assessing motivation and task-focus in actively symptomatic patients. In addition, the effects on dependent measures of neuroleptic medication and institutionalization (often long-term) are not easily teased out. Because of these confounds, research has increasingly turned toward the examination of nonschizophrenic subjects who are at high risk for the disorder. Studying subjects who are schizotypal or hypothetically psychosis-prone has a number of advantages for the identification of psychological, cognitive, and psychophysiological deficits that are vulnerability markers for the disorder. It overcomes the potential confounds mentioned above, as schizotypal subjects are (generally speaking) functionally intact, nonpsychotic, unmedicated, and unhospitalized. Furthermore, replication in schizotypals of deficits found in schizophrenics lends additional support to the hypothesis that such deficits are etiological factors, possibly with a genetic basis. Thus, research utilizing schizotypal subjects represents an important and rapidly growing area of schizophrenia research.

The study of cognitive and neuropsychological deficits constitutes an area in which research on schizotypals can be particularly useful. Studies on schizophrenics have tended to show across-the-board deficits on tasks that exceed a threshold of difficulty (e.g., Spaulding, Garbin, & Dras, 1989), and the identification of differential deficits is rather difficult (Chapman & Chapman, 1978). If schizotypals share (at least some of) the same genetic vulnerability, and that vulnerability is manifested as a neurodevelopmental abnormality, then it can be expected that schizotypals may exhibit more isolable cognitive and neuropsychological deficits related to the specific areas under the influence of the defective gene(s).

Neuropathology

Since the theory holds that the genetic liability is expressed as a central nervous system deficit, it seems reasonable to begin with a brief review of the neuropathology of schizophrenia. A recent review (Bilder & Degreef, 1991) of neurodevelopmental processes in schizophrenia suggested that there may be three independent brain morphological abnormalities implicated in the etiology of the disorder. On the basis of the extensive neuroimaging and neuropsychological literature in schizophrenia, Bilder and Degreef proposed that the three affected systems include (1) the periventricular region, (2) the frontolimbic system, and (3) the development of cerebral specialization, particularly the normal differentiation of the right and left hemispheres. According to this review, the pathophysiological disturbances in each of these systems have their own distinct etiologies and are manifested in different functional deficits.

Of these three neurodevelopmental disturbances, only the latter two are believed to be based on a primarily genetic etiology; they are thought to reflect malfunctions of the genes controlling normal neuronal migration (cf. Cannon, Mednick, & Parnas, 1989; Crow et al., 1989; Weinberger, 1987). Thus, they constitute likely prospects for investigations of subjects genetically related to schizophrenics – that is, schizotypals. Neuropsychological performance on tests measuring frontolimbic deficits and abnormalities of cerebral asymmetry has been studied extensively in schizotypy. It should be noted that most of the neuropsychological studies of schizotypals were not necessarily conducted under the tripartite neurodevelopmental theory outlined above; nevertheless, the frontolimbic and cerebral asymmetry hypotheses serve as useful guides for much of the published literature in this area.

Factors of schizotypy

The notion of separable pathophysiologies of schizophrenia raises an important conceptual issue to be addressed by schizotypal research: Are there separate syndromes of schizophrenia (and schizotypy) with distinct etiologies and correlates? A number of factor-analytic studies (Venables, Chapter 6, this volume) have demonstrated that there are at least two or three factors that underlie scores on conventional schizotypy scales. Of particular interest is a recent study by Raine and colleagues (1994), which used confirmatory factor analysis to identify that DSM-III-R schizotypal personality criteria are best fit to a three-factor solution featuring cognitive–perceptual, social–interpersonal, and disorganized symptom factors. This three-factor solution is consistent with the most recent factor-analytic studies in schizophrenia (Venables, Chapter 6, this volume). It may be the case that each of these factors is differentially correlated with these major pathophysiological processes.

Some researchers who have examined schizotypy from a biological/genetic perspective argue that the "negative" or social–interpersonal factor of schizotypy reflects the primary genetic liability and that these symptoms should therefore be correlated with tests of central nervous system functioning (Siever, 1985). As can be seen from the studies reviewed below, this hypothesis is not cleanly borne out by the data; the cognitive abnormalities reported here correlate differentially with a variety of schizotypal scales which are orthogonal in some cases and partially overlapping in others. Most frequently, and perhaps not surprisingly, cognitive abnormalities are related to traits and symptoms of the cognitive–perceptual factor.

Neuropsychological studies

With these points in mind, this chapter first reviews studies tapping frontolimbic deficits. It should be noted that the term "frontolimbic" is quite broad and can refer to a number of hypothesized circuits. It is used here as an umbrella term to refer to studies that examine learning and executive functions such as the filtering of information and the maintenance of cognitive focus or the shifting of cognitive set. These executive and learning systems are believed to be subserved by frontolimbic circuitry, including specifically the prefrontal lobes (Stuss & Benson, 1986) and the hippocampus (Venables, 1992). As

Frith and Done (1988) note, there are several circuits connecting prefrontal and limbic cortex, and different deficits would be expected from breakdowns at different points in the circuit. As will be seen, the published results are not sufficiently specific to make such delineations. Consequently, the term "frontolimbic" will be employed to include all findings potentially pertaining to functions of this circuit.

A wide variety of experimental manipulations of learning, selective attention, and cognitive flexibility have been devised which in some way tap the ability of the subject to limit or inhibit the contents of consciousness in order to successfully perform a task. This chapter reviews only those that require subjects to perform a task. Psychophysiological measures of cognitive inhibition, such as the startle-blink paradigm, are discussed elsewhere (Dawson, Schell, Hazlett, Filion, & Nuechterlein, Chapter 11, this volume). Findings from such studies, detailed below, address the frequently mentioned hypothesis (Braff, 1993; Frith, 1979; McGhie & Chapman, 1961) that the core deficit in schizophrenia is an inability to focus attention, to inhibit irrelevant stimuli, and thereby to control the contents of consciousness.

This hypothesis rests on the fact that the normal process of attending to a particular stimulus involves the active inhibition of competing stimuli. The failure to inhibit is in turn hypothesized to give rise to hallucinations, explanatory delusions, and formal thought disorder in schizophrenia. The cognitive disinhibition hypothesis of schizophrenia was extended by Beech and Claridge (1987) as an explanation for the symptoms of schizotypy. After a summary and discussion of the literature which explicitly or implicitly addresses this hypothesis, we then turn to the cerebral asymmetries literature.

Tests of cognitive inhibition

Just as the term "frontolimbic" is used here as an umbrella term, it is fair to say that "cognitive inhibition" is an umbrella term, since many of the processes of the brain can be characterized as inhibitory. Four types of neuropsychological tests examining different facets of cognitive inhibition have been utilized in studies of schizotypy. In order of increasing processing demands, these four include (1) perceptual/sustained attention tasks, (2) priming tasks, (3) learning tasks, and (4) conceptual inhibition tasks measuring perseveration. In the review of this literature, several key issues will be highlighted, including the types of information processing involved (automatic vs. controlled); the timing of information processing; and the specificity of findings to particular factors of schizotypy.

Sustained attention

One well-researched cognitive test that involves the ability to ignore irrelevant stimuli and focus on a particular type of stimulus is the Continuous Performance Test (CPT). There are different versions of the CPT, but in all, the subject is presented with a series of numbers very rapidly (100-ms presentation time) and is required to press a button in response to a particular number or sequence of numbers. The subject must filter out irrelevant stimuli (nontargets) to focus in on the task requirement and respond at the right time. Positron emission tomography (PET) studies of the CPT have shown that performance of this task activates the frontal lobes, particularly in the right hemisphere, in normal subjects (Buchsbaum et al., 1990). The CPT is well studied in schizophrenia (Cornblatt & Keilp 1994), and performance deficits are found in schizophrenics regardless of symptom status.

To date, four studies have examined CPT performance in relation to schizotypy (Condray & Steinhauer, 1992; Grove, Lebow, Clementz, Cerri, Medus, & Iacono, 1991; Lenzenweger, Cornblatt, & Putnick, 1991; Venables, 1990). All of these studies found that increased errors were related to cognitive–perceptual symptoms of schizotypy as measured by self-report questionnaire. Relationship of performance to anhedonia (an analogue of interpersonal symptoms) was mixed. Finally, in a unique analysis, Grove et al. determined that CPT accuracy had high heritability ($h^2 = .79$) and significant genetic correlations with the Chapmans' scales of Perceptual Aberration (PerAb, Chapman, Chapman, & Raulin, 1978) and Physical Anhedonia (PA, Chapman, Chapman, & Raulin, 1976) as well as an interview measure of social–interpersonal schizotypal symptoms.

The Span of Apprehension test (SOA) is similar to the CPT, insofar as it requires subjects to pick out a particular stimulus from an array of nontargets. However, the SOA presents the target and the distractors simultaneously, rather than in succession. Subjects must pick out a "T" or "F" from a field of 12 letters with each display presented for only 40 ms. In two studies, SOA performance was significantly related to cognitive–perceptual symptoms but was unrelated to anhedonia (Asarnow, Nuechterlein, & Marder, 1983; Venables, 1990).

Discussion. The nature of stimulus presentation in the SOA allows us to address an important conceptual issue: Which component of information processing is affected in schizotypy? The SOA is the only information processing measure in which the distractors are presented simultaneous with the target rather than serially, and the presentation time is extremely brief (40 ms). As such, it defines one end of the process of sorting information. The strength of the relationship between the SOA and schizotypy lends support to the hypothesis that there is a deficit in automatic, preconscious information processing (Dawson et al., Chapter 11, this volume). Such automatic processing is hypothesized to be the first step in filtering the contents of consciousness. In evaluating the results from the further studies described below, it should be remembered that information processing is a *process,* and the nature of the relationship of preconscious filtering to conscious awareness changes over the course of a second. Further studies are needed, utilizing tasks tapping different stages in the process of filtering information, in order to tease out different cognitive mechanisms with differential correlates at early and late stages of information processing.

Negative priming

In an explicit test of the cognitive disinhibition hypothesis, Beech and his colleagues (Beech & Claridge, 1987; Beech, Baylis, Smithson, & Claridge, 1989; Beech, Powell, McWilliam, & Claridge, 1989) examined deficits in negative priming in schizophrenics and schizotypals. Negative priming refers to the delay in responding that occurs in response to a target stimulus that was actively ignored on a previous trial (Tipper, 1985). In this paradigm, the ignored stimulus is viewed as being actively inhibited rather than simply passively decaying. The active inhibition causes the delay in responding on the subsequent trial.

The methodology for negative priming experiments is described elsewhere (Claridge & Beech, Chapter 9, this volume). In their first experiment (Beech & Claridge, 1987), these researchers found that low scorers on the STA scale of schizotypy (Claridge & Broks, 1984) showed a significant negative priming effect, whereas for subjects in the high STA group, the priming effect was abolished. In fact, the high STA scorers showed a slight facilitation (decrease in RT) on trials following a priming distractor.

This finding is significant for a number of reasons. First, this result shows that in normals (low STA scorers), the ignored stimulus is processed, and it exercises an active effect on conscious processing of subsequent stimuli. Both the negative priming effect and the facilitation effect support the notion that conscious processing involves active inhibition of competing stimuli, and that this inhibition is a form of preconscious processing. Second, it demonstrates a significant relationship between schizotypy and information processing; it should be noted that the STA taps primarily cognitive–perceptual symptoms. Finally, it reveals a situation in which schizotypal performance is improved as a result of a cognitive "failure"; reaction time is uninhibited and therefore faster on the second trial.

Beech et al. (1989a) next tested groups of high and low STA scorers in the same paradigm using different stimulus presentation times: 100, 250, and 500 ms. The negative priming was found in the low STA scorers at 100 and 250 ms, but not at 500 ms. In high STA scorers, the facilitation effect was found only at 100 ms, whereas normal negative priming occurred at 250 ms. No effect was found for either group at 500 ms. Beech et al. concluded that the affected mechanism in schizotypals was a preconscious attentional disinhibition.

Beech et al. (1989a) also predicted that there would be an inverse relationship between negative priming and the well-known Stroop interference effect. It was expected that as cognitive inhibition (negative priming) decreased in proportion to schizotypy, interference would increase. The predicted negative correlation between negative priming and interference was found. However, STA scores were not significantly correlated with interference scores, even though STA was significantly correlated with negative priming at 100 ms. The authors concluded that the attentional process involved several different, overlapping components operating in stages over time, and that only the earliest preconscious processing components were implicated in schizotypy (see Figure 13.1).

Semantic priming

Three studies of semantic priming, in which words or letters are primed by semantically related words or letters, produced mixed results. Fisher and Weinman (1989) asked subjects to identify words of ambiguous meaning that were tachistoscopically presented just below the subject's threshold. Along with target words, two priming stimuli were presented at a much higher intensity. The priming stimuli were both semantically related to the target, but were either concordant or discordant relative to the ambiguous target. As predicted, subjects showed inhibition (increased number of presentations required for identification of the target) in the discordant condition. No significant correlations emerged, however, between this inhibition and the STA. Bullen, Hemsley, and Dixon (1987) found that semantic priming for simple, letter-pair stimuli was significantly correlated with hallucinatory tendencies (LSHS; Launay & Slade, 1981) but not with the STA, the Psychoticism (P; Eysenck & Eysenck, 1975), or the Chapmans' scales of Magical Ideation (MI; Eckblad & Chapman, 1983) and PerAb.

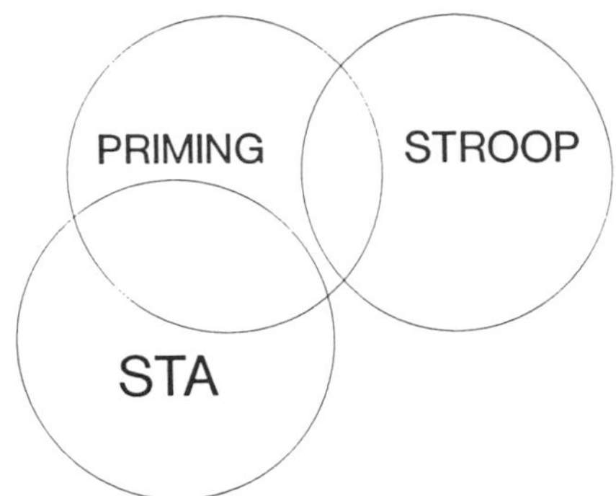

Fig. 13.1. Venn diagram depicting overlap (significant correlation) between negative priming and both schizotypy (as measured by the STA) and the Stroop effect, while there is no significant correlation between the Stroop effect and the STA.

Discussion. In the Fisher and Weinman study, the priming stimuli were each presented for 500 ms. That is the same duration at which Beech et al. (1989a) found no significant relationship between performance and schizotypy. The negative findings suggest the need for future studies of priming to use a variety of stimulus durations and interstimulus intervals, in order to tease out differential effects. This issue clouds the interpretation of negative findings in this area, and alerts researchers in general cognitive psychology to distinctions that may not have been apparent without schizotypal research. In the negative priming studies, Beech and colleagues determined that early, preconscious information processing was the affected system in schizotypy.

Although results are mixed, the above studies explicitly address the hypothesis that schizophrenia (and, by implication, schizotypy) reflects a failure to limit the contents of consciousness. Although most of the studies below do not explicitly refer to the disinhibitory hypothesis, it will be apparent that they are all tap processes that are related to this notion of cognitive disinhibition.

Learning tasks

Latent inhibition

Studies using a variety of experimental paradigms have found schizotypy to be related to abnormalities in learning, which is traditionally associated with the limbic system (Venables, 1992) as well as prefrontal cortex (Goldman-

Rakic, 1987). For example, Baruch, Hemsley, and Gray, (1988a,b) studied cognitive processes in schizotypy using the latent inhibition paradigm. Latent inhibition refers to the phenomenon by which classical conditioning is impaired following repeated exposure to the CS in a neutral (unpaired) context; it is thought to be mediated by the hippocampus (Lubow, 1973). Baruch et al. (1988a) demonstrated that latent inhibition was not exhibited by schizophrenic patients in an acute episode.

Baruch et al. (1988b) examined the relationship between latent inhibition and scales of psychosis proneness in their control group. High scorers on the STA had a marginally significant reduction in latent inhibition compared to low scorers. Interestingly, this reduction was observed more strongly for subjects scoring high on the Eysenck P scale, but not at all for those scoring high on the LSHS. This pattern of findings is notable, as it has been suggested that the P scale does not reflect schizotypy per se but rather a more nonspecific factor that may predispose to antisocial behavior as well as psychosis (Claridge & Broks, 1984). In the experiments by Beech and colleagues, the P scale was not related to measures of negative priming and interference. Still, the P scale is theorized to represent a form of behavioral and cognitive disinhibition that may lead to antisocial behavior (Baruch et al., 1988b; Eysenck & Eysenck, 1975). Thus, the latent inhibition experiments again tap the broad cognitive processes described in the above sections. However, just as the negative priming and Stroop interference effects appear to reflect distinct yet overlapping processes, the latent inhibition paradigm appears to reflect yet another facet of the normal process of focusing awareness. It is important to note that there is a large difference between negative priming and latent inhibition in terms of the presentation of the stimuli. In the former paradigm, the to-be-ignored stimulus is presented only once for a fraction of a second, whereas in latent inhibition the ignored stimulus is presented repeatedly for as long as 1.25 seconds on each trial.

Once again, this study shows that there may be many subcomponents of the process by which material enters, or is blocked from entering, consciousness. These subcomponents may be differentiated by such factors as their place in the time course of information processing and the nature of the stimuli, and may have differential correlates among different aspects of schizotypy. In the studies reported so far, no clear trends emerge; mixed results are found for the LSHS, STA, and P.

The importance of separating out factors of schizotypy was illustrated in experiments by Jones, Gray, and Hemsley (1990, 1992). The researchers examined two more learning processes similar to the latent inhibition paradigm: the Kamin blocking task and incidental learning. In the former, the learning of a pairing of stimuli is inhibited by a preexposure of the target paired with a distractor stimulus. Incidental learning was measured as the number of stimuli (in a list-learning task) remembered outside the bounds of the instructions.

In their first study (Jones et al., 1990), these researchers failed to find any difference in the Kamin blocking effect or incidental learning between high and low STA scorers. In a reanalysis (Jones et al., 1992), the STA was submitted to a factor analysis, yielding a three-factor solution: magical ideation, unusual perceptual experience, and paranoia. High scorers on the first two factors showed a trend ($p < .10$) toward significant reduction in the Kamin blocking effect. Factor analysis led to a similar shift in results for two incidental learning tasks. These are two more examples in which a "failure" to inhibit leads to better learning.

Inhibition of cognitive set

A final neuropsychological test of frontal lobe functioning that has been studied in relation to schizotypy is the Wisconsin Card Sorting Test (WCST), which involves shifting cognitive set in addition to maintaining a cognitive set against distractors (Heaton, 1981). Although this task is superficially quite different from those reported above, it also taps the ability of subjects to inhibit the contents of consciousness. In this task, the rules for sorting the cards constantly change, so subjects must inhibit a response that has previously been correct in order to adapt to the new rules of the game. It is hypothesized that schizotypals, like schizophrenics, may have difficulties in inhibiting the previously correct response, and so have an increased number of perseverative errors. Numerous studies of neurological patients have validated the WCST (perseverative errors) as an index of prefrontal functioning (Milner, 1963). Additionally, the WCST has been shown to activate prefrontal cortex in a study of regional cerebral blood flow (Weinberger, Berman, & Zec, 1986).

While increased perseverative errors are a relatively robust finding in schizophrenics (Weinberger, 1987), findings in schizotypals have been mixed. Raine, Sheard, Reynolds, and Lencz (1992a), examining 17 subjects who had been selected as SES- and education-matched controls for schizophrenics, found a significant correlation between WCST perseverative errors and scores on the STA, as well as the Venables Schizophrenism and Social Anhedonia scales. Non-prefrontal cognitive measures were not correlated with schizotypal scales. However, in a study of 14 undergraduates with DSM-III-R-diagnosed schizotypal personality disorder (SPD), Raine et al.

(1992b) failed to find any significant deficit on the WCST. One possible explanation for this negative finding is the type of sample used; there may have been a restriction of range in the undergraduate sample since students are preselected on the basis of cognitive abilities. This explanation is doubtful, however, as two other studies of undergraduates (Lyons, Merla, Young, & Kremen, 1991; Spaulding et al., 1989) did find significant differences in perseverative errors between groups identified as schizotypal (on the basis of MMPI scores and diagnostic interviews, respectively) and controls. Additionally, a study by Condray and Steinhauer (1992) failed to find WCST deficits in their community samples of schizotypals with and without schizophrenic relatives. Interestingly, the study by Lyons et al. had only 9 schizotypal subjects, as compared to 14 in the study by Raine et al. (1992b) and 25 in the study by Condray and Steinhauer (1992), so the negative findings of the latter are not necessarily attributable to a failure of power.

Summary and general discussion

In summary, the most important point to be made about the literature reviewed above, and summarized in Table 13.1, is simply that virtually all of the neuropsychological studies of frontolimbic inhibitory mechanisms showed significant relationships to schizotypy. In most of these studies, schizotypy was related to decreased inhibition of the contents of consciousness, measured across a gamut of different tasks. Only five of the 22 entries in Table 13.1 reveal exclusively negative findings. This is particularly salient, given the fact that none of the subjects were inpatients or showed gross functional deficits, indicating that these neuropsychological abnormalities might be indices of a relatively more subtle pathology. Viewed this way, it is quite striking that scores on a personality questionnaire would be so strongly correlated with a neurocognitive abnormality.

The robust quality of these findings has two implications. First, these data represent a strong validation of the schizotypy concept; schizotypals showed abnormalities that paralleled those found in schizophrenics. All of the tasks presented here have been validated against schizophrenic samples. At the risk of circularity, it also helps clarify the nature of the deficits shown by schizophrenics. Given that schizotypy is related in some way to schizophrenia, these findings help specify the "core" neurocognitive impairment in schizophrenia, which has been difficult owing to the generalized nature of functional deficits in schizophrenia (Chapman & Chapman, 1978).

The second implication is that the broad range of tests that showed significant effects makes it difficult to tease out which mechanism or stage of infor-

Table 13.1. *Summary of findings in studies of fronto-limbic functioning in schizotypals*

Type of task	Authors (year)	Subject pool	Measure	Findings
Negative priming	Beech & Claridge (1987)	community all-male	STA	No negative priming in high STA group
	Beech et al. (1989a)	community	STA	No negative priming in high STA group at 100 ms No correlation with Stroop
Semantic priming	Fisher & Weinman (1989)	med/nursing students	STA	No correlation of priming with STA
Latent inhibition	Baruch et al. (1988b)	community	STA, P LSHS	Reduced LI in high P group, high STA group, no effect for LSHS
	Bullen et al. (1987)	community	LSHS, STA P, MI, PAb	Inhibition negatively correlated with LSHS, not others
Verbal transformation effect	Bullen et al. (1987)	community	same	Total number of words significantly correlated with LSHS
Kamin blocking	Jones et al. (1990)	community	STA	No significant difference between high and low STA groups
	Jones et al. (1992)	community	STA-factors	Trend toward decreased blocking for high-scoring groups on first two factors of STA
Incidental learning	Jones et al. (1990)	community	STA	No significant difference between high and low STA groups
	Jones et al. (1992)	community	STA-factors	Significant correlation between STA factors and increased incidental recall, decreased ordered recall
Continuous Performance Test (CPT)	Venables (1990)	Mauritius	Szophrenism Anhedonia	Low CPT scorers (high errors) had higher Schizophrenism, but not Anhedonia, scores
	Lenzenweger et al. (1991)	undergrad	PAb	High PAb scorers showed trend toward lower CPT d'

	Condray & Steinhauer (1992)	relatives community	SID-P	Diagnosed schizotypals, from community and relatives of schizophrenics, had lower d'
	Grove et al. (1991)	relatives	PA, PAb SSP	Lower d' correlated with Chapman scales but not with clinical interview ratings of schizotypy (SSP)
Span of Apprehension (SOA)	Venables (1990)	Mauritius	Szophrenism Anhedonia	Low SOA scores had higher Schizophrenism, but not Anhedonia, scores
	Asarnow et al. (1983)	community	PAb, MI	Poor SOA performers had significantly higher scores on these two Chapman scales
Wisconsin Card Sort (WCST)	Raine et al. (1992a)	community	STA Szophrenism Anhedonia	Significant correlation between perseverative errors and STA as well as with schizophrenism and anhedonia
	Raine et al. (1992b)	undergrads	SCID-II	No significant difference between diagnosed schizotypals, controls
	Condray & Steinhauer (1992)	relatives	SID-P	No significant difference between diagnosed schizotypals, controls
	Spaulding et al. (1989)	undergrads	MMPI 8	Significantly more perseverative errors in high schizotypal group
	Lyons et al. (1991)	undergrads	SID-P	Significantly more perseverative errors in diagnosed schizotypals
Combined Index (WCST, CPT)	Kendler et al. (1991)	community twins	SIS, PAb MI, PA, SA	Significant correlation between frontal deficits and negative-symptom schizotypy (SIS); no correlation with self-report

Key: STA, Claridge's STA; P, Eysenck's Psychoticism Scale; PAb, Chapmans' Perceptal Aberration Scale; PA, Chapmans' Physical Anhedonia Scale; SA, Chapmans' Social Anhedonia Scale; MI, Chapmans' Magical Ideation Scale; LSHS, Launay–Slade Hallucinatory Scale; Szophrenism, Venables's Schizophrenism Scale; Anhedonia, Venables's Anhedonia Scale; SIS, Schedule for Interviewing Schizotypals; SID-P, Structured Interview for DSM-III Personality Disorders; SCID-II, Structured Clinical Interview for DSM-III-R, Axis II; SSP, Structured Scale for Schizotypy; MMPI-8, Scale 8 of the Minnesota Multiphasic Personality Inventory.

mation processing is most affected by this cognitive disinhibition. The strongest results were found for the SOA test, which has the shortest stimulus presentation time (40 ms). For the negative priming tasks, relation to schizotypy was significant only with the shortest stimulus presentation time (100 ms). The weakest (most mixed) findings were reported for the Wisconsin Card Sort, which is untimed and involves conscious conceptual processing. Given a serial processing view of preconscious/conscious interactions, these findings lend some support to the view that the abnormality involves very early, preconscious processing. However, there may be multiple, partially overlapping inhibitory processes that are all affected, to some degree, in schizotypals.

The preceding interpretation assumes a serial model of information processing and attention. However, recent research in cognitive psychology suggests that an allocation of resources model may be more appropriate (Nuechterlein & Dawson, 1984). According to this model, deficits in schizophrenia are related to automatic, parallel processing impairments that reduce the available processing capacity. Nuechterlein and Dawson (1984) present four factors that may potentially cause this reduction: (1) defective executive functioning fails to conform to task demands despite a normal pool of resources; (2) increased attention to task-irrelevant stimuli; (3) conscious processing devoted to operations that should be handled preconsciously; and (4) reduction in the overall pool of processing resources.

Owing to the wide array of positive findings in the schizotypy literature, specifying the root cause of the deficit is difficult. Results of the WCST (increased perseveration) tend to support the first interpretation, insofar as this task is generally thought to tap executive functioning. Increased incidental learning in schizotypy may reflect process 2, although the negative priming results suggest that task focus can be improved by failure to inhibit a response. The broad range of effects found on such a variety of tasks (perceptual, semantic, visual, conceptual) lends some support to hypothesis 4. These hypotheses are not mutually exclusive, and further studies are needed to make stronger interpretations of the findings.

The fact that so many tasks measuring cognitive inhibition are implicated leads to a final possible interpretation: There may be a single defect in cognitive inhibition, mediated by frontolimbic circuitry, that underlies all of these partially overlapping tasks. As depicted in Figure 13.2, such a defect might account for disinhibition on tasks such as the SOA, latent inhibition, and negative priming (tasks 1, 2, and 3 in the figure), which are all correlated with schizotypy. At the same time, the defect does not account for abnormalities on other tasks – such as the Stroop interference measure (task 4) – that do not

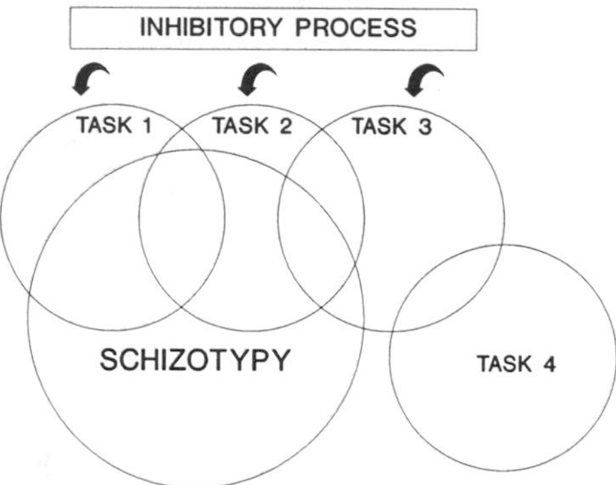

Fig. 13.2. An extension of the Venn diagram in Figure 13.1, this figure illustrates the hypothesis that there may be several partially overlapping cognitive processes (measured by tasks 1–3) implicated in schizotypy. These tasks may share a single underlying cause, a defect in cognitive inhibition.

correlate with schizotypy, even though such measures may correlate with other tasks that *are* implicated in schizotypy. This model is supported by a study by Kendler and colleagues (1991), which examined the relationship between schizotypy and performance on a battery of tests putatively related to frontolimbic performance. A principal components analysis revealed that the CPT and the WCST, though seemingly quite different, both significantly loaded on the first principal component. This component was significantly correlated with negative-symptom schizotypy.

Two methodological points concerning studies of frontolimbic functioning should be noted. First, although most studies utilized subjects drawn as volunteers from the community, five studies utilized undergraduate or postgraduate students. Two of these studies had negative findings, one had a trend toward significance, and only two of the five had clear-cut significant findings. It is possible that these samples, pre-selected on the basis of intellectual functioning, may present a problem of restricted range. Future studies may be more able to avoid Type II errors by utilizing a broader sampling strategy.

Second, several studies have found dissociations by utilizing factor analyses and/or multiple measures of the schizotypy construct. Table 13.1 reveals that these results are too mixed to allow for clear interpretation. However, it is clear that future schizotypal research would be well-advised to utilize a broad range of measures so that differential correlates of separable schizotypy factors can be teased out. This would improve not only our understanding of schizotypy and schizophrenia, but also our understanding of the differences between seemingly similar tests of information processing.

As noted in the introduction to this section, most of the studies presented were limited by the fact that they examined only one neuropsychological measure of interest. Consequently, dissociations of effects, or the discovery of differential deficits, were not possible. As such, the studies to date may be seen as constituting a "first wave" of research, which has served to validate the use of a neuropsychological approach to the underpinnings of nonpsychotic disorders of personality. The next wave of research must be designed so as to find dissociations and differential deficits, in order to identify which subcomponents of frontolimbic inhibitory mechanisms are specifically affected. Such research should employ multiple measures of partially overlapping neuropsychological constructs, as was begun in the studies of Beech et al. (1989a,b). Figure 13.1 shows that dissociations between superficially similar tests can be made. To this end, recent suggestions for neuropsychological studies of schizophrenia (Serper & Harvey, 1994; Strauss & Summerfelt, 1994) can be applied to schizotypal research. Serper and Harvey (1994) suggest that neuropsychological researchers should utilize fine-grained distinctions developed in (nonclinical) cognitive psychology; for example, they suggest that learning and memory should be broken down into subcomponents such as encoding, recall, and recognition. Strauss and Summerfelt (1994) recommend the use of experimental manipulations of tasks, such as matching subjects and controls on performance and observing differences in brain activation using functional brain imaging. In sum, future studies should be designed to compare and contrast specific models of the neurocognitive substrate of schizotypy.

Cerebral hemispheric asymmetries

As was the case in the review of frontolimbic deficits, many studies of abnormal cerebral asymmetries in schizotypy are limited by inclusion of only one dependent measure. However, a comprehensive review of the literature may allow for comparison of competing models to explain these abnormalities. The purpose of this half of the chapter is to attempt such a comparison.

Asymmetries in normals and schizophrenics

The study of cerebral asymmetries has been an important area of schizophrenia research since Flor-Henry's (1969) demonstration of a link between schizophrenia-like psychosis and epilepsy with a left temporal lobe focus. Studies that have examined left/right hemisphere differences in information processing in schizophrenia have produced mixed results (Flor-Henry, 1987). However, reviews do indicate that, at both the neuroanatomical level (Bilder & Degreef, 1991; Crow et al., 1989) and the functional level (Flor-Henry, 1987), schizophrenics tend to show a reduction of the asymmetries found in normal subjects. For example, normal subjects tend to have a larger left than right planum temporale, whereas schizophrenics do not show this difference (Crow et al., 1989). At the functional level, of course, the left hemisphere (LH) in normals is specialized for processing verbal material (Hellige, 1993). Numerous studies of schizophrenics show an increased incidence of left- and mixed-handedness, indicating some abnormality of the normal development of speech lateralization (Green & Kotenko, 1980). Another relatively common finding in the schizophrenia literature is that, when verbal information is presented to each hemisphere in isolation (e.g., in a dichotic listening task), there is a reduction in the normal left-hemisphere (right ear) advantage in processing verbal material (Wexler, Giller, & Southwick, 1991). Such neuropsychological findings are generally interpreted as reflecting LH dysfunction, due to either underactivation (Flor-Henry, 1987) or overactivation (Venables, 1980). However, an alternate theory, based on findings of structural abnormalities of the corpus callosum (Rosenthal & Bigelow, 1972), posits faulty interhemispheric transfer mechanisms as the basis of these performance abnormalities. These competing theories will be examined with respect to the schizotypal literature reviewed below.

Another conceptual issue derived from the schizophrenia literature on hemispheric processing that will also be discussed below concerns the factor structure of the disorder. Regrettably, many studies of schizophrenia do not distinguish subtypes in their patient sample. However, some comparative studies of the syndromes of schizophrenia have identified different hemispheric asymmetry patterns in patients with predominant positive symptoms compared to those with predominant negative features (Gruzelier, 1984). Specifically, negative-symptom schizophrenia may be more related to LH underactivation described above, whereas positive-symptom schizophrenics tend to show signs of LH overactivation, which is hypothesized to underlie symptoms such as auditory hallucinations. Discussion of this issue in the schizotypy literature will be limited by the fact that only two of the cerebral asymmetry studies explicitly examine these dissociations.

Divided visual field and dichotic listening tasks in schizotypals

Claridge and his colleagues (Broks, 1984; Broks, Claridge, Matheson, & Hargreaves, 1984; Claridge & Broks, 1984; Rawlings & Borge, 1987;

Rawlings & Claridge, 1984) at Oxford performed a series of experiments designed to test the relative functioning of the two cerebral hemispheres in volunteer subjects and the relationship of performance asymmetries to individual differences in self-report schizotypy. Generally, in the divided visual field (DVF) and dichotic listening (DL) paradigms, stimuli are presented separately to each visual field or ear that have predominantly contralateral connections to the cerebral hemispheres. The relative functioning of the hemispheres is compared by examining the reaction time or accuracy in reporting the stimuli for each hemisphere. If different stimuli are presented to each hemisphere simultaneously, performance is gauged by which stimulus is reported. In normals, relative left versus right performance on these tasks reflects normal asymmetries of the brain; that is, the left hemisphere is dominant for verbal stimuli (words and word fragments), whereas the right hemisphere is dominant for nonverbal stimuli (shapes and tones).

Claridge and colleagues hypothesized that schizotypals would show performance abnormalities parallel to those found in schizophrenics. Specifically, they predicted that normal functional asymmetries would be attenuated in subjects scoring high on the STA. This hypothesis was borne out for males but not for females in all the studies listed above. Reduction of normal asymmetries was unrelated to overall performance (accuracy on the tasks), which was not significantly correlated with STA scores. Further, in Rawlings and Claridge's (1984) study, the LVF (RH) reaction times to verbal stimuli of high STA scorers were faster than the RVF (LH) reaction times in the low STA group. This finding reveals an advantage in performance in those scoring high in schizotypy, as was found in the latent inhibition and incidental learning results described above.

Interpretation and discussion

The studies reviewed above were all conducted at Oxford University under the same general paradigm. However, even from this limited number of DVF and dichotic listening studies of schizotypals, the findings are subject to a host of potential interpretations. Before completing the review of empirical studies in this area, it is useful to raise some conceptual issues to provide a framework for understanding the meaning of these findings.

As can be seen from the first five entries in Table 13.2, all of these studies showed a decrease in the normal asymmetry on verbal tasks for schizotypal subjects, at least for males. There are at least three potential interpretations of these data, drawn from neurocognitive theories of schizophrenia: (1) left hemisphere processing deficiencies in schizotypy due to simple underactivation; (2) LH dysfunction due to overactivation; and (3) abnormalities of interhemispheric transfer (IHT). In addition, three conceptual issues from the general information processing literature impinge upon any attempt to interpret laterality data: (1) alternate processing strategies (lateral preference) in schizotypals; (2) lateralized attention deficits; and (3) decreased lateralization of function (without lateralized damage) as a dimension of individual difference in neurodevelopment. The three interpretations (some of which may overlap) are considered in turn, and additional empirical studies will be introduced. Finally, a fourth hypothesis is advanced: Schizotypal abnormalities are accounted for by a reduction in lateralization of function. Evidence concerning sex differences in this literature is used to support this hypothesis.

An important methodological point must be noted before proceeding with this comparison. In research on cerebral asymmetries, there are several unknown variables that are in question, including LH performance, RH performance, and corpus callosum performance (interhemispheric transfer, IHT). In order to tease out the role of these three systems, several pieces of data are needed. If only a single laterality coefficient is reported, as in Broks (1984), the source of the effect cannot be discovered. This is analogous to the rules of basic algebra, in which a single equation with two or more unknowns (e.g., $x + y = 5$) cannot be solved uniquely without more information. Thus, it is necessary for future research in this area to report the LH and RH scores separately, as a comparison of these scores can help rule out certain interpretations, as discussed below in reference to the Raine and Manders (1988) study. This review aims to utilize all the data available to draw the most sound inferences from the data.

LH dysfunction or overactivation

One straightforward interpretation of these findings is that schizotypals show a left hemisphere dysfunction, resulting in deficient LH performance and hence decreased linguistic performance asymmetry. However, an LH deficit theory cannot account for the superior RH performance in the studies of Rawlings and Claridge (1984) and Broks et al. (1984). The fit of this theory to the data can be improved by adding the hypothesis that the RH in schizotypals is superior to that of controls as a form of neurodevelopmental compensation for early LH insult. Still, even this theory cannot explain the superior overall performance of the male schizotypals in Rawlings and Borge (1987).

Similarly, these findings of superior RH performance do not mesh with an LH overactivation theory, especially given Venables's (1980) speculation that LH overactivation is a developmental response to early RH damage. In this

Table 13.2. *Summary of findings in studies of cerebral asymmetries in schizotypals*

Type of task	Authors (year)	Subject pool	Measure
Divided Visual Field (DVF)	Broks (1984)	community	STA
	Rawlings & Claridge (1984)	community	STA
	Rawlings & Claridge (1984)	community	STA
Dichotic Listening	Broks et al. (1984)	community	STA
	Rawlings & Borge (1987)	community	STA
	Raine & Manders (1988)	community	index[a]
	Mills & Raine (1993)	delinquents	index[b]
Intermanual Tactile/ Motor	Raine & Manders (1988)	community	index[a]
	Kelley & Coursey (1992)	undergrad	index[c]
	Mills & Raine (1993)	delinquents	index[b]
Warrington Memory Test	Gruzelier et al. (in press)	med school	SPQ factor
	Benishay et al. (1993)	undergrad	SCID
Visual search strategy	Jutai (1988)	undergrad	PA, SA, PM, IN
DVF negative priming	Claridge et al. (1992)	community	STA

Key: STA, Claridge's STA; PA, Chapmans' Physical Anhedonia; SA, Chapmans' Social Anhedonia; PM, Chapmans' Perceptual Aberration (PAb)/Magical Ideation (MI) combined; IN, Chapmans' Impulsive Nonconformity; SPQ, Raine's Schizotypal Personality Questionnaire; SCID-II, Structured Clinical Interview DSM-III-R (Axis II); N/A, not applicable.
[a]index: First principal component of 7 scales: STA, Claridge's STB,

context, it should be noted that an EEG study was performed to test directly the LH overactivation theory at the psychophysiological level (Kidd & Powell, 1993). In this study, alpha power for the left and right hemispheres was compared between schizotypals (identified by STA and SPQ) and controls during a number of lateralized tasks. A decrease in LH alpha ("idling") power, indicating increased active processing, was predicted and found in the schizotypals. However, a significant decrease in alpha power was also obtained for the schizotypals' right hemisphere, indicating increased processing bilaterally. This bilateral hyperactivation parallels the bilaterally superior

Table 13.2. (*cont.*)

Sex effects?	Findings
yes	STA scores inversely correlated with laterality coefficient for males only
no	Superior LVF performance for single-letter stimuli in high STA group
no	Reversed asymmetries in high STA group in local vs. global processing
yes	Improved left ear and binaural recall for stories in high STA males
yes	High STA male group showed improved left ear performance; high STA females showed lower right ear performance
no	Enhanced right ear advantage (increased asymmetry) correlated with schizotypy
N/A	Male delinquents with high schizotypy scores had increased asymmetry
no	No significant correlation of interhemispheric transfer with schizotypy
N/A	No significant difference between high and low schizotypy groups on lateralized motor
N/A	Male delinquents with high schizotypy scores had interhemispheric deficits
N/A	Subjects with LH (word) > RH (faces) memory had increased active symptoms Others had more withdrawn symptoms
no	Subjects scoring high in cognitive–perceptual symptoms had decreased asymmetry due to improved RH memory
N/A	Increased frequency of unsystematic searching in high PA and PM groups
yes	Abolition of negative priming in LVF of male high STA group

Schizophrenism, MI, PAb, LSHS, Disordered Thinking.
[b]index: Subjects identified by cluster analysis, with high scores on Schizophrenism, SA, and MI.
[c]index: First unrotated component of 11 scales: PA, PAb, MI, IN, Intense Ambivalence, Cognitive Slippage, Social Fear, Schizoidia, Schizophrenism, STA, MMPI 2-7-8.

performance found for male schizotypals in the Rawlings and Borge study. Contrary to the authors' interpretation, these findings contradict the LH overactivation theory, and are more compatible with a model of generalized overactivation. Interestingly, this EEG study utilized only male subjects. The significance of the sex of subjects is discussed in a later section.

To address this issue of source of the effects, it is useful to call attention to one study that used multiple measures in an attempt to compare the strengths of competing hypotheses. In the Raine and Manders (1988) study, subjects' scores on a composite schizotypal index, measuring cognitive–perceptual schizotypal traits, were compared with a variety of measures of asymmetry. Subjects were tested on both verbal and nonverbal dichotic listening tasks. The laterality coefficient for the verbal task was significantly positively correlated with schizotypy scores, indicating an enhanced right ear (LH) advantage in schizotypals. This correlation held for males and females equally. Interestingly, the finding of an exaggerated asymmetry runs counter to the rest of the studies described above. Performance on the nonverbal task was not significantly correlated with schizotypy for either males or females.

Given their finding of increased right ear advantage for verbal material, Raine and Manders (1988) rejected the simple LH damage hypothesis. Raine and colleagues (1989) sought to validate this hypothesis further by repeating these experiments on a sample of 13 schizophrenics. Compared to schizotypals, schizophrenics showed significant LH deficits on the verbal dichotic listening task. This finding lends partial support to the hypothesis of Raine and Manders that patterns of LH activation follow an inverted-U shaped curve. Thus, the slight overactivation found in schizotypals leads to an exaggerated right ear advantage compared to normals, whereas extreme overactivation leads to overload, causing the performance deficits seen in schizophrenics.

Though the findings of Raine and Manders are the reverse of those described in the five studies above, their rejection of the simple LH deficit theory is consistent with the preceding analysis of those studies. However, the conclusion by Raine and Manders that LH overactivation underlies schizotypy is at odds with the previous findings of the Oxford group. There are several possible methodological reasons for this discrepancy, including measurement of schizotypy, subject selection, and type of stimuli used in the task. First, the Oxford studies utilized the STA exclusively, whereas Raine and Manders utilized a composite score of seven scales. This is unlikely to be responsible for the difference, as both indices tap the same type of schizotypal traits, namely the cognitive–perceptual abnormalities ("positive" symptoms). Second, the Oxford studies drew subjects from the community, whereas Raine and Manders's subjects were undergraduates. It has been suggested (Lencz & Raine, Chapter 18, this volume) that patterns of cognitive findings from undergraduate schizotypals may differ from those obtained for community schizotypals, since the undergraduates are preselected on the basis of superior (or at least intact) cognitive functioning. Third, there are differences in the type of stimuli (consonant-vowel vs. story or word-pairs) used for the dichotic listening task. Raine and Manders suggest that constant–vowel stimuli are to be preferred because they can be repeated rapidly so that responses to these stimuli are unaffected by directed attention. Further studies, manipulating the type of stimuli used in the task, are needed to assess this possibility.

A final piece of evidence that needs to be examined in consideration of the LH overactivation theory was not addressed by Raine and Manders. Part of the LH overactivation theory, as described by Venables (1980), holds that early RH insult is the cause of this phenomenon. In the Raine and Manders study, this prediction could be tested on the tone contour (nonverbal) dichotic listening task. This study revealed no significant correlation between the laterality coefficient for this task and scores on the schizotypal index. Both groups showed the expected left ear (RH) advantage, indicating no RH deficit, although there was no increase in RH performance as was found in the Oxford studies. Thus, this aspect of the LH overactivation theory was not confirmed, thereby weakening the authors' conclusion. We now turn to consideration of an alternate explanation for these findings.

Interhemispheric transfer

Based on the previous schizophrenia research, Raine and Manders also considered the possibility that their findings could be explained by IHT impairment: The right ear advantage is magnified owing to a problem in transmitting information from the left ear (RH) over to the LH for processing. In order to test this hypothesis, they administered an intramanual and intermanual tactile recognition task, and compared scores in these two conditions. Increased time and decreased accuracy in performing the latter task, which requires the passing of information from one hemisphere to the other, are signs of IHT processing time. Raine and Manders found no significant correlation between these indices of IHT processing and schizotypy scores for either males or females.

Raine and Manders concluded that these results rule out the IHT-deficit interpretation of their dichotic listening task findings. However, it is possible that the intermanual task of Raine and Manders was not in the appropriate modality or did not place sufficient processing demands on the subjects to produce a significant effect. The inability of lateralized manual/motor performance tasks to discriminate between schizotypals and controls was reported by Kelley and Coursey (1992). Schizotypals and controls did not differ on any of a series of neuromotor tasks (finger-tapping, grip strength test, Purdue Pegboard) testing the performance of either or both hands.

Further, the correlation coefficients for both males and females, though nonsignificant, are in the opposite direction from that predicted. This result suggests another possible interpretation: improved IHT performance in schizotypals. A reexamination of the Oxford studies reveals that several of their findings are consistent with an IHT advantage hypothesis. The decrease in normal asymmetry reported by Broks (1984) could be the result of faster and improved transmission from the RH to the LH, so that the left ear performance is increased. Broks et al. (1984) found that improved binaural performance was associated with higher levels of schizotypy. Improved binaural performance relative to single ear performance strongly suggests a more efficient IHT process. Finally, the improved bilateral performance for male schizotypals reported by Rawlings and Borge (1987) is perhaps better explained by an IHT hypothesis as opposed to a explanation confined to one hemisphere. Further studies comparing schizotypals and schizophrenics are needed to test the possibility that IHT performance in normals, schizotypals, and schizophrenics follows an inverted-U pattern. If this is so, (male) schizotypals may show optimal balance of functioning between cerebral hemispheres, whereas normals and schizophrenics show poorer performance based on too much and too little lateralization, respectively. Future studies should utilize data from all three subject groups across several modalities, as in Raine et al. (1989), so as to provide enough data to solve the algebraic puzzle.

New studies of hemispheric asymmetries and IHT

Two new studies reported from our lab also address the issue of interhemispheric transfer and lateralization of function, with differing results for different populations of subjects. In the first study, Benishay, Raine, Lencz, and Bird (1993) examined performance on the Warrington Recognition Memory Test, which compares memory for words (an indicator of LH performance) with memory for faces (RH). Normal subjects tend to show better memory for words (see Gruzelier, Chapter 14, this volume). Benishay et al. utilized a sample of 46 unselected undergraduates, who were median-split into high- and low-scoring groups for each of the three factors of DSM-III-R SPD (as measured by the Structured Clinical Interview for DSM-III-R Personality Disorders, SCID). As shown in Figure 13.3, a significant Group x Hemisphere interaction effect was found for those scoring high on cognitive–perceptual symptoms ($F = 8.29$, $p = .007$); these subjects did not show the normal asymmetry due to improved memory for faces, which almost equaled their memory for words. There were no significant effects for interpersonal or disorganized symptom factors, and no interaction effects of sex. These results could be interpreted as showing that subjects with cognitive–perceptual symptoms (similar to high scorers on the STA) show less lateralization or greater integration of hemispheric performance leading to improved overall performance.

In a study of 40 delinquent males Mills and Raine (1993), found somewhat different effects using a dichotic listening task. Cluster analysis was used to identify three groups defined by scores on a variety of self-report measures of psychopathy and schizotypy (including Venables's schizophrenism and anhedonia scales and the STA). Subjects in the first cluster had high scores on the schizotypal scales (but not psychopathy scales), subjects in the second cluster had high scores on the psychopathy scales, and subjects in the third cluster had low scores on both sets of tests. As shown in Figure 13.4, subjects in both the psychopathic cluster and schizotypal cluster showed an increase of the normal asymmetry (right ear advantage) on a verbal dichotic listening task ($p = .008$ on a repeated-measures ANOVA); effects were most pronounced for the schizotypals. In addition, the schizotypals performed significantly worse than the other two groups on a finger-tapping task requiring interhemispheric processing, while performing normally on an equivalent, intrahemispheric task (Figure 13.5). The authors concluded that impaired interhemispheric transfer might account for the reduced left ear performance on the dichotic listening task. While the finding of IHT impairments contrasts with the earlier suggestion of an IHT advantage for schizotypals, this discrepancy may be due to the unusual sample used in this study. In any event, both of these recent studies call attention to the need to move beyond single-hemisphere explanations of abnormalities in schizotypals.

Processing preferences and factors of schizotypy

The above discussion of the competing hypothesized mechanisms underlying abnormal asymmetries in schizotypals contains two implicit assumptions. The first assumption is that schizotypals utilize the same processing strategies as normals, relying on the left hemisphere to analyze semantic stimuli and localized stimuli, and the right hemisphere for the processing of visual and global stimuli. It is assumed, for example, that the single-letter stimuli in Rawlings and Claridge (1984) were processed more as verbal stimuli, and a right visual-field preference was expected. The second assumption is that schizotypy is a unitary concept. Two recent studies present evidence challenging both these assumptions, and again shed more light on the puzzle of hemispheric processes in schizotypy.

Gruzelier and colleagues (Gruzelier, Burgess, Stygall, Irving, & Raine, in press) sought to test the hypothesis that syndromes of schizotypy showed dissociations in hemispheric preference parallel to those found in positive versus negative schizophrenia. Specifically, he hypothesized that schizotypals with more "active" symptoms, such as odd speech and behavior, would show a processing imbalance, with LH capacity > RH capacity. Conversely, "withdrawn" (negative symptoms, such as no close friends, blunted affect, and

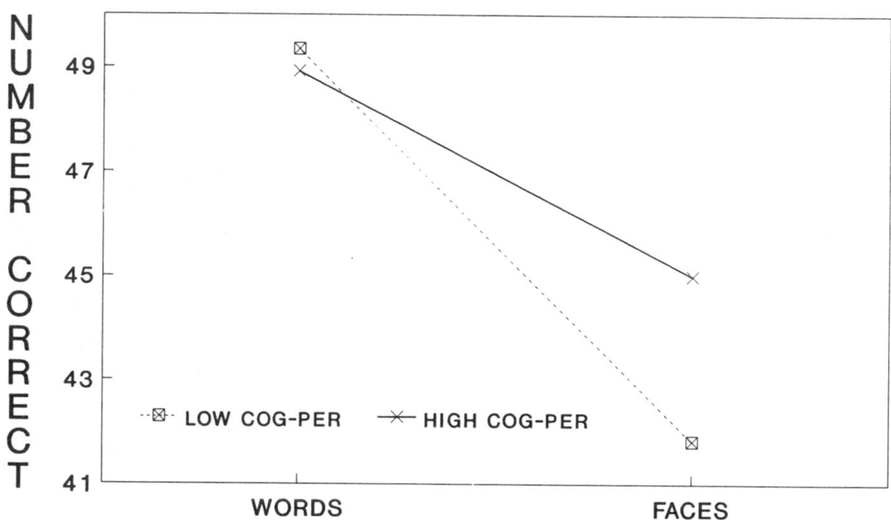

Fig. 13.3. Warrington recognition memory performance for subjects scoring high and low on cognitive–perceptual symptoms of schizotypy. Subjects high in schizotypy have reduced asymmetry due to improved memory for faces. (From Benishay et al., 1993.)

social anxiety) schizotypals were expected to show RH performance > LH performance. These hypotheses were confirmed in a sample of students who were administered the Warrington Recognition Memory Test (cf. Gruzelier, Chapter 14, this volume).

His results conflict with those of the Oxford group, to the extent that the latter group used the STA, a measure of cognitive–perceptual schizotypal features, which Gruzelier argues are nonlateralizing. Still, his findings affect interpretation of these studies, as well as that of Raine and Manders (1988), insofar as he raises the potential confound of hemispheric preference.

Jutai (1989) also considered heterogeneity of schizotypal syndromes by comparing spatial attention performance in undergraduates selected on the basis of high scores on one (and only one) of four schizotypal indices: Physical Anhedonia (PA), Social Anhedonia (SA), Perceptual Aberration/Magical Ideation (PM), and Impulsive Nonconformity (IN). These

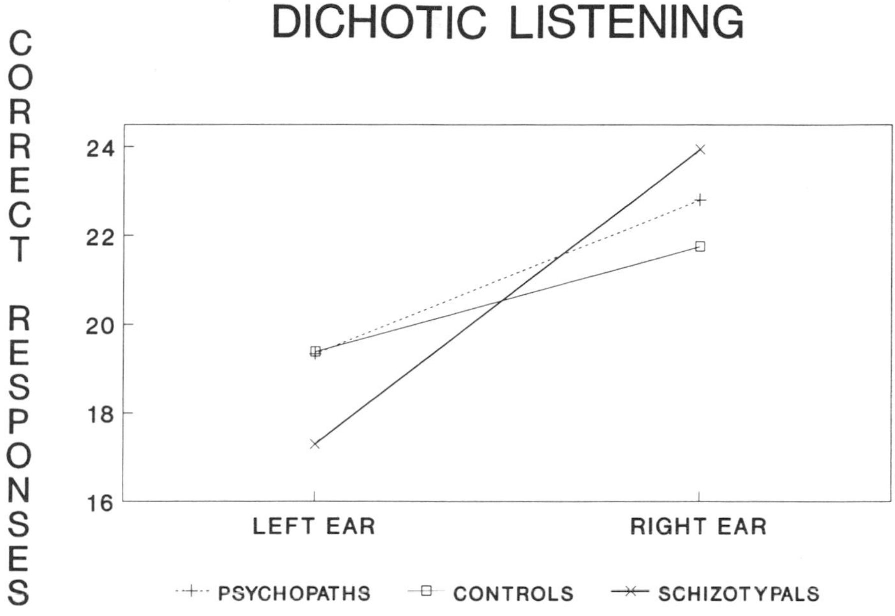

Fig. 13.4. Dichotic listening test scores for schizotypals, psychopaths, and controls. Schizotypals show increased asymmetries favoring the right ear (left hemisphere). (From Mills & Raine, 1993.)

four groups of subjects, as well as a group of controls, were tested on four versions of a paper-and-pen spatial search task. In all versions, they were required to draw a continuous line on the page and track from one target stimulus to another out of a field of distractors. In the four conditions, stimuli were either verbal (letters) or nonverbal (shapes), and the distractor field was either patterned (in straight rows and columns) or random. Performance was scored as either "systematic" (if the subject chose an efficient strategy of drawing relatively straight lines) or "unsystematic," and chi-square analyses were performed to compare the percentage of subjects in each group who performed systematically in each condition. Unsystematic processing was interpreted as revealing an information processing deficit.

Significantly more subjects in the PA and PM, but not SA and IN, groups were found to use unsystematic (disordered) strategies, compared to controls. These abnormalities were particularly evident in the random nonverbal condition; this effect was not a result of task difficulty. Jutai posited that the search strategy was dictated by RH mechanisms of visuomotor control, and interpreted schizotypal processing abnormalities as reflecting a disruption of these

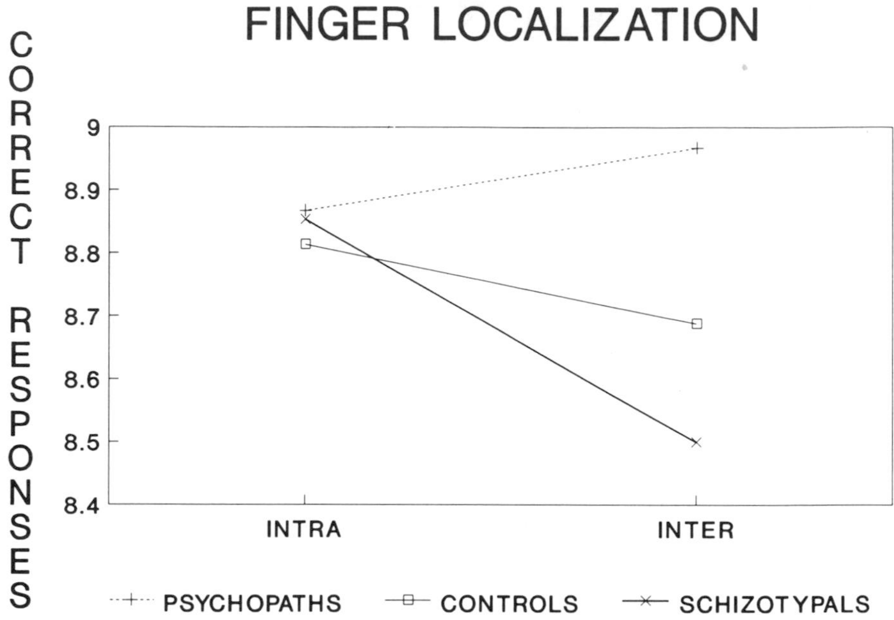

Fig. 13.5. Finger localization task results for schizotypals, psychopaths, and controls. Schizotypals show a deficit in interhemispheric processing, which may account for their increased asymmetry in the dichotic listening test. (From Mills & Raine, 1993.)

RH processes, consistent with Venables's (1980) articulation of the LH overactivation theory.

However, another interpretation of these findings is possible, based on a more detailed analysis of his design. It is likely that the verbal and nonverbal versions tapped LH and RH functioning, respectively, but Jutai does not interpret the differential impact on performance of the structured versus unstructured distractor pattern. It is possible that the structured field of rows and columns utilized the global, gestalt processing strategies of the RH, whereas the random field required more minute, local processing of the LH. If so, then the structured nonverbal and the random verbal tapped RH and LH performance, respectively, whereas the structured verbal and random nonverbal tasks required interhemispheric linkage. Given the preceding analysis, deficits shown by both PA and PM groups on the random nonverbal version of the task can be interpreted as evidence of an IHT impairment, rather than a strictly RH impairment. Further, the PA group also showed deficits on the other mixed condition, structured verbal, lending further evidence of IHT impairment. The PM group showed deficits on the random verbal task, indicating impaired LH performance. These interpretations run counter to those offered by Jutai, as well as to the findings of the previous studies, perhaps owing to the unusual nature of the task. However, they do highlight the issue of syndrome heterogeneity, with a dissociation found between schizotypals with "negative" symptoms (PA), linked to IHT deficits, and those with "positive" symptoms (PM) linked to LH processing impairments.

Hemispheres and attention

As stated above, Jutai (1989) draws the conclusion that schizotypal performance was impaired owing to damage to the right hemisphere. Contrary to the other studies, however, he focuses on the attentional mechanisms directed by the right hemisphere, specifically the scanning of visual space. While it is true that visuomotor scanning is directed primarily by the RH (Kolb & Whishaw, 1990), the attentional circuit underlying this process is considerably more complex, involving links among the frontal lobes, subcortical structures, and the right parietal region (Posner, Early, Reiman, Parod, & Dhawan, 1988). This brings us full circle to the frontolimbic attentional tasks discussed in the first half of this paper.

In this light, it can be seen that the results of Jutai (1989) are not necessarily explicable strictly in terms of lateralized processes. The task employed in that study appears analogous to the Span of Apprehension task (SOA), in which a letter serves as a target stimulus that must be selected out from a distractor field. Although the presentation method of the two tasks is vastly different, the search strategy abnormalities identified in the Jutai study might help explain deficient performance on the SOA. By the same token, the cognitive disinhibition hypothesis can be used as an explanatory framework for the deficits in Jutai's study. Specifically, Jutai suggests that disinhibitory processes may underlie erratic search strategies.

This linkage of hemispheric abnormalities with attentional deficits in schizotypals was studied directly in only one study (Claridge, Clark, & Beech, 1992). These researchers performed a replication of the negative priming study of Beech and Claridge (1987), except that the priming stimuli were presented to either the left or right visual field alone. The target stimulus (a Stroop color-word) was presented in the center of the screen. A negative priming index was computed by subtracting mean RT following neutral primes from mean RT when the priming stimulus was a distractor. Subjects were 101 volunteers from the community divided into high and low STA groups; analyses were divided by gender.

In this study, there was a significant Field x STA interaction effect for males. Low STA males showed strong negative priming in both visual fields. High STA males showed normal negative priming when the distractor was shown to the RVF (LH) only. The result of the earlier study (abolition of negative priming) was obtained for the LVF (RH) only. As in earlier studies, this effect was found for males only. Female subjects did not show this visual Field x STA interaction effect. Both high and low STA females demonstrated significant negative priming for both visual fields, though the effect was smaller in magnitude than for males.

Similarly to Jutai (1989), the authors link attentional dyscontrol and disinhibition in male schizotypals to an abnormality in the RH. Again, the RH abnormality cannot be interpreted simply as a localized deficit. Since the Stroop stimuli are linguistic in nature, and the significant effect was found in the right (nonlinguistic) hemisphere, this may reveal an abnormality of interhemispheric transfer. Specifically, the priming stimulus may not be transferred from the RH to the LH strongly enough for it to have an inhibitory (negative priming) effect. However, even this explanation may be too simple. The dissociation between male and female subjects, one that has been found in many of the studies reviewed above, suggests a related, yet different, interpretation of the data. Schizotypal abnormalities may be the result of a reduced lateralization of function, not due to hemispheric damage per se, but as an individual difference in normal brain development.

Reduced lateralization and gender effects

Table 13.2 reveals that four of the eight studies examining sex differences in hemispheric processes in schizotypals have found significant dissociations of effects between males and females. In these studies, female schizotypals failed to show the abnormalities (generally, a lack of normal asymmetry) in lateralized tasks exhibited by male schizotypals. There are two possible explanations for this dissociation, one coming from the individual differences point of view and the other stemming from research on gender differences in schizophrenia.

Sex differences in schizotypal performance on tests tapping cerebral asymmetries cannot be divorced from the literature on sex differences in cerebral organization in normals. In a seminal paper, McGlone (1980) demonstrated evidence that, in the general population, females were less lateralized for functions such as language and spatial ability than were males. Given this widely accepted finding, the lack of asymmetry exhibited by schizotypal males might be interpreted as reflecting that they also show a reduction in the normal lateralization. This reduction need not be due to damage, as suggested by the LH overactivation theory, for example. Rather, this is a function of normal variation, individual differences, in brain development.

This hypothesis is supported by an examination of the data of Rawlings and Borge (1987) and Claridge et al. (1992). In Rawlings and Borge (1987), low STA males showed the expected right ear advantage. Their high STA counterparts showed no performance asymmetry, with both ears performing as well as the low STA subjects' right (preferred) ear. For females, low STA subjects showed good performance in each ear, whereas high STA subjects had poor performance in each ear. A reordering of their data reveals that high STA males show patterns of performance that closely parallel performance in low STA females. The suggestion that decreased lateralization of function is at the heart of (at least cognitive–perceptual) schizotypy is also supported by the fact that Claridge and Hewitt (1987) reported consistently higher scores on the STA in females compared to males. Raine (1992) also found higher self-report cognitive–perceptual symptoms in women.

In these studies, furthermore, high STA females not only lack asymmetry in performance, they also show a generalized decrease of performance. Conversely, in several of the studies reviewed above, male schizotypals showed improved performance relative to controls (e.g., Broks et al., 1984; Kidd & Powell, 1993; Rawlings & Borge, 1987). It may be that lateralization of function follows an inverted-U curve, with optimal performance occurring when there is some sharing of function between the hemispheres, as in high STA males and low STA females. Thus, as this sharing is carried to an extreme, as in high STA females, performance deteriorates owing to interference of redundant, inefficient, and possibly conflictual processing.

The second explanation of these findings derives from well-replicated findings in schizophrenics. The schizophrenia literature suggests that females show differences in the rate, transmission, and expression of schizophrenia (e.g., Goldstein, Tsuang, & Faraone, 1989). Females tend to show less genetic transmission of schizophrenia, and a more acute onset with fewer premorbid symptoms compared to male schizophrenics. This is paralleled by Claridge and Hewitt's (1987) finding of a decreased heritability for schizotypy in females as compared to males. Lack of significant findings in schizotypal females, not only in the cerebral asymmetry area but also in the attentional tasks described above, may reflect a difference in the etiology of schizotypy in males versus females. In males, the schizotypy construct may be revealing root antecedents of the schizophrenic syndrome(s), whereas for females, high schizotypy may be caused by social/environmental factors that are not reflected in neurocognitive studies. Further research, comparing male and female schizotypals with and without schizophrenic relatives, is required to examine this hypothesis. From this analysis, it would be predicted that female schizotypals would have fewer schizophrenic relatives, but those who did would show performance abnormalities similar to those of male schizotypals.

Summary

The first noteworthy point to emerge from this review of the cerebral asymmetries literature in schizotypy, as with the frontolimbic literature, is that the findings are overwhelmingly positive. Only 2 of the 11 studies reported in Table 13.2 failed to show significant relationships between schizotypal personality scores and hemispheric performance. As always, it is possible that this ratio is biased, owing to the publication biases of journals and the file-drawer problem. Still, this bias cannot account for the sheer preponderance of positive findings reported.

The relative consistency of the findings in this area sheds light on a major conceptual issue, namely whether such studies should be done at all. Cohen (1982) argued that findings of hemispheric imbalances in schizophrenia were the result of state factors, which caused transient changes in the relative arousal of each hemisphere. Cohen suggested that research into hemisyndromes in schizophrenia be performed at the physiological level tapping ongoing processes, rather than searching for fixed structural effects. However, the studies reviewed here tend to support a role for structural effects, while not ruling out the possibility of transient effects. Further research explicitly addressing this question is needed to examine potential interactions, and to determine if the attentional issues raised by Jutai (1989) reflect transient, functional properties or more stable traits.

In this chapter, evidence of hemispheric abnormalities in schizotypals has been presented in the context of three potential explanatory theories: left hemisphere deficit, left hemisphere overactivation, and interhemispheric transfer (IHT) abnormality. The majority of the studies can be interpreted as supporting the IHT hypothesis, with an unexpected twist. The results suggested improved IHT in schizotypals, and it was speculated that this effect may indicate an inverted-U–shaped curve of interhemispheric performance. A number of schizophrenia researchers have rejected the IHT hypothesis for schizophrenia (e.g., Raine, Harrison, Reynolds, Sheard, Cooper, & Medley, 1990; Walker & McGuire, 1982). It is recommended that this issue be reopened.

Finally, it should be noted that these IHT effects are impossible to distinguish, at this point, from a reduction of normal lateralization of function in male schizotypals. This hypothesis conforms to the data equally well, and accounts for differences between nonschizotypal males and females as well as for increased levels of positive-symptom traits in females. Indeed, reduced lateralization and improved IHT may go hand in hand as a single neurodevelopmental process.

Methodological issues

Subject selection appears to be less of an issue in this area as compared to the frontolimbic literature. Table 13.2 reveals that only one study of a student population (Kelley & Coursey, 1992) failed to find significant effects, whereas the other two studies drawing from this population did report significant relationships between schizotypy and laterality. This may indicate that the hemispheric tasks are less relevant to school performance or require a smaller processing load.

There were several pieces of evidence reviewed which indicated that neurocognitive abnormalities may actually result in performance advantages in schizotypals on tasks such as dichotic listening and negative priming. It was suggested that on these tasks, schizotypals may lie at the top of an inverted-U curve of performance. Alternatively, it is possible that schizotypals lie at one end of an inverted U, whereas subjects scoring low in schizotypy are at the other extreme. In any event, caution should be used in applying the word "normals" to subjects scoring low on schizotypy scales. If schizotypals are marked by an inability to limit the contents of consciousness, then subjects scoring abnormally low on scales such as the STA might be expected to display an extreme degree of cognitive rigidity. Subjects hovering around the mean of the distribution of schizotypal scale scores might make a more appropriate control group; however, this was performed in only one study (Jutai, 1989).

Another issue affecting subject selection concerns handedness of the subjects. All of the cerebral asymmetry studies reviewed in this paper utilized right-handed subjects only. This procedure is standard in the neuropsychological literature, for it is felt that left-handers, having abnormal cerebral organization, pose a confound for interpretation of results. However, a number of studies (Chapman et al., 1978; Kelley & Coursey, 1992; Kim, Raine, Triphon, & Green, 1992) have demonstrated that schizotypals show a significant increase in left- and/or mixed-handedness. Selection of right-handers only as a method of "controlling" for handedness may artificially bias the schizotypal sample in the direction of less impairment, thereby increasing the risk of type II errors. As Lord (1969) demonstrates, if two traits naturally covary, the attempt to separate them out artificially may lead to distorted results.

The method of hypothesis comparison employed in the cerebral asymmetries review clearly indicates the need for future studies to employ multiple methods of assessment of laterality. It is useful for a study to have more results than unknowns in question. To this end, future researchers should note that laterality coefficients do not provide as much information as providing the raw scores. In addition, studies employing several different tasks, as in Raine and Manders (1988), allow for the examination of dissociations needed to reach firm conclusions about the mechanisms underlying performance abnormalities. Assessment of lateral preference or strategy (by simply asking the subjects whether they employed verbal or visual strategies) also facilitates this process.

As with the frontolimbic studies above, the question of factors or syndromes of schizotypy remains an issue. Only two of the studies reviewed in this section consider dissociations of different scales or factors of schizotypy, and these found significant effects. Given the evidence of different lateralization of positive versus negative schizophrenia (Gruzelier, 1984), such investigations in the area of schizotypy are required. The one study to date that examined this question (Gruzelier, Burgess, Stygall, Irving, & Raine, in press) obtained results parallel to those found for schizophrenics. If indeed there are separate schizotypies, just as there may be separate pathophysiologies for the schizophrenias (Bilder & Degreef, 1991), research in this area will risk Type I errors, owing to a confounded (mixed) sample.

Directions for future research

A number of suggestions for future research have already been discussed throughout the body of this chapter. These include (1) the use of multiple, converging tests with slightly different stimulus parameters (e.g., stimulus presentation time); (2) experimental manipulations of the task to isolate the source of deficits; (3) the use of multiple measures of schizotypy with a goal of identifying subsyndromes with distinct pathophysiologies; and (4) the careful examination of gender and handedness effects. The most important goal is the use of multiple measures of neuropsychological functioning and schizotypy to allow for the identification of dissociations of deficits.

Future research needs to be directed to consider the specificity of the neuropsychological abnormalities found in schizotypals. Raine (1993) reviews evidence of frontolimbic neuropsychological deficits associated with criminal behavior that are parallel to those of schizotypals. Further, psychopaths may show some evidence of abnormal lateralization of language. Csernansky, Leiderman, and Goldman (1990) reported an increased incidence of schizotypy in temporal lobe epilepsy patients. Given these parallels in other disorders, research must be conducted to identify the differences, as well as potential overlap, between schizotypals and, for example, psychopaths. In addition, further studies of schizotypy in epileptics and other neurological patients (e.g., agenesis of the corpus callosum) may shed more light on the neurodevelopmental issues underlying the cognitive performance abnormalities.

Neuroimaging is a rapidly growing field that will prove extremely useful in identifying brain structure–function relationships in schizotypals. For example, Raine et al. (1992a) found correlations between schizotypy and frontal lobe structure (smaller) as well as frontal lobe performance [increased perseverative Wisconsin Card Sorting Test (WCST) performance]. Future MRI studies are needed to replicate and extend these findings to important brain regions such as the hippocampus and corpus callosum. Functional imaging (such as positron emission tomography, PET) can identify which areas of the brain are activated during task performance. This technique can be extremely useful in solving the puzzle of cerebral asymmetries by its ability to assess directly, for example, left hemisphere overactivation.

A final consideration for future researchers involves what kind of effects researchers are looking for. The popular model of schizotypy is implicitly linked to a disease model of schizophrenia. In this model, schizotypals have a faulty gene(s) or some other neurodevelopmental abnormality that constitutes an increased risk for the disease of schizophrenia given sufficient environmental stress. The logical converse of this statement is that schizotypals who do not develop schizophrenia must have some protective factors – special strengths relative to normal controls either that are indicators of a lack of environmental stress or that serve to compensate for the deficits inherent in schizotypy. An example of the former is the finding of Mednick, Parnas, and Schulsinger (1987) that schizotypal subjects actually had smaller ventricles and fewer birth complications compared to normal controls. According to Cannon et al. (1989), periventricular damage and ventricular enlargement are the result of birth complications (primed by a genetic liability to such insult). Schizotypals are individuals who share the genetic liability but lack the obstetrical insult; in order to remain compensated, schizotypals must show an abnormal lack of certain stressors that individuals without the genetic liability would have been able to cope with. Neuropsychological research into schizotypy has not explicitly searched for protective factors. Future studies following the disease model should utilize schizotypal subjects who are beyond the age of risk for schizophrenia (50 years old or so), and compare them to a group of age-matched controls. Subjects still within the risk years would have a tendency to confound the search for protective factors, because some may yet become schizophrenic. Finally, studies that search for deficits in schizotypals but obtain negative results should be cautious in their interpretation of the findings. Such results may simply indicate a mechanism that is uninvolved in schizotypy, but they may indicate a protective factor of some significance.

Acknowledgments

Research described in this chapter was supported by a National Institute of Mental Health (NIMH) Shared Instrumentation Grant and by BRSG S07 RR07012-21 awarded by the Biomedical Research Support Grant Program, Division of Research Sources, the National Institute of Health. The authors are grateful to Mike Dawson, Sarnoff Mednick, David Walsh, Bill McClure, and Tony Beech, who provided helpful comments.

References

American Psychiatric Association. (1987). *Diagnostic and statistical manual of mental disorders* (3rd edition, rev). Washington, D.C.: APA.

Arndt, S., Alliger, R. J., Andreasen, N. C. (1991). The distinction of positive and negative symptoms: The failure of a two-dimensional model. *British Journal of Psychiatry, 158,* 317–322.

Asarnow, R. F., Nuechterlein, K. H., & Marder, S. R. (1983). Span of apprehension performance, neuropsychological functioning, and indices of psychosis proneness. *Journal of Nervous and Mental Disease, 171,* 662–669.

Baruch, I., Hemsley, D. R., & Gray, J. A. (1988a). Differential performance of acute and chronic schizophrenics in a latent inhibition task. *Journal of Nervous and Mental Disease, 176,* 598–606.

Baruch, I., Hemsley, D. R., & Gray, J. A. (1988b). Latent inhibition and "psychotic proneness" in normal subjects. *Personality and Individual Differences, 9,* 777–783.

Beech, A., & Claridge, G. (1987) Individual differences in negative priming: Relations with schizotypal personality traits. *British Journal of Psychology, 78,* 349–356.

Beech, A., Baylis, G. C., Smithson, P., & Claridge, G. (1989a). Individual differences in schizotypy as reflected in measures of cognitive inhibition. *British Journal of Clinical Psychology, 28,* 117–129.

Beech, A., Powell, T., McWilliam, J., & Claridge, G. (1989b). Evidence of reduced 'cognitive inhibition' in schizophrenia. *British Journal of Clinical Psychology, 28,* 109–116.

Benishay, D. S., Raine, A., Lencz, T., & Bird, L. (1993). Dissociations between schizotypal factors on measures of cerebral asymmetry. Poster presented at the 1993 meeting of the Society for Research in Psychopathology, Chicago, Ill.

Bilder, R. M., & Degreef, G. (1991). Morphologic markers of neurodevelopmental paths to schizophrenia. In S. A. Mednick (Ed.), *Developmental neuropathology of schizophrenia.* New York: Plenum.

Braff, D. L. (1993). Information processing and attention dysfunctions in schizophrenia. *Schizophrenia Bulletin, 19,* 233–259.

Broks, P. (1984). Schizotypy and hemisphere function – II: Performance asymmetry on a verbal divided visual field task. *Personality and Individual Differences, 5(6),* 649–656.

Broks, P., Claridge, G., Matheson, J., & Hargreaves, J. (1984). Schizotypy and hemisphere function – IV: Story comprehension under binaural and monaural listening conditions. *Personality and Individual Differences, 5,* 665–670.

Buchsbaum, M. S., Nuechterlein, K. H., Haier, R. J., Wu, J., Sicotte, N., Hazlett, E., Asarnow, R., Potkin, S., & Guich, S. (1990). Glucose metabolic rate in normals and schizophrenics during the continuous performance test assessed by positron emission tomography. *British Journal of Psychiatry, 156,* 216–227.

Bullen, J. G., Hemsley, D. R., & Dixon, N. F. (1987). Inhibition, unusual perceptual experiences and psychoticism. *Personality and Individual Differences, 8,* 687–691.

Cannon, T. D., Mednick, S. A., & Parnas, J. (1989). Genetic and perinatal determinants of structural brain deficits in schizophrenia. *Archives of General Psychiatry, 46,* 883–889.

Chapman, L. J., & Chapman, J. P. (1978). The measurement of differential deficit. *Journal of Psychiatry Research, 14,* 303–311.

Chapman, L. J., Chapman, J. P., & Raulin, M. L. (1976). Scales for physical and social anhedonia. *Journal of Abnormal Psychology, 85,* 374–382.

Chapman, L. J., Chapman, J. P., & Raulin, M. L. (1978). Body-image aberration in schizophrenia. *Journal of Abnormal Psychology, 87,* 399–407.

Claridge, G., & Broks, P. (1984). Schizotypy and hemisphere function – I. Theoretical considerations and the measurement of schizotypy. *Personality and Individual Differences, 5,* 633–648.

Claridge, G., Clark, K. H., & Beech, A. R. (1992). Lateralization of the 'negative priming' effect: Relationships with schizotypy and with gender. *British Journal of Psychology, 83,* 13–23.

Claridge, G., & Hewitt, J. K. (1987). A biometrical study of schizotypy in a normal population.

Cohen, G. (1982). Theoretical interpretations of lateral asymmetries. In J. G. Beaumont (Ed.), *Divided visual field studies of cerebral organization.* London: Academic Press.

Condray, R., & Steinhauer, S. R. (1992). Schizotypal personality disorder in individuals with and without schizophrenic relatives: Similarities and contrasts in neurocognitive and clinical functioning. *Schizophrenia Research, 7,* 33–41.

Cornblatt, B. A., & Keilp, J. G. (1994). Impaired attention, genetics, and the pathophysiology of schizophrenia. *Schizophrenia Bulletin, 20,* 31–46.

Crow, T. J., Ball, J., Bloom, S.R., Brown, R., Bruton, C. J., Colter, N., Frith, C. D., Johnstone, E. C., Owens, D. G. C., & Roberts, G. W. (1989). Schizophrenia as an anomaly of development of cerebral asymmetry: A post-mortem study and a proposal concerning the genetic basis of the disease. *Archives of General Psychiatry, 46,* 1145–1150.

Csernansky, J. G., Leiderman, D. B., & Goldman, J. (1990). Schizophrenia spectrum disorder and limbic epilepsy. [letter] *Journal of Neuropsychiatry and Clinical Neurosciences, 2,* 236.

Eckblad, M., & Chapman, L. J. (1983). Magical ideation as an indicator of schizotypy. *Journal of Consulting and Clinical Psychology, 51,* 215–225.

Eysenck, H. J., & Eysenck, S. B. G. (1975). *Manual of the Eysenck Personality Questionnaire.* Hodder & Stoughton.

Fisher, M., & Weinman, J. (1989). Priming, word recognition, and psychotic tendencies. *Personality and Individual Differences, 10,* 185–189.

Flor-Henry, P. (1969). Psychoses and temporal lobe epilepsy: A controlled investigation. *Epilepsia, 19,* 363.

Flor-Henry, P. (1987). Cerebral dynamics, laterality, and psychopathology: A commentary. In R. Takahashi, P. Flor-Henry, J. Gruzelier, & S. I. Niwa (Eds.), *Cerebral dynamics, laterality, and psychopathology,* 3–22. Amsterdam: Elsevier.

Fowles, D. C. (1992). Schizophrenia: Diathesis–stress revisited. *Annual Review of Psychology, 43,* 303–336.

Frith, C. D. (1979). Consciousness, information processing, and schizophrenia. *British Journal of Psychiatry, 134,* 225–235.

Frith, C. D., & Done, D. J. (1988). Towards a neuropsychology of schizophrenia. *British Journal of Psychiatry, 153,* 437–443.

Goldman-Rakic, P. (1987). Development of cortical circuitry and cognitive function. *Child Development, 58,* 601–622.

Goldstein, J. M., Tsuang, M. T., & Faraone, S. V. (1989) Gender and schizophrenia: Understanding the heterogeneity of the illness. *Psychiatry Research, 27,* 243–253.

Green, P., Hallett, S., & Hunter, M. (1983). Abnormal interhemispheric integration and hemispheric specialisation in schizophrenics and high-risk children. In P. Flor-Henry & J. Gruzelier (Eds.), *Laterality and psychopathology.* Amsterdam: Elsevier.

Green, P., & Kotenko, V. (1980). Superior speech comprehension in schizophrenics under monaural versus binaural listening conditions. *Journal of Abnormal Psychology, 89,* 399–408.

Grove, W. M., Lebow, B. S., Clementz, B. A., Cerri, A., Medus, C., & Iacono, W. G. (1991). Familial prevalence and coaggregation of schizotypy indicators: A multitrait family study. *Journal of Abnormal Psychology, 100,* 115–121.

Gruzelier, J. (1984). Hemispheric imbalances in schizophrenia. *International Journal of Psychophysiology, 1,* 227–240.

Gruzelier, J., Burgess, A., Stygall, J., Irving, G., & Raine, A. (in press). Hemisphere imbalance and syndrome of schizotypal personality. *British Journal of Psychiatry.*

Heaton, R. K. (1981). *The Wisconsin Card Sorting Test manual.* Odessa, Fla.: Psychological Assessment Resources.

Hellige, J. B. (1993). *Hemispheric asymmetry: What's right and what's left.* Cambridge, Mass.: Harvard University Press.

Jones, S. H., Gray, J. A., & Hemsley, D. R. (1990). The Kamin blocking effect, incidental learning, and psychoticism. *British Journal of Psychology, 81,* 95–110.

Jones, S. H., Gray, J. A., & Hemsley, D. R. (1992). The Kamin blocking effect, incidental learning, and schizotypy (a reanalysis). *Personality and Individual Differences, 13,* 57–60.

Jutai, J. W. (1989). Spatial attention in hypothetically psychosis-prone college students. *Psychiatry Research, 27,* 207–215.

Kelley, M. P., & Coursey, R. D. (1992). Lateral preference and neuropsychological correlates of schizotypy. *Psychiatry Research, 41,* 115–135.

Kendler, K. S., Ochs, A. L., Gorman, A. M., Hewitt, J. K., Ross, D. E., & Mirsky, A. F. (1991). The structure of schizotypy: A pilot multitrait twin study. *Psychiatry Research, 36,* 19–36.

Kidd, R. T., & Powell, G. E. (1993). Raised left hemisphere activation in the nonclinical schizotypal personality. *Personality and Individual Differences, 14*(5), 723–731.

Kim, D., Raine, A., Triphon, N., & Green, M. F. (1992). Mixed handedness and features of schizotypal personality in a nonclinical sample. *Journal of Nervous and Mental Disease, 180,* 133–135.

Kolb, B., & Whishaw, I. Q. (1990). *Fundamentals of human neuropsychology.* New York: W. H. Freeman.

Launay, G., & Slade, P. (1981). The measurement of hallucination predisposition in male and female prisoners. *Personality and Individual Differences, 2,* 221–234.

Lenzenweger, M. F., Cornblatt, B. A., & Putnick, M. (1991). Schizotypy and sustained attention. *Journal of Abnormal Psychology, 100,* 84–89.

Liddle, P. (1987). The symptoms of chronic schizophrenia: A re-examination of the positive-negative dichotomy. *British Journal of Psychiatry, 151,* 145–151.

Lord, F. M. (1969). Statistical adjustments when comparing pre-existing groups. *Psychological Bulletin, 72,* 336–337.

Lubow, R. E. (1973). Latent inhibition. *Psychological Bulletin, 79,* 398–407.

Lyons, M. J., Merla, M. E., Young, L., & Kremen, W. S. (1991). Impaired neuropsychological functioning in symptomatic volunteers with schizotypy: Preliminary findings. *Biological Psychiatry, 30,* 424–426.

McGhie, A., & Chapman, J. (1961). Disorders of attention and perception in early schizophrenia. *British Journal of Medical Psychology, 34,* 103–115.

McGlone, J. (1980). Sex differences in human brain asymmetry. *Behavioral and Brain Sciences, 3,* 215–263.

Mednick, S. A., Parnas, J., & Schulsinger, F. (1987). The Copenhagen High-Risk Project, 1962–1986. *Schizophrenia Bulletin, 13,* 485–495.

Meehl, P. E. (1976). Psychodiagnosis: Selected papers. New York: Raven Press.

Meehl, P. E. (1990). Toward an integrated theory of schizotaxia, schizotypy, and schizophrenia. *Journal of Personality Disorders, 4,* 1–99.

Mills, S., & Raine, A. (1993). Right ear advantage in delinquent schizotypals. Poster presented at the 1993 meeting of the Society for Research in Psychopathology, Chicago, Ill.

Milner, B. (1963). Effects of different brain lesions on card sorting. *Archives of Neurology, 9,* 90–100.

Nuechterlein, K. H., & Dawson, M. E. (1984). A heuristic vulnerability/stress model of schizophrenic episodes. *Schizophrenia Bulletin, 10,* 300–312.

Posner, M. I., Early, T. S., Reiman, E., Parod, P. J., & Dhawan, M. (1988). Asymmetries in hemispheric control of attention in schizophrenia. *Archives of General Psychiatry, 45,* 814–821.

Raine, A. (1992). Sex differences in schizotypal personality in a nonclinical population. *Journal of Abnormal Psychology, 101,* 361–364.

Raine, A. (1993). *The psychopathology of crime: Criminal behavior as a clinical disorder.* San Diego: Academic Press.

Raine, A., Andrews, H., Sheard, C., Walder, C., & Manders, D. (1989). Interhemispheric transfer in schizophrenics, depressives and normals with schizoid tendencies. *Journal of Abnormal Psychology, 98* (1), 35–41.

Raine, A., Harrison, G. N., Reynolds, G. P., Sheard, C., Cooper, J. E., & Medley, I. (1990). Structural and functional characteristics of the corpus callosum in schizophrenics, psychiatric controls, and normal controls: A magnetic resonance imaging and neuropsychological evaluation. *Archives of General Psychiatry, 47,* 1060–1064.

Raine, A., & Manders, D. (1988). Schizoid personality, inter-hemispheric transfer, and left hemisphere over-activation. *British Journal of Clinical Psychology, 27,* 333–347.

Raine, A., Reynolds, C., Lencz, T., Scerbo, A., Triphon, N., & Kim, D. (1994). Cognitive–perceptual, interpersonal, and disorganized features of schizotypal personality. *Schizophrenia Bulletin, 20,* 191–201.

Raine, A., Sheard, C., Reynolds, G. P., & Lencz, T. (1992a). Prefrontal structural and functional deficits associated with individual differences in schizotypal personality. *Schizophrenia Research, 7,* 237–247.

Raine, A., Triphon, N., Kim, D., Hesler, A., Bird, L., Lencz, T., Redmon, M., & Scerbo, A. (1992b). Schizotypal personality: Factor structure, sex differences, psychiatric differences, genetics, psychophysiology, and neuropsychology. Paper presented at the 1992 Western Psychological Association meeting, Portland, Ore.

Rawlings, D., & Borge, A. (1987). Personality and hemisphere function: Two experiments using the dichotic shadowing technique. *Personality and Individual Differences, 8(4)*, 483–488.

Rawlings, D., & Claridge, G. (1984). Schizotypy and hemisphere function – III: Performance asymmetries on tasks of letter recognition and local–global processing. *Personality and Individual Differences, 5,* 657–663.

Rosenthal, R., & Bigelow, L. B. (1972). Quantitative brain measures in chronic schizophrenia. *British Journal of Psychiatry, 121,* 259–264.

Serper, M. R., & Harvey, P. D. (1994). The need to integrate neuropsychological and experimental schizophrenia research. *Schizophrenia Bulletin, 20,* 1–11.

Siever, L. J. (1985). Biological markers in schizotypal personality disorder. *Schizophrenia Bulletin, 11,* 564–574.

Spaulding, W., Garbin, C. P., & Dras, S. R. (1989). Cognitive abnormalities in schizophrenic patients and schizotypal college students. *Journal of Nervous and Mental Disease, 177,* 717–728.

Strauss, M. E., & Summerfelt, A. (1994). The need to integrate neuropsychological and experimental schizophrenia research: Response. *Schizophrenia Bulletin, 20,* 13–21.

Stuss, D. T., & Benson, D. F. (1986). *The frontal lobes.* New York: Raven Press.

Tipper, S. P. (1985). The negative priming effect: Inhibitory priming by ignored objects. *Quarterly Journal of Experimental Psychology, 37a,* 571–590.

Venables, P. H. (1980). Primary dysfunction and cortical lateralization in schizophrenia. In M. Koukkou, D. Lehmann, & J. Angst (Eds.), *Functional states of the brain: Their determinants.* Amsterdam: Elsevier.

Venables, P. H. (1990). The measurement of schizotypy in Mauritius. *Personality and Individual Differences, 11,* 965–971.

Venables, P. H. (1992). Hippocampal function and schizophrenia: Experimental psychological evidence. *Annals of the New York Academy of Science,* 111–126.

Walker, E., & McGuire, M. (1982). Intra- and interhemispheric information processing in schizophrenia. *Psychological Bulletin, 92,* 701–725.

Weinberger, D. R. (1987). Implications of normal brain development for the pathogenesis of schizophrenia. *Archives of General Psychiatry, 44,* 660–669.

Weinberger, D. R., Berman, K. F., & Zec, R. F. (1986). Physiologic dysfunction of dorsolateral prefrontal cortex in schizophrenia. *Archives of General Psychiatry, 43,* 114–124.

Wexler, B. E., Giller, E. L., & Southwick, S. (1991). Cerebral laterality, symptoms, and diagnosis of psychotic patients. *Biological Psychiatry, 29,* 103–116.

14

Syndromes of schizotypy: patterns of cognitive asymmetry, arousal, and gender

JOHN GRUZELIER

In this chapter we describe two experiments in which we approach the nature and central nervous system basis of the schizotypal personality from the perspective of schizophrenia. From a series of experiments (Gruzelier, 1991b; 1994) we have evolved a three-syndrome neuropsychophysiological model of acute schizophrenia, two syndromes of which have a basis in imbalances in hemispheric activation, whereas the third is not consistently associated with lateral asymmetry. Here we show that schizotypy has a similar three-syndrome structure of core features, and we provide preliminary evidence of a similar basis in hemispheric asymmetry as found in schizophrenia. This account provides unambiguous evidence of a dimensional rather than categorical view of the relationship between schizotypy and schizophrenia, in keeping with genetic evidence (Claridge, 1985), and, given that our results were obtained from healthy, high achieving medical students, provides support for the dimensional view of schizotypy and normality. It describes a syndromal model of schizotypy that offers a theoretical framework for the nature and neuropsychophysiological basis of the syndromes, too often investigated from an operational or atheoretical perspective. Finally, by monitoring arousal and stress levels from self-report questionnaires, and by utilizing an ecologically valid stressor, test anxiety, we gain insights about how schizotypy may progress to schizophrenia, results that endorse the importance of extremes of arousal in the dynamics of schizotypy and schizophrenia.

Three-syndrome model of schizophrenia

In acute schizophrenia we have found three syndromes derived from a comprehensive clinical evaluation with the Present State Evaluation (Wing,

Cooper, & Satorius, 1974) and the Brief Psychiatric Rating Scale (BPRS) (Overall & Gorham, 1962). Two of the syndromes were related to a behavioral and physiological activation dimension, and were associated with opposite patterns of hemispheric activation (Gruzelier, 1981; Gruzelier & Manchanda, 1982). The Active syndrome was characterized by affective delusions, positive or labile affect, together with raised levels of cognitive activity, speech, and motor activity generally, as seen in overactivity on the ward. This was in contrast to the Withdrawn syndrome, which consisted of negative-symptom features such as social and emotional withdrawal, blunted affect, poverty of speech, and motor retardation. The two syndromes were delineated originally on the basis of opposite patterns of lateral asymmetry in electrodermal orienting responses to moderate intensity and loud tones. The nature of the two syndromes could be seen to be at opposite extremes of an arousal dimension involving cognition, mood valence, and behavioral activity. Both syndromes coexisted with a third Unreality syndrome, consisting of Schneiderian symptoms of first rank, which provided a second positive-symptom syndrome.

A similar three-syndrome approach in schizophrenia has arisen from factor analyses of ratings in which two positive and one negative syndrome have been delineated. Liddle and colleagues (e.g., Liddle, 1987) have described three overlapping syndromes in mostly chronic patients: (1) "psychomotor poverty," akin to the Withdrawn syndrome, above; (2) "disorganization," largely composed of various speech and thought disorders, incongruous affect, distractability, and self neglect, and having affinities with the Active syndrome; (3) "reality distortion," consisting of hallucinations and delusions, similar to the third syndrome above but not distinguishing between Schneiderian and non-Schneiderian delusions. Arndt, Alliger, and Andreasen (1991), pooling ratings from three studies (N = 207), found one negative-syndrome factor; four positive-symptom clusters were subdivided into two factors, one containing positive thought disorder and bizarre behavior and also loading on alogia, and the second consisting of delusions and hallucinations. Gur et al. (1991), using scales that overlapped with those of Arndt et al., obtained three factors, one consisting of hallucinations and delusions, one of negative symptoms, and a third of bizarre behavior, positive thought disorder, and attentional disturbance. An affinity between the last factor and the Active syndrome was endorsed by a correlation with the activity factor of the BPRS. Bilder et al. (1985) also report three syndromes in chronic schizophrenic patients.

Syndromes and patterns of cerebral asymmetry

In our investigations the syndrome model first arose from psychophysiological considerations (Gruzelier, 1984). Patients were subdivided on the basis of the direction of the lateral asymmetry of electrodermal orienting responses. Those with a dominance of left hemispheric influences delineated the Active syndrome. This pattern of asymmetry is in keeping neuropsychologically with the increased verbal and motor activity of the syndrome and of its positive mood valence through activation of the left hemisphere. Those with a dominance of right hemispheric influences delineated the Withdrawn syndrome. This pattern of asymmetry is in keeping neuropsychologically with the opposite state of hemispheric imbalance; poverty of speech is compatible with underactivation of the left hemisphere, whereas social withdrawal and negative emotional valence have been associated with activation of the right hemisphere.

A review of the literature on cerebral asymmetry and schizophrenia disclosed evidence of both patterns of asymmetry. Descriptions of the type of patients in the various studies showed a consistency between the direction of asymmetry and clinical features similar to, or commonly associated with, what were to be called the Active and Withdrawn syndromes (Gruzelier, 1983, 1991). Subsequently, the model has been validated using subjects classified with a rating scale devised to measure the syndromes and with dependent variables including lateralized neuropsychological tests of learning and memory (Gruzelier, Seymour, Wilson, Jolley, & Hirsch, 1988), Warrington's (1984) test of recognition memory for words compared with unfamiliar faces (Gruzelier, 1990; Gruzelier & Wilson, 1995), and an EEG spectrum analysis of visual evoked response–stimulus intensity relationships (Gruzelier, Jutai, & Connolly, 1993).

Cerebral laterality and the schizotypal personality

Evidence has also been reviewed for the involvement of cerebral laterality in investigations of the schizotypal personality (Gruzelier, 1991; Lencz & Raine, Chapter 18, this volume). Notably Claridge and collaborators (Broks, 1984; Broks, Claridge, Matheson, & Hargreaves, 1984; Rawlings & Borge, 1987; Rawlings & Claridge, 1984), in a series of studies, have found an impairment in left hemispheric processing using their scale, which has strong associations with perceptual distortions and magical thinking (Hewitt & Claridge, 1989; Kelley & Coursey, 1992). Results with a divided visual-field letter identification task were similar to those for our medical students the day before an examination as compared with their performance on a less stressful occasion, in a closely similar tachistoscopic study (Gruzelier & Phelan, 1991). This may imply the coexistence of anxiety in the Claridge schizotypes and a functional lability of the pattern of asymmetry. Their results with a dichotic shadowing, story comprehension test produced laterality effects more commonly associated with chronic or negative-symptom schizophrenic patients (Gruzelier, 1991b).

In an attempt to elucidate further the nature of the lateralized abnormality, Claridge, Clark, and Beech (1991) examined negative priming in a divided field paradigm (see Claridge & Beech, Chapter 9, this volume). They found that the priming effect in high scoring schizotypes was enhanced in the left hemisphere but absent in the right hemisphere. This result may be interpreted as reflecting an imbalance in excitation–inhibition processes: the right hemisphere an excitatory valence and the left hemisphere inhibitory. Right hemispheric overactivation has also been shown in schizotypy with measurement of conjugate lateral eye movements (Raine & Manders, 1988; Winterbotham, 1979, using the Eysenck Psychoticism Scale and MMPI Schizophrenia Scale, respectively). These were predominantly in a leftward direction, which is indicative of greater right than left hemispheric activation of the frontal eye fields. The leftward asymmetry pattern is less commonly reported in schizophrenia and has been found in less florid schizophrenics and in depressive patients (Gruzelier, 1983).

The opposite state of imbalance has also been reported in schizotypy. Raine and Manders (1988) found positive correlations between schizotypy and left hemispheric activation or processing strategies. They used a composite schizotypy measure which could perhaps be conceptualized as having a broad positive-symptom character including features having affinities with the Active and Unreality syndromes described above in schizophrenia. Evidence in keeping with right hemispheric impairments, and thereby an imbalance also favoring the left hemisphere, was reported by Jutai (1988), who measured schizotypy with several scales developed by Chapman and Chapman and colleagues. The results were particularly definitive on Magical Ideation; with respect to the other significant subscale, Physical Anhedonia, bilateral impairments were noted. Thus two states of hemispheric imbalances of function have been reported in schizotypy. Measures of both laterality and schizotypy have varied across studies. We advocated a syndromal approach to the measurement of schizotypy to determine whether the inconsistencies could be reconciled such that opposite patterns of asymmetry may be aligned with different syndromes.

We set out to test this hypothesis using our three-syndrome model of schizophrenia (see also Gruzelier & Richardson, 1994, for a more recent approach).

Experiment I: three-syndrome model of schizotypy

Experimental predictions

In the first investigation (Gruzelier, Burgess, Stygall, & Raine, 1995) we examined, prior to its publication, a new scale devised by Raine (1991) called the Schizotypal Personality Questionnaire (SPQ) and composed of nine subscales based on the nine features of the schizotypal personality in DSM-III-R. We hypothesized a correspondence between our three-syndrome model of schizophrenia and the factor structure of the scale that we administered to British medical students. In addition, we hypothesized that the two factors having affinities with the Active and Withdrawn syndromes in schizophrenia would have identical patterns of cognitive asymmetry on the Warrington Recognition Memory Test (WRMT), and would be differentiated by arousal levels as measured with the Thayer (1967, 1989) Activation–Deactivation scales: Tension, Energy, Calmness, Tiredness. Specifically, high scorers on the Active factor would have superior memory for words compared with faces, whereas those scoring highly on the Withdrawn factor would have superior memory for faces compared with words. Further, self-report measures of level of arousal or alertness would indicate higher scores on the Active factor, whereas lower levels of arousal would characterize high scorers on the Withdrawn factor. These predictions would hold for strongly right-handed subjects. Those scoring highly on the third factor, termed the Unreality factor, would show no consistent pattern of asymmetry.

We predicted that the essential features of the three factors would involve the following subscales: (1) Withdrawn factor – no close friends, constricted affect, and social anxiety; (2) Active factor – eccentricity and odd speech; (3) Unreality factor – unusual perceptual experiences, magical thinking, ideas of reference, and suspiciousness. These predictions were based on the following considerations:

1. The Withdrawn factor: No close friends would reflect social withdrawal; constricted affect was akin to the blunted affect of patients; and social anxiety could be seen as a precursor to social withdrawal.

2. The Active factor: Both eccentricity and odd speech reflected acting-out behavior underpinned by left hemispheric motoric and speech production processes.
3. The Unreality factor: Unusual perceptual experience could be seen as a precursor of Schneiderian symptoms, as with magical thinking, whereas paranoid features such as ideas of reference and suspiciousness could be related to delusions. Paranoid features were not consistently related to cerebral asymmetry in our schizophrenic patients.

Schizotypy factor structure

Subjects – 63 men and 77 women – of average age 22 years were investigated in two half classes divided alphabetically and examined at the same time of day. The factor structure of the SPQ after varimax rotation, shown in Table 14.1, indicates that three factors had eigenvalues greater than one. Factor 1 was composed of the three hypothesized Withdrawn subscales: no close friends, social anxiety, and blunted affect, together with suspiciousness. Factor 2 consisted mostly of the hypothesized Unreality subscales: unusual perceptual experiences, magical thinking, ideas of reference, and suspiciousness. Factor 3 consisted of the Active features of eccentricity and odd speech.

Patterns of lateral asymmetry, schizotypy, and activation

The 79 dextral subjects, defined as those with scores above 69 on the Edinburgh scale (–100 – +100), were subdivided on the basis of a median split on word–face memory discrepancy scores after z transformation: that is, $N = 40$ faces superior to words (F/W); $N = 39$ words superior to faces (W/F). As can be seen in Table 14.2, the group with the faces superiority had higher scores on the Withdrawn factor, whereas the group with the word superiority had higher scores on the Active factor ($F = 5.04$, $df = 1.77$, $p < .027$). On average, the Unreality factor showed a word advantage, but this effect was not significant. Considering individual subscales there were significant effects in the predicted direction for no close friends ($p < .04$) and odd speech ($p < .02$); constricted affect approached significance ($p < .06$). Subjects with a word advantage scored higher on the Thayer Tension Scale ($p < .05$).

Comparison of extreme quartiles (F/W, $N = 20$; W/F, $N = 21$) confirmed the results with the Withdrawn factor ($p < .03$) and the subscales constricted affect ($p < .01$) and no close friends ($p < .09$). There was no difference on the Active factor, though the subscale odd speech showed a tendency in the predicted direction ($p < .1$). Subjects with a word advantage had higher Tension

Table 14.1. *Factor structure of the Schizotypal Personality Questionnaire in experiments 1 and 2*

Scales	Factor I	Factor II	Factor III
Experiment 1			
No close friends	0.73	0.10	0.06
Social anxiety	0.72	0.05	0.10
Blunted affect	0.66	–0.04	0.39
Suspiciousness	0.61	0.58	0.02
Unusual perceptual experiences	0.21	0.78	0.28
Ideas of reference	0.26	0.72	0.11
Odd beliefs	–0.28	0.70	0.06
Eccentricity	0.12	0.12	0.83
Odd speech	0.09	0.20	0.81
Experiment 2			
No close friends	0.78	–0.11	0.18
Social anxiety	0.74	0.16	–0.03
Blunted affect	0.68	–0.09	0.34
Suspiciousness	0.69	0.37	–0.04
Unusual perceptual experiences	0.12	0.80	0.15
Ideas of reference	0.25	0.75	0.01
Odd beliefs	–0.19	0.74	0.15
Eccentricity	0.02	0.09	0.87
Odd speech	0.20	0.18	0.77

scores ($p < .01$), whereas those with a memory-for-faces advantage scored more highly on the Calmness scale ($p < .01$) – results that were compatible with the model.

Replication study

Schizotypy measures and factor solutions

We set out to replicate the results in a second sample of British medical students tested two years after the first sample. In addition to the SPQ and the Thayer scales we included the Physical Anhedonia Scale of Chapman. This aspect was not covered by the SPQ, whereas the Social Anhedonia Scale had

Table 14.2. *The relations among pattern of cognitive asymmetry and schizotypy factors, schizotypy subscales, and activation scales*

	Word advantage		Face advantage	
Scales/Factors	$\bar{X}$	σ	$\bar{X}$	σ
Withdrawn	–0.17	1.06	0.25	0.88
Unreality	0.13	1.09	–0.04	0.93
Active	0.13	0.96	–0.13	0.98
Odd speech	3.43	1.80	2.58	1.61
No close friends	1.08	1.77	1.75	1.69
Blunted affect	1.15	1.31	1.68	1.59
Tension	15.31	6.67	13.05	5.35
Quartile analysis				
Withdrawn	–0.23	1.05	0.37	0.92
Unreality	0.10	1.07	–0.04	0.88
Active	–0.01	0.94	–0.01	0.88
No close friends	1.14	2.01	1.95	1.75
Blunted affect	0.95	1.16	2.05	1.73
Odd speech	3.24	1.79	2.60	1.35
Calmness	12.64	4.56	15.10	4.49
Tension	16.14	6.78	11.69	5.19

close affinities with the Withdrawn factor. We also included the Eysenck Personality Questionnaire (EPQ) (Eysenck & Eysenck, 1975), which measures the personality dimensions of Psychoticism, Extraversion–Introversion, and Neuroticism.

There have been several attempts to factor-analyze schizotypy scales which we detail elsewhere (Gruzelier & Doig, 1995; see also Venables, Chapter 6, this volume). What is perhaps most straightforward is the separation of anhedonia from the positive features of schizotypy. Furthermore, associations with cerebral asymmetry support this conjecture. We examined relations between anhedonia and electrodermal orienting response asymmetries (Gruzelier & Davis, 1995). In unmedicated psychotic patients the Social Anhedonia Scale (Chapman, Chapman, & Raulin, 1976) was associated with the right hemispheric activational dominance pattern of asymmetry. This was compatible with the view that social anhedonia represents a feature of social withdrawal and the Withdrawn syndrome. Anhedonia has more than once been associated with Introversion, a relation that may be understood as integrating the social withdrawal aspects of schizotypy; accordingly both the Social Anhedonia and Introversion scales were predicted to load on our Withdrawn factor. Psychoticism has been described as floating across the various factors from study to study (Bentall, Claridge, & Slade, 1989). In view of its association with noncomformity (Chapman, Chapman, Numbers, Edell, Carpenter, & Bechfield, 1984), social deviancy (Mutaner, Garcia-Sevilla, Fernandez, & Torruba, 1988), and Eysenck's recent theorizing as to its basis in eccentricity and genius (Eysenck, 1994), we predicted that it would load on the Active factor.

Replication sample and schizotypy structure

The replication sample consisted of 151 medical students, 73 men and 78 women, mean age of 21 years, who were tested in two subgroups divided alphabetically by surname. The group K–Z were tested in the afternoon following a midcourse examination. We also examined performance on three cognitive tests: the Mill Hill Vocabulary and Analogies tests and the Hooper Visual Organization Test.

A principal components analysis (PCA) was first performed on the SPQ. The results replicated the three-factor solution found previously (see Table 14.1, where the factors and loadings of the two experiments are compared).

Cognitive asymmetry patterns

Strongly right-handed subjects (N = 78) were subdivided into those with a word recognition memory advantage and those with a faces memory advantage (N = 39 in each group), after z transformation of scores. The two groups were examined on the nine subscales and the three factor scores. The relationship between a faces advantage and withdrawal was confirmed by higher scores on the Withdrawn factor in those with a faces advantage compared with a word advantage ($p < .06$), owing largely to the no close friends subscale ($p < .003$). In contrast to the results of the first experiment, the Active factor did not relate to pattern of asymmetry ($t = 0.28$). In addition, there was a tendency for unusual perceptual experiences to be associated with a word advantage ($p < .09$); differences on the Unreality factor as a whole fell short of significance ($p < .12$).

Subjects were then selected to form high and low scoring groups on the basis of group distributions of factor scores, approximately 15% at each end of the distribution, and examined for differences on the cognitive tests. There was a tendency for verbal memory to be superior in low ($N = 16$) than high ($N = 15$) scorers on the Unreality factor ($p < .06$). This effect on verbal processing was corroborated by analyses of the Vocabulary test ($p < .002$) and the Analogies test ($p < .01$). Male and female subjects were examined separately with median split analyses on the memory discrepancy scores. The relationship between unusual perceptual experiences and word memory superiority was found in females ($\bar{X}3.23$ vs. $\bar{X}2.44$, $p < .035$), but not in males, in whom the means were in the opposite direction ($\bar{X}2.19$ vs. $\bar{X}2.67$). In contrast, males contributed most to the relationship between withdrawal and faces memory advantage (Withdrawn factor: males, $\bar{X}{-0.35}$ vs. $\bar{X}0.42$, $p < .02$; no close friends: males, $\bar{X}0.69$ vs. $\bar{X}2.5$, $p < .0005$; blunted affect: males, $\bar{X}0.81$ vs. $\bar{X}1.52$, $p < .05$).

Activation level

The memory asymmetry groups were examined for differences on the Thayer scales. There was a weak relationship between Energy and a word memory advantage in the direction predicted ($\bar{X}18.92$ vs. $\bar{X}16.87$, $p < .08$) which was found to be due to the male subjects ($\bar{X}20.44$ vs. $\bar{X}16.94$, $p < .06$). There was also a relationship in male subjects between a faces memory advantage and Tension ($\bar{X}10.69$ vs. $\bar{X}13.50$, $p < .05$). There were no significant effects with Calmness and Tiredness in the total group or with gender subgroups.

Subjects were then divided into high and low scorers on the three factors, and compared for self-report arousal ratings. Only on the Active factor were there significant effects, and these were in the direction predicted; that is, high-scoring Active subjects had higher Energy ($\bar{X}21.19$ vs. $\bar{X}16.5$, $p < .013$) and lower Tiredness ($\bar{X}12.8$ vs. $\bar{X}15.7$, $p < .09$) scores.

Test anxiety

The effect of test anxiety in altering hemispheric asymmetry was tested by comparing the two half classes. As predicted, there was a significant difference between the groups in the direction of a word advantage in the nontest group and a faces advantage in the examination group ($p < .05$). This was due largely to an increase in right hemispheric nonverbal processes as seen in lower word memory and higher face memory scores in the exam group ($p < .01$). This interpretation was supported by lower Vocabulary ($p < .002$) and Analogies ($p < .008$) scores and a trend toward superior right hemispheric Visual Organization ($p < .07$) scores in the test group, results which together supported a shift in hemispheric balance.

Anhedonia

High and low scorers on the Withdrawn factor differed significantly in anhedonia ($\bar{X}$50.92 vs. $\bar{X}$45.53, $p < .015$). This was supported by significant Pearson correlations with the Withdrawn factor ($r = .25$, $p < .01$) and its subscales No close friends ($r = .27$, $p < .001$) and Constricted affect ($r = 0.33$, $p < .001$). The correlation between Anhedonia and Odd Beliefs ($r = 0.20$, $p < .01$) was also found to be significant. In keeping with the affinity between anhedonia and withdrawal, Anhedonia was related to a faces memory advantage when comparing groups with a faces advantage ($\bar{X}$48.15) versus a word advantage ($\bar{X}$50.68, $p < .065$), a result largely due to males ($\bar{X}$43.44 vs. $\bar{X}$48.47, $p < .035$).

Psychoticism, neuroticism, and extraversion

A PCA involving the three Eysenck dimensions – Psychoticism, Neuroticism, and Extraversion – and the three SPQ factors and anhedonia produced the factor structure shown in Table 14.3. Three factors with eigenvalues greater than one accounted for 28.6%, 20.8%, and 18.9% of the variance. The first consisted of the Withdrawn SPQ factor together with Introversion and Anhedonia; the second, the Acting Out SPQ factor together with Psychoticism; the third, the Reality SPQ factor together with Neuroticism and Anhedonia, though with a reduced loading (.44) on the latter.

Combined sample (*N* = 300)

Factor structure of schizotypy

In view of their homogeneity, the two samples were combined for further analysis and to explore individual differences of neuropsychological relevance such as handedness and gender. A PCA on the SPQ confirmed the three-factor structure of the previous two experiments, unsurprisingly in view of the almost exact replication. A second PCA included the Eysenck scales, which were obtained on the first sample close to the time of the experiment but not reported on previously (Gruzelier, Burgess, Stygall, & Raine, 1995); and the Physical Anhedonia Scale, which was included only in the second sample. This PCA produced four factors that contributed 24.4%, 15.4%, 11.7%, and 9.0% of the variance: factor 1 [No close friends, (0.84), Extraversion (–0.78), Blunted affect (0.66), Anhedonia (–0.51), and Social anxiety (0.43)]; factor 2: [Unusual perceptions (0.76), Odd beliefs (0.70),

Table 14.3. *Factor structure of the SPQ Withdrawn, Unreality, and Active factors together with Physical Anhedonia, Psychoticism, Extraversion, and Neuroticism*

	Factor 1	Factor 2	Factor 3
Withdrawn	–0.88	0.04	0.03
Unreality	0.29	0.07	0.78
Active	0.15	0.81	0.01
Anhedonia	0.54	–0.24	0.44
Psychoticism	–0.13	0.83	–0.01
Extraversion	0.79	0.13	–0.00
Neuroticism	–0.39	–0.15	0.77

Ideas of reference (0.69), and Suspiciousness (0.42)]; factor 3 [Eccentricity (0.75), Psychoticism (0.72), Odd speech, 0.71)]; factor 4 (Neuroticism (0.74), Social anxiety (0.70), and Suspiciousness (0.48)]. Thus a fourth anxiety factor dissociated Neuroticism from the Unreality factor.

Gender

Females were characterized by higher scores on odd beliefs ($p < .02$), but not on the Unreality factor as a whole. In the second experiment, where evidence on ethnicity was available, females scored higher on the Active factor when non-Europeans were excluded ($p < .05$). Social anxiety, associated with this factor above, tended to be higher ($p < .1$) in females, and in the first sample this was significant ($p < .02$). Consistent with this relationship, Neuroticism was higher in women in both samples (combined sample, $p < .05$).

Males scored higher on the Withdrawn factor ($p < .05$), which was due to subscales of No close friends ($p < .001$), a result that was significant in both experiments ($p < .03$; $p < .008$), together with Blunted affect ($p < .003$), an effect highly significant in the second experiment ($p < .003$) and approaching significance in the first experiment ($p < 0.09$). When just these two subscales alone were considered, the levels of significance were for experiment 1, $p < .06$; and for experiment 2, $p < .004$ (total, $p < .001$). Consistent with the association between withdrawal and anhedonia, males scored higher on Anhedonia ($p < .01$).

Males also tended to score higher on the Active factor ($p < .09$), primarily owing to Eccentricity (exper. 1, $p < .04$; exper. 2, $p < .002$; total, $p < .001$), for only in the second experiment was there a tendency for higher scores on Odd speech ($p < .08$). As has been well established, males also scored higher on Psychoticism (exper. 1, $p < .0001$; exper. 2, $p < .04$; combined, $p < .0001$).

There were no consistent sex differences on the activation scales, though women provided evidence of reduced arousal on Calmness in experiment 1 ($p < .04$) and on Tiredness in experiment 2 ($p < .01$). Men scored higher than women on Energy in experiment 2 ($p < .04$).

We have previously shown, using the WRMT in four samples, that, on average, men show a faces memory advantage and women a word memory advantage (Gruzelier, 1991). Here the memory discrepancy score differed significantly ($p < .025$) in the direction predicted, with men having a faces memory advantage (z score: $x = 0.128$) and women a word memory advantage (z score: $x = -0.117$).

Activation level

In addition to examining the four scales, we carried out a PCA which provided two factors contributing 42.1% and 25.4% of the variance. The first consisted of Tension with a negative loading on Calmness. The second consisted of Tiredness with a negative loading on Energy. The first factor was termed a Stress factor, ranging from tense, fearful, anxious, jittery, stirred up, and tense for high scores; and at rest, still, leisurely, quiescent, quiet, calm, and placid for low scores. The second factor, termed an Arousal factor, ranged from sleepy, tired, drowsy to wide-awake, lively, full of pep, energetic, activated, and vigorous.

Groups were formed by a median split on each of the three SPQ factors. Results are shown in Table 14.4.

1. Withdrawn factor: In the group as a whole, withdrawal was associated with lower scores on Energy ($p < .02$) and the Arousal factor ($p < .05$). There were no sex differences.
2. Unreality factor: In female subjects, high scorers were associated with both extremes of arousal – Tension ($p < .04$) and Tiredness ($p < .006$). In contrast, in males the opposite relationship was found. High scorers were associated with both low Tension ($p < .04$) and low Tiredness ($p < .07$), suggesting moderate levels of arousal in males.
3. The Active factor: As predicted, this factor was associated with high levels of activation for the combined group as shown by high Energy ($p < .02$) and high Arousal factor scores ($p < .06$). In females, there were significant effects with Tension ($p < .008$), low Calmness ($p < .06$), and high Stress factor scores ($p < .05$). In males, the Active factor was associated with high scores on Arousal ($p < .05$).

Table 14.4. *Thayer scores and schizotypy factors*

Factor	Scale	Gender	Factor groups High	Low	p
Withdrawn	Energy	combined	16.17	17.92	0.02
	Arousal	combined	–0.12	0.07	0.05
Unreality	Tension	female	13.49	10.78	0.04
	Tiredness	female	14.60	12.11	0.006
	Tension	male	10.78	13.49	0.04
	Tiredness	male	12.11	14.60	0.07
Active	Energy	combined	18.00	16.17	0.02
	Arousal	combined	0.07	–0.12	0.06
	Tension	female	14.88	12.40	0.008
	Calmness	female	14.88	16.50	0.06
	Stress	female	0.08	–0.19	0.05
	Arousal	male	0.18	–0.11	0.05

Handedness

Subjects were classified as right-handed (>69: N = 189), mixed (0–69: N = 81), and left-handed (–1 to –100: N = 19). The groups were compared by analysis of variance (ANOVA). There was a significant group effect for the Active factor ($p < .045$) owing to the higher scores of the left handers. These effects were consistent for both Active subscales: Eccentricity ($p < .10$); and Odd speech ($p < .08$). In addition, although there was no group effect for the Withdrawn factor, there was a significant group effect for No close friends ($p < .05$) and an effect approaching significance for Constricted affect ($p < .08$). In the case of No close friends, the difference lay between right handers and both mixed and left handers, who were the more withdrawn. On Constricted affect, it was the left handers who were distinguished from the other groups by their higher scores.

Right handers were subdivided into those with a family history of left handedness (N = 57) and those without (N = 125). Subjects with familial left handedness showed tendencies to higher scores on Constricted affect ($p < .09$) and Anhedonia ($p < .10$). Left handers were also divided according to familial sinistrality: 5 with and 11 without. There was a tendency toward a difference between them in memory discrepancy scores ($p < .06$), which was due to a word advantage in those with familial sinistrality (z score: –0.22) and a faces advantage in those without ($\bar{X}$0.51). Separate comparisons of words and faces scores indicated that this difference was due to a highly significant reduction in memory for words in those without familial sinistrality ($\bar{X}42.46$) as compared with superior performance in those with familial sinistrality ($\bar{X}49$). Those without familial sinistrality had higher scores ($p < .04$) on the Unreality factor ($\bar{X}7.58$ vs. $\bar{X}4.71$ without), largely as a result of the Odd beliefs subscale ($p < .003$: $\bar{X}2.58$ vs. $\bar{X}0.57$ without). In keeping with the results from the right handers, this was coupled with higher scores on Neuroticism ($p < .009$: $\bar{X}12.142$ vs. $\bar{X}6.86$).

Vulnerability: high scores on two or more factors

When considering how schizotypy may lead to schizophrenia, we reasoned that subjects scoring high on two or more schizotypy factors, and thereby those with higher total schizotypy scores, may be particularly at risk. Given also long-standing theories on the importance of high or low arousal in the etiology of schizophrenia, we used the Thayer arousal scales to compare those whose summated scores were in approximately the top 10% of the class on two or more schizotypy factors, with the remainder. Significant effects, which are summarized in Table 14.5, were found only when the sexes were considered separately.

Males scoring high on the Unreality factor in combination with the Withdrawn or Active factor scored lower, not higher, on the Tension/Stress factor, yet at the same time scored lower on Tiredness. In other words, male schizotypes could be seen to be at moderate rather than extreme levels of arousal. It was the female schizotypes who were at extremes of arousal, with both extremes being represented when the Unreality factor was involved. They scored higher on Tension in all three pairs of syndromes, and when the Active factor was paired with Withdrawn, parallels were also found with Tension/Stress and Tiredness, all in the direction of higher arousal in female schizotypes. However, when the Withdrawn factor was paired with Unreality, in addition to Tension, female schizotypes showed lower scores on the Arousal factor and scored more highly on Tiredness. Similarly, in pairing Active with Unreality, aside from evidence of Tension, female schizotypes were more likely to be represented in the upper quartile of Calmness and Tiredness ($p < .04$).

Discussion

The results with the SPQ provided confirmation of the proposed three-syndrome structure of schizotypy. The three factors were here described as

Table 14.5. *Examination of high-scoring schizotypes on two or more factors with the Thayer arousal scales*

Schizotypy factors	Gender	Variable	Schizotype	Normal	*p*
Withdrawn/ Unreality	Male	Stress	0.47	–0.05	.03
	Female	Tension			
		Arousal	–0.41	–0.04	.03
		Tiredness	17.71	14.92	.03
Active Unreality	Male	Tiredness	11.50	14.54	.05
		Stress	–0.55	0.05	.01
	Female	Tension	17.25	15.00	.10
Active/ Withdrawn	Female	Tension	16.47	14.31	.01
		Stress	0.14	–0.17	.04
		Calmness	14.31	16.47	.01
Active/ Withdrawn/ Unreality	Male	Stress	–0.50	–0.06	.03
	Female	Arousal	–0.42	–0.06	.10

Withdrawn, Unreality, and Active factors, and they had a composition not dissimilar to the three-factor structure of Mutaner et al. (1988). The structure was shown to be reliable through the almost exact replication of results in our two samples. The structure was mostly retained with the addition of scales of Physical Anhedonia, Psychoticism, Introversion, and Neuroticism. The combination of psychometry and neuropsychology helped define what may be considered core features of the syndromes and has assisted in clarifying the nature of schizotypy and its factorial structure. Both domains of measurement had strong parallels in three-syndrome accounts of schizophrenia and its neuropsychophysiological basis.

Withdrawn, Unreality, and Active factors

Essential features of the Withdrawn factor were the absence of close friends, which is akin to the social withdrawal seen in schizophrenia, and constricted affect, which may be akin to the blunted affect of schizophrenia. Suspiciousness loaded on this factor, and to a lesser extent, on Unreality, suggesting a nonspecific relationship. Social anxiety was found to load more strongly on a separate Anxiety factor when the other scales were included. The dimension of Introversion, developed from a global personality perspective, was also found to load on the Withdrawn factor, a result in keeping with social withdrawal aspects of introversion. Physical Anhedonia also loaded on the Withdrawn factor, and correlations with subscales of this factor were significant in the case of Constricted affect and No close friends, attesting to their central importance.

The Unreality factor would appear to have as cardinal features Unusual perceptual experiences and Odd beliefs, akin to aspects of hallucinations and delusions seen in schizophrenia. The subscale Ideas of reference did not share the relations with the cognitive, handedness, or gender variables found with the other two subscales. Similarly, Suspiciousness, which correlated with Ideas of reference ($r = 0.43$, $p < .001$), had a lesser loading on this factor ($r = .37$) and also loaded on Withdrawn. In schizophrenia we had also found that paranoid features were not consistently related to Active or Withdrawn syndromes or lateral asymmetry. Similarly, Suspiciousness was not related here to the neuropsychological variables.

The third – Active – factor consisted unambiguously of Odd speech and Eccentricity. In keeping with an Active character, Psychoticism, often described as representing impulsive nonconformity, showed similar high loadings on this factor. Nevertheless, Psychoticism did not share the same relationships with laterality or handedness as did the Active factor.

Support was found for the relationship of Withdrawn and Active factors to activation and arousal with the Thayer scales. Through a factor analysis these self-report measures of activation were found to represent two dimensions, one conceptualized as representing Tension/Stress, with items ranging from sluggishness to tension and feeling jittery, and so on, and the other factor an energy/arousal dimension ranging from sleepiness to alertness. In support of the schizophrenia model, the Withdrawn schizotypy factor was associated with lower scores on Energy (alert, etc.), and on Arousal, whereas the Active factor was associated with opposite effects: higher scores on Energy and on the Energy/Arousal factor.

Cerebral laterality and the schizotypy factors

Turning to patterns of cognitive asymmetry, parallel relations were found between asymmetry and those syndromes that were associated with lateral asymmetry in schizophrenia. In both experiments, the Withdrawn factor was associated with superior faces compared with word memory, representing higher functional activity in the right hemisphere. In the first experiment, the Active factor was associated with superior word than faces memory, representing higher functional activity in the left hemisphere.

As shown previously, test anxiety can reverse asymmetry to favor the right hemisphere and thereby compromise a left hemispheric advantage (Gruzelier & Phelan, 1991). In the second sample where half the class completed an examination a few hours before, we found in this subgroup the predicted right-hemisphere, faces-memory advantage, whereas in the subgroup that had not undergone the examination, there was a left-hemisphere, verbal-memory advantage. The effects of stress may have compromised relations between the Active syndrome and left hemispheric functions, effects corroborated not only by the inferior word memory of the exam group but also by lower scores on vocabulary and analogies. The effect of stress was not just to compromise left hemispheric functions but also to alter hemispheric balance (Gruzelier & Phelan, 1991), as supported by the superior performance on the spatial visual organization test as well as the faces memory advantage over verbal memory in the exam group, particularly in females.

Relations between cerebral laterality and arousal were further supported by the Thayer scales. In experiment 1, Tension was associated with a word-memory–left-hemisphere advantage, whereas, Calmness was associated with a faces-memory–right-hemisphere advantage. In experiment 2, high Energy was associated with a word advantage in males, but, in keeping with a shift in lateralization with stress, high scores on Tension were associated with a faces memory advantage.

Serendipitously a single case validated our predictions about pattern of asymmetry and predisposition to schizophrenic syndrome. A student characterized as an outlier by virtue of an extreme faces memory advantage, due to chance performance with word memory, sometime later had the first of several schizophrenic breakdowns. He presented with Withdrawn and Unreality syndromes as would be predicted by his face/word discrepancy.

Relations between the schizotypy factors and asymmetry were corroborated by measures of handedness. "Sinistrality," or mixed handedness, has been reported to be higher in schizotypes (Chapman et al., 1984; Kim, Raine, Triphon, & Green, 1992). Here there was support for this as relationships were found with the two syndromes that have been associated with cerebral asymmetry and not with the putative inconsistently lateralized syndrome. Left-handers as a group scored higher on the Active factor. Left handers together with mixed handers also scored higher on the core aspect of the Withdrawn factor – No close friends – and there was a tendency for left handers to score higher on Constricted affect. The latter effect was endorsed by the finding that right handers with sinistrality in the family tended to have more Constricted affect as well as Anhedonia.

Left handedness is, however, a heterogeneous condition, with opinion divided on the number of sinistrals who have left-hemisphere, right-hemisphere, or bilateral language (Herron, 1980). One guide is thought to be whether there is evidence of familial sinistrality. If there is none, one possibility is that nongenetic factors such as perinatal trauma have affected the left hemisphere and are responsible for the reorganization of both language and handedness with relocation of language to the right hemisphere. Our patterns of asymmetry in sinistrals with and without familial sinistrality supports this contention. The left-hander group without familial sinistrality – the putative pathological group – had a highly significant reduction in memory for words, whereas in marked contrast the sinistral group with familial sinistrality had superior word memory. Pathology, if it occurs at an early stage of development, will involve subcortical structures. It follows that if, as we hypothesize, the Unreality factor involves subcortical limbic mechanisms, then left handers without familial sinistrality – the pathological group – will have higher Unreality factor scores. Although this was not entirely the case, they did score significantly higher on the Odd Beliefs subscale ($p < .009$).

It was our prediction that the Unreality factor was not associated with asymmetry or, rather, that the relationship was an inconsistent one. In the first sample, there was no relation between asymmetry and the Unreality factor, though the mean results favored the left hemisphere. In the second sample, there was no relation for the sample as a whole; however, the subscale Unusual Perceptual Experiences was associated with a left hemisphere advantage in females. Odd Beliefs, on the other hand, showed some indirect relation with the right hemisphere. Notably this subscale was correlated with Anhedonia, which itself was associated with a faces memory advantage. In left handers without family sinistrality, the two features that characterized them were Odd Beliefs and a faces memory advantage.

Furthermore while in factor-analytic studies of schizotypy scales, negative correlations have been reported between Anhedonia and "unreality" -type scales, as reviewed by Kelley and Coursey (1992); here, we found positive correlations between Physical Anhedonia and Magical Ideation. If we consider the previous research on cerebral asymmetry and schizotypy, this result was compatible with the reports of Claridge and colleagues with the STA scale (a scale that correlates with the Perceptual Aberration and Magical Ideation scales); these authors consistently associated schizotypy with right hemispheric advantages. Jutai (1989), on the other hand, found right hemispheric–like deficits in association with the Magical Ideation scale scores. Similary in schizophrenia, when we examined hallucinating versus nonhallucinating schizophrenics with auditory thresholds, we found a right-ear–left-hemispheric advantage in nonhallucinating patients, who also scored higher on ratings of Tension and Excitement on the Brief Psychiatric Rating Scale (BPRS); hallucinators, in comparison, showed reduced acuity in the right ear and no overall asymmetry. Hallucinators also showed Motor Retardation compatible with a Withdrawn syndrome in contrast to the Active syndrome–like features on the BPRS of the nonhallucinators.

None of the evidence on the Unreality syndrome suggests any consistent relation with cerebral asymmetry, a result recently replicated in a third investigation (Gruzelier & Richardson, 1994). Other variables – such as Neuroticism, activation, and the female gender – did appear persistently related to the Unreality factor. In the second experiment, Neuroticism loaded with the Unreality factor and, in the combined sample, with Social Anxiety and Suspiciousness. Females scored higher on Neuroticism, a well-established finding (Eysenck & Eysenck, 1975), as well as on Odd Beliefs and Social Anxiety. High Activation in the combined sample was associated with the Unreality factor, whereas in women Unreality was associated with both extremes of activation. Given that anxiety can alter and reverse patterns of cerebral laterality (Gruzelier, 1993; Gruzelier & Phelan, 1991), in keeping here with the effect of test anxiety, the Unreality factor may be associated with a lability in lateralized subcortical–cortical influences and hence the inconsistent relationships with patterns of asymmetry.

Gender

Gender had an important bearing on schizotypy, as it does in schizophrenia. In schizophrenia there is a substantive body of evidence that in general, males have an earlier-onset, poorer-prognosis, negative-symptom form of the disorder, whereas females have a later-onset, less characteristic florid schizoaffective disorder (Lewine, 1981). In keeping with this tendency, schizotypy in males was associated with higher scores on the Withdrawn syndrome – in particular, on the No close friends and Constricted affect subscales350 – as well as on Physical Anhedonia, all negative-symptom features. Females scored higher on Odd Beliefs, on the Active factor when ethnicity was taken into account, on the nonspecific subscale Social Anxiety and Neuroticism, all positive-symptom features.

Accordingly, it is perhaps not surprising that gender influenced our attempt to conceptualize putative vulnerability to schizophrenia as indexed by high scores on more than one factor. Men were characterized by the absence of extreme scores on levels of activation and arousal, and with significantly lower scores on the Tension/Stress factor when the Unreality syndrome was included. This profile suggested a state of moderate, quiescent arousal. Women, on the other hand, disclosed high levels of activation in all combinations of syndromes, as well as reduced arousal whenever the Unreality syndrome was included. Thus the role of arousal and stress in schizotypy warrants further investigation. The fact that women, in contrast to men, are characterized by mood swings, by virtue of the menstrual cycle, may endorse the importance of endocrine influences on schizotypy; see also our more detailed report which includes androgyny scales (Gruzelier, 1994; Gruzelier & Doig, 1995).

Conclusions

The results support the applicability of a three-syndrome model of schizophrenic symptoms to the schizotypal personality. They support a dimensional model of the relation between schizotypy and schizophrenia, as well as a dimensional relationship between schizotypy and normality (Claridge, 1985; Meehl, 1962). They endorse the etiological importance of hemispheric asymmetry in both schizotypy and schizophrenia through the relation disclosed between syndromes or personality factors and patterns of cognitive asymmetry, handedness, and gender. The results are of heuristic as well as theoretical importance for research on schizotypy. Heretofore, measurement of aspects of schizotypy has tended to be based on operational considerations such as the popularity and availability of scales, notably of Anhedonia and of Magical Ideation–Perceptual Aberration. Less often have investigators drawn on the implications of the genetic association between schizotypy and schizophrenia, and begun with a model of schizophrenic behavior and applied the framework to elucidate the schizotypal personality. By far the majority of work in the field has assumed a two-syndrome structure, a compliment to the importance of the pioneering work of Chapman and Chapman in filling the void which this concept holds in contemporary thinking in psychiatry at large. Here we have investigated the three-syndrome neuropsychological approach and have found some promise in unraveling some of the complexities and ambiguities surrounding the concept of schizotypy (Gruzelier & Raine, 1993).

References

Arndt, S., Alliger, R. J., & Andreasen, N. (1991). The distinction of positive and negative symptoms: The failure of a two dimensional model. *British Journal of Psychiatry, 158,* 46–50.

Bentall, R. P., Claridge, G. S., & Slade, P. D. (1989) The multidimensional nature of schizotypal traits: A factor analytic study with normal subjects. *British Journal of Clinical Psychology, 28,* 363–375.

Broks, P. (1984). Schizotypy and hemisphere function. II. Performance asymmetry on a verbal divided visual-field task. *Personality and Individual Differences, 5,* 649–656.

Broks, P., Claridge, G. S., Matheson, J., & Hargreaves, J. (1984). Schizotypy and hemisphere function. IV. Story comprehension under binaural and monaural listening conditions. *Personality and Individual Differences, 5,* 665–670.

Chapman, L. J., Chapman, J. P., Numbers, J. S., Edell, W. S., Carpenter, B. N., & Beckfield, D. (1984). Impulsive nonconformity as a trait contributing to the prediction of psychotic-like and schizotypal symptoms. *Journal of Nervous and Mental Disease, 172,* 681–691.

Chapman, L. J., Chapman, J. P., & Raulin, M. L. (1976). Scales for physical and social anhedonia. *Journal of Abnormal Psychology, 85,* 374.

Claridge, G. (1985). *The origins of mental illness.* Oxford: Blackwell.

Claridge, G. S., Clark, K. H., & Beech, A. R. (1991). Lateralisation of the negative priming effect: Relationships with schizotypy and with gender. *British Journal of Psychiatry.*

Eysenck, H. (1967). *The biological basis of personality.* Springfield: Harper.

Eysenck, H. J., & Eysenck, S. B. G. (1975). *Manual of the Eysenck Personality Questionnaire* (*Junior and Adult*). London: Hodder & Stoughton.

Eysenck, H. J. (1994). The psychophysiology of creativity and genius. *Journal of Psychophysiology, 8,* 82 (abstract).

Gruzelier, J. H. (1981). Hemispheric imbalances masquerading as paranoid and nonparanoid syndromes. *Schizophrenia Bulletin, 7,* 662–673.

Gruzelier, J. H. (1983). A critical assessment and integration of lateral asymmetries in schizophrenia. In M. Myslobodsky (Ed.), *Hemisyndromes: Psychobiology, neurology and psychiatry* (pp. 265–326). New York: Academic Press.

Gruzelier, J. H. (1984). Hemispheric imbalances in schizophrenia. *International Journal of Psychophysiology, 1,* 227–240.

Gruzelier, J. H. (1991a). Brain localisation and neuropsychology in schizophrenia: Syndrome and neurodevelopmental implications. In H. Hafner & W. Gattaz (Eds.), *Search for the causes of schizophrenia,* Vol. 2 (pp. 623–629). New York: Springer.

Gruzelier, J. H. (1991b). Hemispheric imbalance: Syndromes of schizophrenia, premorbid personality, and neurodevelopmental influences. *In* S. Steinhauer, J. Gruzelier, & J. Zubin (Eds.), *Handbook of schizophrenia, Vol. IV: Experimental psychopathology, neuropsychology, & psychophysiology* (pp. 599–650).

Gruzelier, J. H. (1994). Syndromes of schizophrenia and schizotypy, hemispheric imbalance and sex differences: Implications for developmental psychopathology. *International Journal of Psychophysiology, 18,* special issue on *Developmental Psychopathology, 18,* 167–178.

Gruzelier, J. H., Burgess, A., Stygall, J., & Raine, A. (1995). Patterns of cerebral asymmetry and syndromes of schizotypal personality. *Psychiatry Research, 56,* 71–79.

Gruzelier, J., & Davis, S. (1995). Social and physical anhedonia in relation to cerebral laterality and electrodermal habituation in unmedicated psychotic patients. *Psychiatry Research,* 56.

Gruzelier, J., & Doig, A. (1995). The factorial structure of schizotypy: Patterns of cognitive asymmetry, arousal, handedness, and gender. (In preparation)

Gruzelier, J. H., Jutai, J., & Connolly, J. (1993). Cerebral asymmetry in EEG spectra in unmedicated schizophrenic patients: Relationships with Active and Withdrawn syndromes. *International Journal of Psychophysiology, 15,* 239–246.

Gruzelier, J. H., & Manchanda, R. (1982). The syndrome of schizophrenia: Relations between electrodermal response lateral asymmetries and clinical ratings. *British Journal of Psychiatry, 141,* 488–495.

Gruzelier, J. H., & Phelan, M. (1991). Laterality-reversal in a lexical divided visual field task under stress. *International Journal of Psychophysiology, 11,* 267–276.
Gruzelier, J., & Raine, A. (1994). Bilateral electrodermal activity and cerebral mechanisms in syndromes of schizophrenia and the schizotypal personality. *International Journal of Psychophysiology, 16,* 1–16.
Gruzelier, J. H., & Richardson, A. (1994). Patterns of cognitive asymmetry and psychosis proneness. *International Journal of Psychophysiology, 18,* 217–225.
Gruzelier, J. H., Seymour, K., Wilson, L., Jolley, T., & Hirsch, S. (1988). Impairments on neuropsychological tests of temporo-hippocampal and fronto-hippocampal function and word fluency in remitting schizophrenia and affective disorders. *Archives of General Psychiatry, 45,* 623–629.
Gruzelier, J., & Wilson, L. (1995). Memory deficits in schizophrenia: Cognitive asymmetry, syndrome relations, sex differences and drugs. (Submitted)
Gur, R. E., Mozley, P. D., Resnick, S. M., Levick, S., Erwin, R., Saykin, A. J., & Gur, R. C. (1991). Relations among clinical scales in schizophrenia. *American Journal of Psychiatry, 148,* 472–478.
Herron, J. (1980). *The neuropsychology of left-handedness.* New York: Academic Press.
Hewitt, J. K., & Claridge, G. S. (1989). The factor structure of schizotypy in a normal population. *Personality and Individual Differences, 10,* 323–330.
Jutai, J. W. (1989). Spatial attention in hypothetically psychosis-prone college students. *Psychiatry Research, 27,* 207–215.
Kelley, M. P., & Coursey, R. D. (1992). Lateral preference and neuropsychological correlates of schizotypy. *Psychiatry Research, 41,* 115–135.
Kim, D., Raine, A., Triphon, N., & Green, M. (1992). Mixed handedness and schizotypal personality. *Journal of Nervous & Mental Disease, 180,* 131–133.
Liddle, P. (1987). Symptoms of chronic schizophrenia: Examination of the positive–negative dichotomy. *British Journal of Psychiatry, 151,* 145–151.
Mathew, V. K., Gruzelier, J. H., & Liddle, P. (1993). Lateral asymmetries in auditory acuity distinguish hallucinating from nonhallucinating schizophrenic patients. *Psychiatry Research, 46,* 127–138.
Meehl, P. (1962). Schizotaxia, schizotypy, schizophrenia. *American Psychologist, 17,* 827–838.
Muntaner, C., Garcia-Sevilla, L., Fernandez, A., & Torruba, R. (1988). Personality dimensions, schizotypal and borderline personality traits and psychosis proneness. *Personality & Individual Differences, 9,* 257–268.
Overall, J. E., & Gorham, D. F. (1962). The Brief Psychiatric Rating Scale. *Psychological Reports, 10,* 799–812.
Raine, A. (1991). The Schizotypal Personality Questionnaire (SPQ). *Schizophrenia Bulletin, 17,* 554–564.
Raine, A., & Manders, D. (1988). Schizoid personality, interhemispheric transfer, and left hemisphere overactivation. *British Journal of Clinical Psychology, 27,* 333–347.
Rawlings, D., & Borge, A. (1987). Personality and hemisphere functions: Two experiments using the dichotic shadowing techniques. *Personality & Individual Differences, 8,* 438–488.
Rawlings, D., & Claridge, G. (1984). Schizotypy and hemispheric function. II. Performance asymmetries on tasks of letter recognition and local–global processing. *Personality & Individual Differences, 5,* 657–663.
Thayer, R. E. (1967). Measurement of activation through self report. *Psychological Reports, 20,* 663–678.

Thayer, R. (1989). *The biopsychology of mood and arousal.* Oxford: Oxford University Press.
Warrington, E. (1984). *Recognition Memory Test.* Windsor: Nelson.
Wing, J. K., Cooper, J. E., & Sartorius, N. (1974). *The measurement and classification of psychiatric symptoms.* Cambridge: Cambridge University Press.
Winterbotham, R. G. (1979). Torque, conjugate lateral eye movements, and scores on the Minnesota Multiphasic Personality Inventory. Unpublished Master's thesis. Simon Fraser University, Burnaby, British Columbia.

15

Working memory deficits, antisaccades, and thought disorder in relation to perceptual aberration

PHILIP S. HOLZMAN, MICHAEL COLEMAN, MARK F. LENZENWEGER, DEBORAH L. LEVY, STEVEN MATTHYSSE, GILLIAN O'DRISCOLL, and SOHEE PARK

The larger than usual number of authors of this paper (listed, except for the first author, alphabetically) indicates that this research was a team effort in which three studies were conducted simultaneously by three teams of investigators. The effort began when Mark Lenzenweger conceived of the idea to study normally functioning college students who, on psychometric examination, showed significant elevations on traits that Loren and Jean Chapman have identified as schizotypal. Lenzenweger thought that it would be informative to determine how these students performed on tests that distinguish schizophrenic patients and their relatives from both the normal population and patients with nonschizophrenic illnesses. The scientists in our laboratory agreed.

Three teams of investigators set out from the Harvard–McLean Hospital laboratory to work at Cornell University, where they completed the testing of 57 people in Lenzenweger's population. Each of the teams completed a report of its own, which has been submitted for publication; these reports are summarized here. In addition, this chapter considers the performance of these college students on all of the tasks, which could not be done in the individual reports. The three tasks are (1) delayed response, from which we assess working memory; (2) antisaccade eye movements, and (3) thought disorder assessed from the Thought Disorder Index (TDI).

Rationale

The measures

For many years, the Psychology Research Laboratory at McLean Hospital has been studying psychological and psychophysiological characteristics that are associated with schizophrenia. Some of these performance measures show a familial aggregation among the relatives of schizophrenic individuals, which enhanced their significance beyond the mere demonstration that performance was deviant in a group of psychotic people. Examples of the behaviors that showed familiality are eye tracking dysfunctions (ETD; e.g., Levy, Holzman, Matthysse, & Mendell, 1993), specific qualities of thought disorder (e.g., Shenton, Solovay, & Holzman, 1987; Solovay, Shenton, & Holzman, 1987), and delayed response performance (e.g., Park & Holzman, 1992).

Some of these performance deviations, like thought disorder, seem obviously phenomenologically related to schizophrenic pathology since most schizophrenic patients show characteristic thought slippage; others, like antisaccade eye movements and delayed response, do not. But the absence of an obvious relation between schizophrenia and a particular task deficit presents an opportunity for probing in greater depth the nature of schizophrenic pathology. In other diseases – phenylketonuria (PKU), for example – such associations are not unusual. In PKU, light skin pigmentation and subnormal intelligence are associated, but that relation became understandable only after it was learned that tyrosine hydroxylase is the key to that puzzle. Therefore, when, in the course of investigating vestibular integrity in schizophrenic patients, we discovered that eye tracking was disordered, we were not dissuaded from investigating the significance of this finding merely because the relation of eye tracking dysfunctions to schizophrenia was not readily apparent.

The population

Most recurrence risk studies record clinical schizophrenia in only about 4% to 10% of the first-degree relatives of schizophrenic patients. The prevalence of schizophrenia in families is thus rather low. But beginning with Kraepelin and Bleuler, there has been a general recognition that schizophrenic pathology is not limited to the psychotic form of the illness. Bleuler, for example, remarked that "[s]ymptoms exist in varying degrees and shadings on the entire scale from pathological to normal; also, the milder cases, latent schizophrenics with far less manifest symptoms, are many times more common than the overt manifest cases." Later in his monograph, he wrote:

> [T]here is also a latent schizophrenia, and I am convinced that this is the most frequent form, although admittedly these people hardly ever come for treatment. . . . In this form, we can see *in nuce* all the symptoms and all the combinations of symptoms which are present in the manifest types of disease. Irritable, odd, moody, withdrawn, or exaggeratedly punctual people arouse, among other things, the suspicion of being schizophrenic. . . . [E]very form of this disease may take a latent course." (*Bleuler, 1911/1950, pp. 13, 239*)

The recognition that the nonpsychotic forms of schizophrenia are more prevalent than the psychotic forms lay behind Rado's (1953), Grinker's (1969), and Meehl's (1962) emphasis on schizotypy. The many modifiers of the term "schizophrenia" that were used in diagnostic practice prior to the introduction of the DSM-III and DSM-III-R, such as "pre-," "latent," "incipient," "remitted," "borderline," and "pseudoneurotic" schizophrenia, and also "schizophrenic character" attempted to tag nonpsychotic forms of schizophrenia.

If the basic pathology of the latent or schizotypal form of the disorder is in crucial aspects the same as that of its psychotic form, investigation of the nonpsychotic manifestations of schizophrenia will be less influenced by the noisy distractions of poor motivation, inattention, medication effects, generalized performance deficits, and social deterioration, which plague most studies of schizophrenic patients. This rationale underlies our laboratory's emphasis on studying "unaffected" first-degree relatives of patients (Holzman & Matthysse, 1990). And it provides the motivation for embarking on this collaboration with the Cornell laboratory in the study of "normal" students identified as psychometrically deviant by one of the scales introduced by Chapman and Chapman (1958). In short, we decided to examine a variety of functions associated with schizophrenia – working memory deficits, antisaccades, thought disorder – among those in the general population who have been selected by a psychometric measure of schizotypy.

Method

The subjects for this study were drawn from a larger, randomly ascertained sample of first-year undergraduates at Cornell University who voluntarily completed a 250-item objective psychological inventory entitled "Attitudes, Feelings, and Experiences Questionnaire" (AFEQ). The AFEQ included the 35-item Perceptual Aberration Scale (PAS; Chapman, Chapman, & Raulin, 1978), the scores on which represented the principal independent variable. We selected a random sample in order to maximize diversity within our pool of potential subjects as well as to minimize the effects of self-selection and group-related test-taking attitudes that are often associated with sampling from students enrolled in introductory psychology courses. Of the 2,000 students who were invited to complete the inventory, 1,684 (51.3% women, 48.7% men) did so. The response rate of 84.2% suggests that we achieved representative sampling of this population. Of the 1,684 subjects, 35 (2.1%) were excluded from our sample as invalid, and an additional 3 subjects were dropped because of extensive missing data. The resulting final sample consisted of 1,646 cases.

Two subject groups were composed for the experiments described below, using the complete pool of 1,646 individuals. Group means and standard deviations on the PAS, computed separately for males and females, served as the basis for group composition. Following Chapman and Chapman (1985), subjects classified as high PAS scorers were required to have scores at least 2.0 standard deviations above the PAS group mean, whereas subjects classified as normal scorers were required to have scores no higher than 0.5 standard deviations above the group mean. By this method we identified 76 (4.6%) students who had high PAS scores and 1,371 (83.3%) students with low PAS scores. From these two groups we randomly selected 31 students (16 female) from the high PAS group and 26 students (14 female) from the low PAS group for the normal control subjects. Table 15.1 presents the demographic characteristics of this final sample.

High and low PAS subjects did not differ with respect to sex ratio, age, ethnicity, or consent rate. All subjects were screened for psychosis, and none had a diagnosis of any psychotic illness at the time of testing. The three measures used are described as follows.

The Perceptual Aberration Scale (PAS)

The PAS is a well-established 35-item true–false self-report measure of disturbances and distortions in perceptions of body image as well as other objects (Chapman et al., 1978). It includes such items as “Occasionally I have felt as though my body did not exist” (keyed *true*), and “I have never felt that my arms or legs have momentarily grown in size” (keyed *false*). The scale is described more fully elsewhere (e.g., see Chapman, Chapman, & Kwapil, Chapter 5, this volume).

We chose the PAS score as the independent variable for this study because of the emphasis given to body-image and perceptual distortions in schizotypy by both Rado and Meehl. Multiple converging lines of evidence show that the PAS is a valid, though fallible, psychometric indicator of traits associated with schizotypy (cf. Cronbach & Meehl, 1955).

Table 15.1. *Demographic characteristics of study subjects*

	Age			Sex	PAS		Ethnic background			
	N	Mean	SD	*N* (%)	Mean	SD	Black	Hispanic/ Latin	Caucasian	Asian
Total sample	57	18.98	.52	30 F (52.6%) 27 M (47.4%)	—	—	1 (1.8%)	7 (12.3%)	37 (64.9%)	12 (21.1%)
High PAS	31	19.00	.52	16 F (51.6%) 15 M (48.4%)	19.77	6.35	1 (3.20%)	5 (16.1%)	19 (61.3%)	6 (19.4%)
Low PAS	26	18.96	.53	14 F (53.8%) 12 M (46.2%)	.77	.99	0	2 (7.7%)	18 (69.2%)	6 (23.1%)

Psychological state measures

The Beck Depression Inventory (BDI; Beck, Ward, Mendelsohn, Mock, & Erbaugh, 1961), a 21-item self-report inventory, was used to measure depressive/dysphoric symptoms. The State–Trait Anxiety Inventory (Form Y; Spielberger, 1983), a 40-item self-report inventory, was used to measure state and trait anxiety.

Intellectual functioning measures

An estimate of general intellectual functioning was obtained from the Digit Symbol subscale of the Wechsler Adult Intelligence Scale – Revised (WAIS-R) (Wechsler, 1981). Furthermore, each subject provided written consent to release the official Scholastic Aptitude Test (SAT) scores, verbal and quantitative, from his or her Cornell record.

The subject groups did not differ significantly on our three measures of intellectual achievement, namely digit Symbol (raw score), SAT Quantitative score, and SAT Verbal score, indicating that the high PAS group did not have a generally lower intellectual capacity. The high PAS subjects displayed significantly greater levels of dysphoric symptoms ($p < .001$, 2-tail), a state anxiety ($p < .01$), and trait anxiety ($p < .001$), as one would expect of such subjects (cf. Meehl, 1990).

Subjects were tested individually in quiet and conventionally lighted laboratory rooms at Cornell University. All procedures were administered by the investigators, who were assisted by trained research staff. Because a complex coding scheme was employed to disguise the group status of the subjects, both study staff and the investigators were blind to group membership throughout recruitment, testing, and scoring. All subjects were paid $50.00 for participating, and all gave written informed consent.

Experiment 1: the delayed response test

One of the several cognitive deficits of schizophrenic conditions appears to be a dysfunction of working memory that leads to a breakdown of behaviors guided by internal representations (Park & Holzman, 1992). Neuroanatomical and neurophysiological observations point out the important role of the prefrontal cortex in working memory deficits (Funahashi, Bruce, & Goldman-Rakic, 1991; Goldman-Rakic, 1991). Surgical and chemical lesions in the dorsolateral prefrontal cortex – in particular, the region of the principal sulcus in the rhesus monkey (roughly equivalent to Brodmann's Area 46) – lead both to severe deficits in working memory as assessed by an oculomotor delayed response task, and to some symptoms that resemble those of schizophrenia, such as distractibility and perseveration.

Park and Holzman (1992) developed a human analogue of the oculomotor spatial delayed-response paradigm in order to test the hypothesis that schizophrenic patients show working memory deficits. They found that schizophrenic inpatients were significantly impaired on memory-guided delayed response tests (DRT), whether the sense modality was visual or haptic, but the same patients showed almost no impairments on a sensory guided DRT. Bipolar patients, in contrast, showed no impairments on the same oculomotor spatial DRT. Park and Holzman (1993) replicated the oculomotor DRT deficit in schizophrenic outpatients, and also found that 40% (6 of 15) of the first-degree relatives of these patients also showed the same oculomotor DRT deficits (Park, Holzman, & Levy, 1993).

Procedure

A total of 50 subjects were tested on the oculomotor DRT; 28 were in the high PAS group and 22 were in the low PAS group. The procedure was identical to that used by Park and Holzman (1992, 1993). Subjects sat with their heads stabilized on a chin and head rest and were asked to look at a stimulus display screen. A red fixation point (a small dot, 0.5° of visual angle) was located in the center of the screen. The target was a small black circle that measured 2° of visual angle. The location of the target varied from trial to trial. There were eight possible target locations, each separated by 45°, on the circumference of an imaginary circle.

In the oculomotor memory task, which assesses working memory, a target (black circle) was flashed on the screen for 200 ms at one of the eight positions. During this brief period, the subject was asked to fixate at the center. Immediately afterward, there was a 10-second delay period, during which the subject performed a distractor task, which prevented rehearsal and kept the subject looking at the location of the fixation point during the 10-second delay period.

After the delay period, the fixation point and eight "reference" circles (empty, rather than black) appeared on the screen. Subjects were required to move their eyes to the position that the target circle had occupied prior to its disappearance. If the subjects did not move their eyes to the correct location within a 10-second time limit, the reference circles disappeared.

A control for the working memory component of the delayed response task was an oculomotor sensory task. This task was identical to the oculomotor memory task in all respects except that the target remained on the screen at all times, and therefore, no working memory was required to perform this task. There were 64 trials in each of the tasks.

Apparatus

An infrared reflected light method recorded eye movements via a video camera that was connected to an ISCAN RK-426 pupil/corneal reflection tracking system. Eye position information was stored on a Macintosh II computer. The system is fully described in Park and Holzman (1992).

Scoring

The dependent variable was accuracy, defined as the percentage of trials that were correct. A response was scored as correct only if the eye moved directly to within 1.5° of the center of the target position. If the eye moved to an incorrect position first and then moved to the correct target position, the trial was counted as incorrect.

Results

Table 15.2 presents the means for the two subject groups with respect to the delayed response memory and sensory tasks. The high PAS group made significantly more errors than the normal control group on the oculomotor memory task, $t(df, 49) = 1.79$, $p < .04$, 1-tail, but the two groups did not differ on the sensory control task. The effect size estimate is .49 (Cohen's *d;* Cohen, 1988), a "medium" effect size.

Figure 15.1 shows a scatter plot of the DRT scores. It is clear from this figure that not every person with a low DRT score had a high PAS score. If one uses an arbitrary cutoff point of 86% accuracy, which is the lowest accuracy score in Park and Holzman's (1992) normal sample, the 12 people with the lowest DRT score consisted of 9 high PAS scorers and 3 low PAS scorers. It is also noteworthy that 5 of these 9 high PAS subjects have first-degree relatives with an DSM-III-R Axis I disorder (Table 15.3).

Mental state variables (anxiety and depression) were not associated with performance on the DRT, indicating that DRT deficits were not likely the result of transient mental state factors. The SAT math and verbal scores were also not associated with DRT performance, whereas the Digit Symbol score was modestly correlated with DRT performance ($r = .30$, $p < .03$, 2-tail), which may reflect the shared motor component of both the DRT and Digit

Table 15.2. *Principal scores (M ± SD) on the delayed response task, antisaccade task, and Thought Disorder Index for high and low PAS students*

	High PAS			Low PAS		
	N	Mean	SD	*N*	Mean	SD
Delayed response task						
Percent correct	28	89.05	7.92	22	93.12	5.29
Antisaccade task						
No. errors	31	3.04	2.90	25	1.16	1.38
Thought Disorder Index						
No. TD responses	30	7.27	10.52	26	3.00	3.32
Total TDI	30	8.83	15.30	26	3.65	4.97
Idiosyncratic verbaliz.	30	4.87	8.39	26	1.69	2.48

Symbol tasks. There was no effect of handedness or sex on performance of the oculomotor delayed response task. These data suggest that the significantly poorer DRT performance of the high PAS subjects was not likely due to an intellectual deficit or to anxiety or depression in the subjects.

Discussion

Subjects with high scores on the PAS made significantly more errors on the oculomotor memory DRT than those with low PAS scores; 75% of the low accuracy DRT subjects were high PAS scorers. This result adds psychometrically ascertained schizotypes (those with high PAS scores) to schizophrenics and first-degree relatives of schizophrenics as showing deficits in working memory.

We note that only a subgroup of the high PAS scorers shows the working memory impairment. Two issues must be considered with respect to these results. First, the PAS screens for endorsement of only a subset of symptoms associated with schizotypy: perceptual aberrations and body image distortions. The PAS is not intended to identify all individuals with schizotypic characteristics, that is, individuals who manifest schizotypic characteristics other than perceptual aberrations and body image distortions. Nor does the PAS claim to exclude individuals whose perceptual aberrations and body image distortions reflect conditions other than schizotypy. Therefore, the optimal expectation for this psychometric instrument is that it identifies a group of individuals, some of whom have circumscribed symptoms associated with

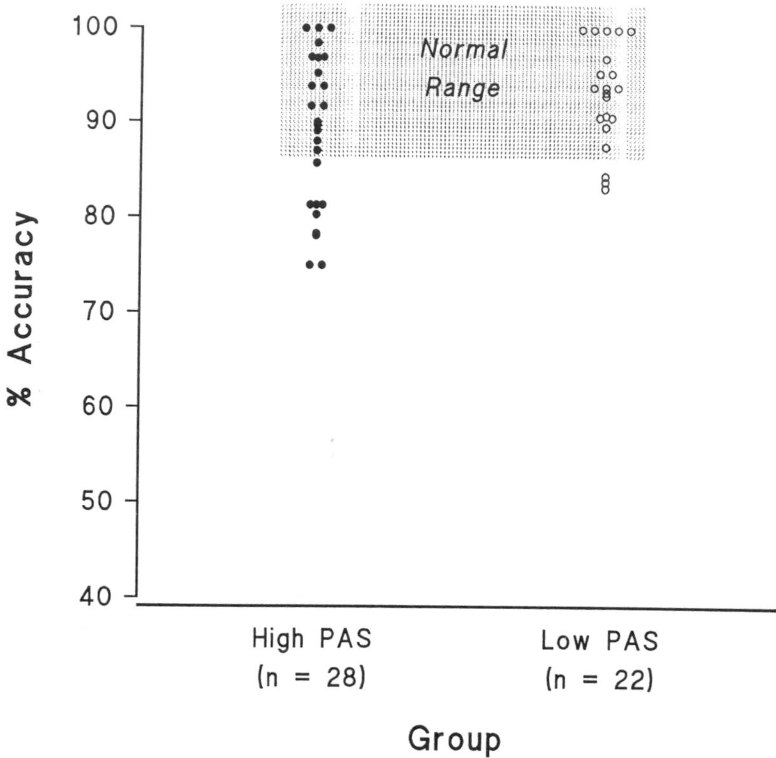

Fig. 15.1. Scatter diagram of percent accuracy scores for high and low PAS students on the delayed response task. The shaded area represents the range of scores by normal subjects in the Park and Holzman (1992) study.

schizotypic pathology. These issues will be further discussed in the final section of this paper.

Second, the DRT is targeted at a specific impairment – working memory deficits – and the DRT will therefore tag those individuals with working memory deficits. DRT deficits are, however, also associated with conditions other than schizophrenia-related pathology, such as clearly diagnosed frontal lobe lesions. Therefore, not everyone with DRT deficits will have a high PAS score, and not everyone with a high PAS score will have schizophrenia-related psychopathology.

These two factors – the imperfect specificity and sensitivity of the PAS measure, and the absence of an exclusive relation between DRT performance deficits and schizophrenia-related pathology – can account for the predicted modest but significant relation found between working memory and PAS scores.

Table 15.3. *List of subjects' relatives with Axis I conditions and their delayed response accuracy score, antisaccade error score, and number of thought-disordered responses*

		Students' scores		
Relative's diagnosis	Student PAS group	DRT (% correct)	Antisaccade (No. errors)	No. TD responses
Major depressive disorder	high	93.8	3	6
Schizophrenia	high	78.3[a]	2	40[a]
Major depressive disorder	high	81.3[a]	1	1
Bipolar disorder	high	81.3[a]	1	0
Major depressive disorder	high	96.8	0	0
Bipolar disorder	high	100.0	0	2
Schizophrenia	high	97.9	0	4
Affective disorder	high	80.3[a]	2	7
Bipolar disorder	high	78.1[a]	9[a]	2

[a]Abnormal scores.

Poor accuracy on the DRT also occurs in about 40% of the otherwise unaffected first-degree relatives of schizophrenic patients, as shown by the results of Park, Holzman, and Levy (1993). In the present study, 9 subjects – all with high PAS scores – have first-degree relatives with major psychopathology, and 5 of these are in the group with low DRT accuracy scores. Four of the 9, however, have very good DRT scores. None of the low PAS scorers had a first-degree relative with major psychopathology (Table 15.3).

In summary, there is a statistically significant association between high PAS scores and low accuracy on the DRT, and these same high PAS individuals tend to have relatives with an Axis I psychiatric disorder. The high scorers on the PAS account for three times as many of the students with working memory deficits as do the normal students.

Experiment 2: antisaccade performance

Schizophrenic patients can shift their eyes to a target as rapidly and accurately as normal people can. When these rapid shifts of gaze, called "saccadic eye movements," are under 10° amplitude, the latency, accuracy, and velocity of the saccade made by a schizophrenic patient are indistinguishable from those made by a normal person (Iacono, Tuason, & Johnson, 1981; Levin, Holzman, Rothenberg, & Lipton, 1981). For saccadic amplitudes of greater than 10°, however, Levin and colleagues (Levin, Jones, Stark, Merrin, &

Holzman, 1982) reported that schizophrenic patients show longer latencies than do normal controls.

On an antisaccade task, in contrast, individuals are instructed not to look at the target when it moves, but instead to look as quickly as possible in the opposite direction. Thus, a saccade and an antisaccade task differ both in the location to which the person makes an eye movement in response to target movement and in whether the eyes move in response to a foveated target. Studies of antisaccade performance in schizophrenics show that these patients have higher error rates and longer latencies than do normal individuals (Fukushima, Fukushima, Chiba, Tanaka, & Yamshita, 1988; Fukushima, Fukushima, Morita, & Yamashita, 1990; Fukushima, Morita, Fukushima, Chiba, Tanaka, & Yamashita, 1990; Thaker, Nguyen, & Tamminga, 1989). The nature of the performance deficit shown by schizophrenic patients differs from that seen in patients with frontal lesions, however. Frontal lobe patients are unable both to suppress reflexive glances to the target and to make an antisaccade even after making an incorrect saccade to the target; schizophrenic patients make more reflexive saccades to the target than do control subjects, but their initial errors are corrected by appropriate antisaccades (Levy, in press). We chose this task to discover whether high PAS scorers also show a performance deficit on this task.

Procedure

Data were collected from 56 students, 25 of whom had low PAS scores and 31 of whom had high PAS scores. Horizontal eye movements were recorded from both eyes, by an infrared reflection system mounted on eye glass frames. Eye position was calibrated using six target positions on the screen. Sampling rate was 5 ms. Data were recorded on a computer that generated position and velocity tracings and provided automated analysis of saccade direction, amplitude, peak velocity, and duration.

At the beginning of each trial, a small solid square, $1° \times 1°$, appeared at the center of the screen for 800, 1,000, or 1,200 ms. The period was unpredictable, but each time interval was represented equally often in every testing block. Coinciding with the offset of the fixation point, a peripheral target of the same size flashed for 100 ms 15° to the left or right of the fixation point. The direction of the target was pseudorandom, with the restriction that the target appear an equal number of times on the right and the left, and that it appear a maximum of three times consecutively on the same side. After the peripheral target flashed, the screen remained blank for 1 second to allow the subject to make a saccade to the mirror position on the screen (antisaccade). After making the antisaccade, subjects were not to wait at the periphery, but to return their eyes immediately to the center to await the reappearance of the fixation point.

Data were collected for three blocks of 15 trials each, for a total of 45 trials. Data were entered automatically into a computer program that codes eye movements.

Antisaccades were scored as right or wrong solely on the basis of the first saccade following offset of the fixation point. Saccades of greater than 1° in the direction opposite that of the target were considered correct responses. Data from all three blocks of trials were included in the data analysis. All antisaccade errors were immediately corrected by the subject, indicating that all people understood the task and were attempting to comply.

Results

The high PAS students made significantly more errors (mean of 2.84 errors) than the low PAS students (mean of 1.16 errors) in the 45 trials ($t = 2.66$, $df = 54$, $p < .01$, 1-tail). The effect size (Cohen's *d;* Cohen, 1988) is .69, a "large" effect size. Table 15.2 presents these data. Figure 15.2 shows a scattergram of the error scores for the two subject groups. Eight high PAS students (about 26% of this group) made 5 or more errors on the 45 trials – that is, more errors than were made by any of the low PAS students. A Pearson correlation coefficient indicates that this association between high antisaccade errors (5 or more) and high PAS scores is statistically significant and accounts for almost 14% of the variance in antisaccade error scores ($r = .367$, $p = .005$).

The eight high PAS students with high antisaccade error scores were not necessarily the same subjects who made high numbers of delayed response errors. Although only three high PAS students performed abnormally on both the DRT and antisaccade tasks, the Pearson correlation between antisaccade errors and DRT errors, however, is statistically significant ($r = .276$; $p = .05$, 2-tail), indicating that those with poor DRT accuracy tended to make more antisaccade errors.

There was virtually no relation between number of antisaccade errors and Axis I psychopathology in first-degree family members ($r = .024$, ns). Only one person with more than five antisaccade errors had a first-degree relative with an Axis I diagnosis (Table 15.3). This person also had a high number of DRT errors. All other subjects with a first-degree relative with an Axis 1 diagnosis performed normally on the antisaccade task. Tests of intellectual functioning and aptitude, such as the WAIS and the SAT, showed no relation to antisaccade performance. Neither the Beck Depression Inventory nor the anxiety measures showed any significant relation to antisaccade performance.

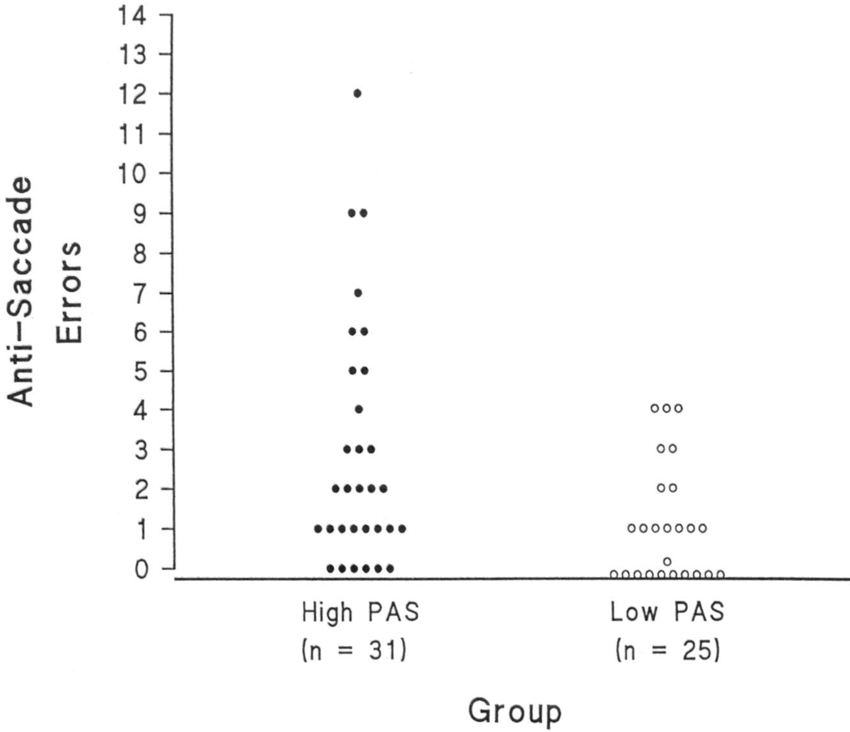

Fig. 15.2. Scatter diagram of the number of errors made by high and low PAS students on the antisaccade task.

Discussion

Interest in antisaccades first emerged from studies of patients with frontal lesions. In a series of papers, Guitton, Buchtel, and Douglas (1982, 1985) reported that patients with unilateral lesions of the dorsolateral and mesial regions of the frontal lobes had difficulty suppressing reflexive saccades to a target and initiating voluntary saccades to the side opposite that of the target. The poor performance of schizophrenic patients on antisaccade tasks has usually been discussed in terms of frontal dysfunctions – particularly of the dorsolateral prefrontal area.

The antisaccade task, however, is not specific for damage to any single brain area, including specific areas of the frontal lobes, or to any specific central nervous system disease. Not only the dorsolateral prefrontal cortex but also the mesial frontal cortex have been implicated in impaired antisaccade performance (Guitton et al., 1982, 1985). Patients with Huntington's disease, progressive supranuclear palsy, and Alzheimer's disease show antisaccade deficits. Data from our own laboratory indicate that both schizophrenic patients and patients with bipolar affective disorders show similar performance deficits on the antisaccade task (O'Driscoll, 1993; Sereno & Holzman, 1991).

In spite of its lack of specificity, the antisaccade task has been used rather widely in studies of the oculomotor functioning of schizophrenic patients. The present results, then, indicate that a subgroup of the high PAS students show high antisaccade error rates. The significance of this finding is, nevertheless, unclear, because antisaccade errors are spontaneously corrected by all of the groups except the patients with frontal lesions, as noted above.

Experiment 3: thought disorder

Schizophrenic patients think in peculiar and sometimes bizarre ways. This observation, systematically presented as early as Kraepelin's (1896/1919) descriptive efforts and Bleuler's (1911/1950) attempts to characterize the nature of the thought disorder, remains one of the most conspicuous and salient diagnostic symptoms of schizophrenia. Since Kraepelin's and Bleuler's descriptions of schizophrenic thought disorder, there have been many efforts to define the essence of the thought disorder. The nature of schizophrenic thinking eludes a simple categorization or dimensionality. The deviancies in schizophrenic thinking are multifactorial and multidimensional, in that autistic logic, neologistic word formations, confabulatory tendencies, confusion, among many others, all occur, and in varying degrees. Schizophrenic thinking also differs from the thinking disorders of other pathological conditions such as mania, delusional states, and dementias associated with various brain disorders.

Observers such as Rado (1953) and Meehl (1973) have noted that people with very mild forms of schizophrenia manifest a thought disorder that resembles, in attenuated form, that observed in schizophrenic psychoses. These observations require validation, and validation requires a reliable measuring instrument.

Although there are several instruments for assessing thought disorder, we chose the Thought Disorder Index (TDI; Johnston & Holzman, 1979), which is a psychometric tool for identifying and measuring disturbances in thinking. The TDI has been validated on a variety of groups, including those with and without psychiatric illness, and relatives of psychiatric patients. It has a high degree of interrater reliability (Coleman et al., 1993). The TDI yields qualitative and quantitative indexes of the ways in which ideational and perceptual organization and verbalizations can be distorted in psychopathological and neuropathological conditions.

Johnston and Holzman, the developers of the TDI, attempted to refine and extend Kraepelin's (1896/1919) clinical observations, which were, to a large extent, incorporated and described by Rapaport, Gill, and Schafer (1946/1968) in their work on diagnostic psychological testing. Rapaport, Gill, and Schafer's (1946/1968) qualitative descriptions of thought slippage were subsequently quantified by Watkins and Stauffacher (1952) in the Delta Index, a predecessor of the TDI (Johnston & Holzman, 1979).

Previous studies have shown that elevated levels of thought disorder are found not only in psychotic patients, both schizophrenic and bipolar (Shenton et al., 1987; Solovay et al., 1987), but also in a significant number of their otherwise unaffected first-degree relatives (Johnston & Holzman, 1979; Shenton, Holzman, & Solovay, 1989), including children (Arboleda & Holzman, 1985), and in borderline and schizotypic patients (Edell, 1987). Although the amount and severity of thought disorder, as measured by the TDI, are significantly reduced by neuroleptic treatment (Hurt, Holzman, & Davis, 1983; Patterson, Spohn, Bogia, & Hayes, 1986), the thought disorder detected at any particular time reflects both a propensity for thought slippage (a trait characteristic) and adventitious events (state variables, such as clinical state and medication variables).

The hypothesis in the present study is that there will be higher than normal levels of thought disorder in subjects with high PAS scores, and that this propensity for manifesting thought disorder represents a feature of the thinking of these high PAS students.

Method

Thirty high PAS and 26 low PAS subjects were tested by two examiners. All subjects were administered a 10-card Rorschach test (Rorschach, 1921), from which the TDI is assessed. Administration of each Rorschach protocol followed the procedures described by Rapaport et al. (1946/1968). All sessions were audiotaped and subsequently transcribed verbatim. The protocols were scored for thought disorder by consensus decision by three trained scorers, according to the TDI manual (Solovay, Shenton, & Holzman, 1986). Both Rorschach administration and TDI scoring were performed without knowledge of the PAS status of the subjects.

Instrument: description and scoring

The 23 TDI categories represent most of the types of deviant verbalizations encountered as disordered thought of a formal nature, such as idiosyncratic speech, combinatory thinking, associative thinking, and disorganized thinking. The TDI manual contains complete descriptions of the categories as well as the psychometric characteristics of the instrument (Johnston & Holzman, 1979; Solovay et al., 1986).

The total TDI score is computed as the number of instances of thought disorder tagged by the TDI, multiplied by its category weight (e.g., .25, .50, .75, or 1.0), divided by the number of Rorschach responses to control for verbal productivity, and multiplied by 100 to express the value as a percent.

Results

High PAS subjects had a significantly higher mean total TDI score (8.83) than low PAS subjects (3.65) ($t = 1.75$, $df = 54$, $p < .045$, 1-tail). High PAS students also had a significantly higher *mean number* of responses that were scored as disordered (7.27) than low PAS students (3.00) ($t = 2.10$, $df = 54$, $p = .02$, 1-tail). In addition, the high PAS group showed a significantly higher mean number of idiosyncratic verbalizations (i.e., peculiar and queer verbalizations and absurd responses) (4.87 vs. 1.69; $t = 1.98$, $df = 54$, $p < .028$, 1-tail; see Table 15.2). The effect sizes for all three TDI variables range between .46 and .55 (Cohen's *d*; Cohen, 1988), considered to be "medium" effect sizes. Four individuals showed very high levels of idiosyncratic verbalizations, and all four of them were in the high PAS group. None of the other TDI categories distinguished the two groups of students. Figure 15.3 shows the distribution of the number of thought-disordered responses for the two groups of students.

Only one of the high PAS students with high TDI scores had a first-degree relative with an Axis I psychiatric disorder (Table 15.3). One of the four high PAS students who showed a high level of idiosyncratic verbalizations also had poor DRT scores. There were no significant relations between the total number of thought-disordered responses, the TDI score, or number of idiosyncratic verbalizations and the anxiety measures, SAT scores, or the Digit Symbol Tests. The total number of thought-disordered responses showed a marginally significant tendency to be related to scores on the Beck Depression Inventory, although the total TDI score and idiosyncratic verbalizations were not at all related to the Beck scores.

All three TDI scores were significantly associated with antisaccade performance at moderate levels, such that those with higher amounts of thought disorder, however measured by the TDI, made more antisaccade errors. The correlations between antisaccade errors and the three TDI scores ranged from .35 to .47, all of which are statistically significant at <.005.

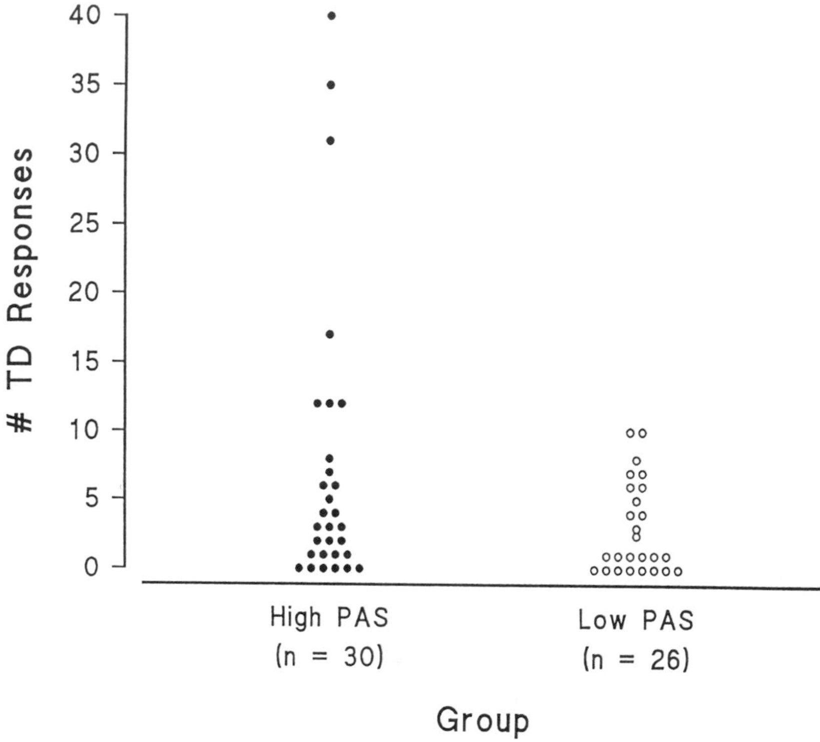

Fig. 15.3. Scatter diagram of the number of thought-disordered responses made by high and low PAS students on the Rorschach test, as scored according to the Thought Disorder Index.

Discussion

The high and low PAS groups differ in the amount of thought slippage detected by the TDI, with the high PAS group producing a significantly greater number of thought-disordered responses. The principal type of thought disorder that characterized the high PAS group was idiosyncratic verbalizations – the mild peculiarities of speech that indicate an ellipsis, a failed effort to self-edit, or even an autistic idea. Nine of 30 high PAS students (30%) showed significant elevations on the TDI, compared with 4 of 27 students with low PAS (18%) scores. The high PAS group showed not only peculiar and queer verbalizations, but in several instances incoherence, autistic logic, and ideational looseness occurred as well. These features of thought disorder in the high PAS group are also characteristic of clinical populations, particularly schizophrenics. These results are compatible with those reported by Edell and Chapman (1979) using the Delta Index. Combinatory ideational activity accounted for the slippage shown by the low PAS group and was also present in the high PAS group.

Reflections and speculations

The principal findings of this investigation show that some college students who were selected for proneness to perceptual aberrations and body image disturbances show performance patterns like those seen in schizophrenic patients and in some of their first-degree biological family members. Nine of 28 (32%) of the students with high PAS scores, compared with 3 of 22 (14%) of students with low PAS scores, had DRT accuracy of less than 86%, which was also the lowest score obtained by the normal group tested by Park and Holzman (1992). On the antisaccade task, eight students (26%) made more than five antisaccade errors, and all were identified as having high PAS scores. Higher levels of thought disorder were also detected among the students with high PAS scores. Our sample of psychometric "schizotypes" was identified on the basis of perceptual aberrations and body image distortions. Thought disorder may also accompany other characteristics of schizotypy, such as magical thinking, odd speech, and cold, aloof affect.

Although a substantial proportion of the high PAS students performed deviantly on each of the three tasks, the students who performed poorly on the DRT were not necessarily the same ones who performed poorly on the antisaccade task or who showed significant amounts of thought disorder. Each task identifies approximately the same proportion of high PAS students – between 20% and 30% – as having schizophrenia-related deficits. Of students with high PAS scores, 60% had deviant scores on at least one of the dependent measures, compared with 22% of the students with low PAS scores.

The PAS identifies many more people as deviant than do the DRT, the antisaccade task, or the TDI. Further, the PAS probably fails to identify some people who have schizotypic traits other than perceptual aberrations or body image distortions, such as those that accompany impaired interpersonal relatedness, social isolation, or odd appearance. Therefore, only a subgroup of schizotypic individuals will be identified by the PAS, yielding an indeterminate false negative and false positive rate of detection. This psychometric method, then, poses several questions, which we attempt to address here.

1. How diagnostic of schizotypy is the PAS? Our data suggest that there are many students with high PAS scores who probably do not have schizophrenia-related performance deficits. This yield is expectable both epidemiologically and clinically, since many of the traits tapped by the PAS are associated

with many other disorders. Consider the symptom of body image distortion, which is an aspect of depersonalization. Depersonalization refers to a feeling of unreality about oneself, a sense of unconnectedness with one's own body and thoughts, emotional numbness, a sense that one's voice, actions, or feelings are not under one's control. All of these experiences can occur among people in the general population who have not identified themselves as in need of treatment (Dixon, 1963), and they range on a continuum from very mild and transient to the severe and chronic. They can occur as a consequence of sleep deprivation, acute intoxications, being in strange places, and serious accidents (Noyes et al., 1977). Various organic conditions are associated with these conditions, such as temporal lobe epilepsy, brain tumors, and migraine aura. Depersonalization experiences may also occur with anxiety, panic, depression, schizophrenia, and personality disorders, and, of course, as the identifying characteristic of depersonalization disorder. Mayer-Gross regarded depersonalization as a nonspecific brain response that is built into the CNS, much like a fever response to an organic insult (Mayer-Gross, 1935). It is therefore to be expected that the PAS will cast a very wide net and detect people who share certain symptoms that reflect disparate psychiatric conditions, and thus produce a number of false positive detections.

As we have already remarked, the PAS concentrates on experiences of perceptual and body distortions, and thus does not focus at all on the other defining dimensions of schizotypy, such as disturbed social interactions, magical or referential thinking, behavioral eccentricities, or odd speech. As a consequence, the PAS will fail to identify people who possess other identifying characteristics of schizotypy, but who do not experience perceptual and bodily distortions. A number of false negative identifications will thus occur in the low PAS or normal group, thereby misclassifying some valid schizotypic individuals. In this connection, it is noteworthy that six students in the low PAS group had either low accuracy DRT ($n = 3$), high levels of thought disorder ($n = 3$), or both ($n = 1$). A more intensive clinical examination of these students would shed light on whether they also have schizotypal symptoms not captured by the PAS.

Similar heterogeneity of schizotypal symptoms and traits was shown by Kendler et al. (Kendler, Ochs, Gorman, Hewitt, Ross, & Mirsky, 1991), who studied 29 pairs of twins, monozygotic (MZ) and dizygotic (DZ), selected from a population registry. Several measures of schizotypy were obtained, including schizotypal symptoms (from the Structured Interview for Schizotypy), schizotypal personality traits (from a self-report questionnaire which included the Chapmans' PAS scale), and a neuropsychological attentional battery. A factor analysis of the schizotypy measures showed two independent factors. The first factor had high loadings on "positive symptoms" such as speech oddities, avoidant traits, and social anxiety. The second factor had high loadings on poor modulation of affect, and oddness in social behavior, including social isolation. The attentional battery summary score correlated significantly with this second schizotypy factor, a result that is similar to that of Asarnow, Nuechterlein, and Marder (1985), who reported a significant association between scores on the Span of Apprehension test and only a subset of symptoms of schizotypy.

2. Does this psychometric method of selecting schizotypes reveal more than knowing that a person is a biological relative of a schizophrenic person? Contemporary research studies of populations at risk for schizophrenic conditions have selected their subjects in three different ways. The first is to focus on the biological first-degree relatives of schizophrenic patients; the second is to select patients with a clinical diagnosis of a schizophrenia-spectrum disorder, such as schizotypal, paranoid, or schizoid personality disorder; the third, the method used in this study, is to select members of the general population who perform in a deviant way on certain psychometric or physiological indices associated with schizophrenia.

The first two methods have been generally successful in finding deviance on several measures that parallel the abnormalities found in schizophrenic patients. For example, eye tracking dysfunction (ETD) is as prevalent in patients with schizophrenia-spectrum disorders as it is in first-degree relatives of schizophrenic patients and in patients with schizophrenia (Holzman, Proctor, Levy, Yasillo, Meltzer, & Hurt, 1974; Siever et al., 1990; Smeraldi et al., 1987).

The psychometric method employed in this study identified all nine students who have a first-degree relative with an Axis I psychiatric disorder (Table 15.3). Five of these nine students performed in a deviant way on at least 1 of the 3 dependent measures. It therefore appears that the psychometric method and the tests used in this study may indeed validly identify those who may be gene carriers, although there is a price to be paid in an unknown rate of false positive and false negative identifications.

3. Does the presence of perceptual aberrations, body image distortions, or other "schizotypic" characteristics identify people who have a greater than base rate probability for developing schizophrenia?

This question shelters two different issues. The first would ask whether the PAS identifies "gene carriers," who, by virtue of a genetic endowment, inherit the schizotypic characteristics that can be considered phenotypic expressions of the schizophrenia genotype. Only some of these schizotypic people would, sooner or later, become clinically schizophrenic. Others may be able to maintain a state of compensated adaptation, but this adaptation probably exacts a toll on the functional efficiency of various psychological processes. The term "risk" in these instances seems better replaced by the term "liability" or "vulnerability," since the issue is one of a diathesis that represents a necessary but not sufficient condition for the two clinical outcomes described above. Still other people, some with and some without the schizophrenia genotype, may show schizotypic characteristics but do not succumb to psychosis or show deviant performance on relevant psychological tasks. In this instance, the presence of schizotypic characteristics, determined psychometrically, may or may not be an expression of vulnerability. Given only the psychometric information concerning the presence of schizotypic characteristics, one cannot tell for any specific individual whether these schizotypic traits represent a necessary condition for a schizophrenic condition.

The second issue implicit in the question involves a different model, one in which perceptual aberrations and body image distortions are not an outcome of a schizophrenia diathesis, but are independent of it. These characteristics may function as a potentiator of schizophrenia-like pathology in those who inherit the hypothesized schizophrenia diathesis, but they are not exclusively coupled with the diathesis. In this sense, behaviors like those identified by the PAS could, if present, predispose a person to develop schizophrenia, just as high dietary cholesterol, smoking, and obesity can place a person at risk for developing cardiovascular disease. "Risk" in this model is a statistical term that refers to an increase in the probability for developing the disease. (See Holzman, 1982, for a discussion of the issues of vulnerability and risk.) For clarity, we have diagramed the three causal models discussed in this section. The first, a "risk" model, is presented in Figure 15.4.

Although we require data for our preference, we regard the PAS as an identifier of vulnerability for schizophrenia. If one keeps in mind the fallibility of the instrument, the traits that characterize the high PAS scorers can be viewed as some of the phenotypic expressions of a schizophrenia diathesis, which has many manifestations. These symptoms can be considered as another expression of a latent trait, along with ETD and schizophrenia (Matthysse, Holzman, & Lange, 1986). Figure 15.5 presents this model.

The psychometric method, as we have noted, identifies a number of false positives and false negatives, and does not include a principal vulnerability factor: whether a person is a gene carrier. It therefore approaches the issue of risk from a side not yet addressed by the "genetic high risk method." It asks whether the possession of certain personality traits is significantly associated with schizophrenic (or perhaps other psychotic) conditions, as well as the compromises in psychological functioning associated with those conditions.

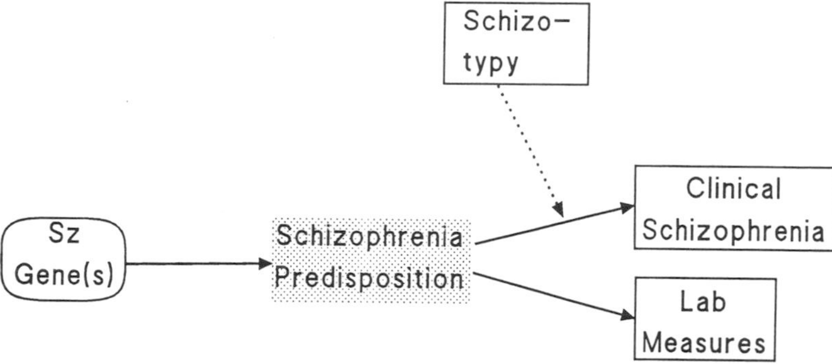

Fig. 15.4. Diagram of the hypothetical causal model in which a gene (or genes) for schizophrenia gives rise to a predisposition, which is not directly observable (the shaded rectangle denotes the hypothetical entity). The predisposition can give rise to schizophrenia and to deviant behaviors on measures such as those investigated in this study. These two outcomes are independent of each other and conditioned on the presence of the hypothetical predisposition. Schizotypy, an observable constellation of cognitive, perceptual, affective, and interpersonal deviances, is not caused by the gene or genes that give rise to the schizophrenia disposition, but independently acts to potentiate the predisposition to lead to a schizophrenic outcome.

The method provides the opportunity to examine conditions that protect a person from developing the disease. These conditions may be intrapersonal, interpersonal, biological, and social. The genetic risk method also affords such opportunities, but they have rarely been exploited for this purpose.

4. Why are the differences between the groups not greater? We anticipated relatively subtle, but statistically reliable, differences between the groups for reasons related to our subject selection strategy. We selected our experimental group using the PAS, a fallible psychometric marker, that most likely generated an admixture of people, some of whom may be compensated schizotypes (only a subset of whom will ever decompensate), an unknown proportion of false positives who represent a variety of personality types, and an unknown number of false negatives whose schizotypic symptoms differ from those identified by the PAS. Thus, we most likely identified individuals representing a diversity of liabilities.

Finding subtle differences between groups on such tasks is consistent with the usual results from "high-risk" studies (Cornblatt & Erlenmeyer-Kimling, 1985; cf. Hanson, Gottesman, & Meehl, 1977). Clearly, the goal of the high-risk approach in psychopathology research is the isolation of reliable objective behaviors that might aid in more efficient identification of schizophrenia (or psychosis) liability. Even if individual objective markers reflect relatively

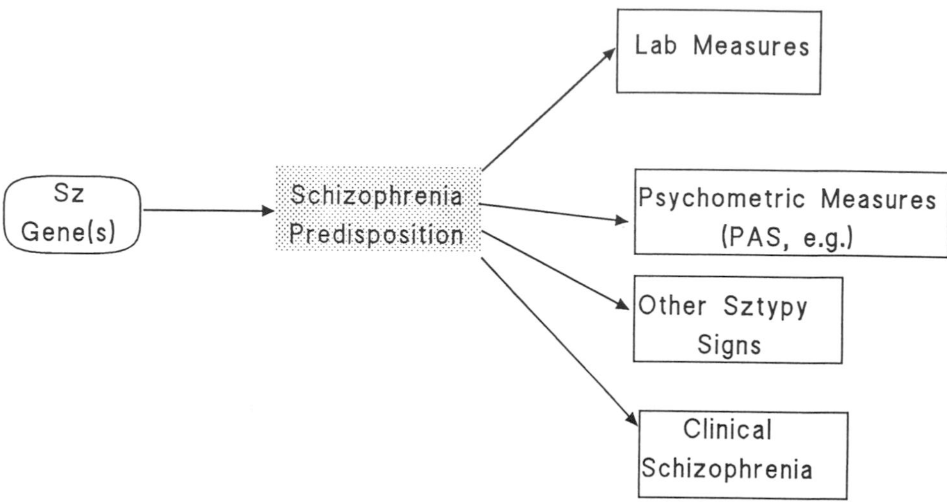

Fig. 15.5. The latent trait model is essentially equivalent to the causal chain depicted in this figure. The gene or genes give rise to a schizophrenia predisposition, which Matthysse et al. (1986) called a latent trait [shaded to indicate it is not (yet) an observable entity]. The predisposition can independently give rise to schizotypy (measured psychometrically or clinically observed), clinical schizophrenia, and deviance on laboratory measures. These outcomes are independent of one another, but conditioned on the presence of the schizophrenia predisposition (latent trait).

subtle deviance, in aggregate they may help to reduce the imprecision in detecting liability that is characteristic of the clinical method of identifying symptoms. Efficient detection of true liability might ultimately provide clues to etiology and pathophysiology as well as to protective factors.

5. How can we interpret the finding that different tests identify different people in the schizotypy group? One model that seems reasonable is that of some pleiotropic disorders, such as neurofibromatosis or osteogenesis imperfecta, in which there is one genotype but several phenotypes. In these instances, a parent may have particular manifestations of the disorder, but the offspring may have different ones. Thus, in a case of osteogenesis imperfecta described by Pignatti and Turco (1992), the mother's symptoms included blue sclerae, deafness, and osteoporosis; the child's symptoms included multiple bone fractures that necessitated the placing of steel rods in the bones. In the case of schizotypy, one could postulate that the genotype, as yet undefined, unfolds as several phenotypes, which we measure only imperfectly with our tests and with clinical assessment.

6. How should this set of findings be integrated with the family studies of

schizophrenia? Since the psychometric method has identified a significant number of persons with schizophrenic-like traits, and since a significant proportion of these people show deficit performance on some cognitive tasks associated with schizophrenia, these people should be followed longitudinally, as the Chapmans (Chapman & Chapman, in press) and as Lenzenweger are doing.

This method alone cannot address one important issue, however: Is schizotypy the inevitable route to schizophrenia? This psychometric method must be used in conjunction with longitudinal and familial studies of schizophrenia. The study of MZ twins would be especially useful for answering this question. We would ask whether, in MZ twins discordant for schizophrenia, schizotypy always occurs in the well twin and must always precede the development of schizophrenia in the affected twin. Do schizotypic traits in the well twin increase the risk for eye movement dysfunctions, working memory deficits, antisaccade errors, and thought disorder? If they do, one must then entertain a model of the transmission of schizophrenia that postulates that schizotypy is the channel through which these traits must pass (see Figure 15.6, which depicts this model). If, however, these performance deficits are only modestly associated with schizotypic characteristics, as appears to be the case in this study's population, then support is given for another kind of model that is more consistent with the Mendelian latent structure model proposed by Matthysse et al. (1986; see Figure 15.5).

Acknowledgments

This research was supported in part by U.S. Public Health Service grants MH 31340, MH 31154, MH 49487, MH 44876, MH 44866, MH 01021, MH-45448, a Stanley Foundation Fellowship Grant, and a Special Projects Fund Grant from Cornell University. Computer resources for this study were provided in part by the Cornell Institute for Social and Economic Research, which is funded jointly by Cornell University and the National Science Foundation.

We thank Sylvia Emmerich, Natasha Frangopoulos, and Jill Salem for their assistance in testing study subjects. We also thank Lauren Korfine, who was our psychometric screening project coordinator, and Kim Altman, Seth Axelrod, Sarah Cho, Jennifer Cohen, Christine Duncan, Natasha Frangopoulos, Eliotte Hirshberg, Lori Isman, James Murray, Michael Remacle, Kenneth Robin, Jill Salem, Timothy Sheahan, Suzanne Sheirr, and Tara White for their help during the screening data collection procedure. Clara Lajonchere and Charlotte Stimpson helped with data analysis.

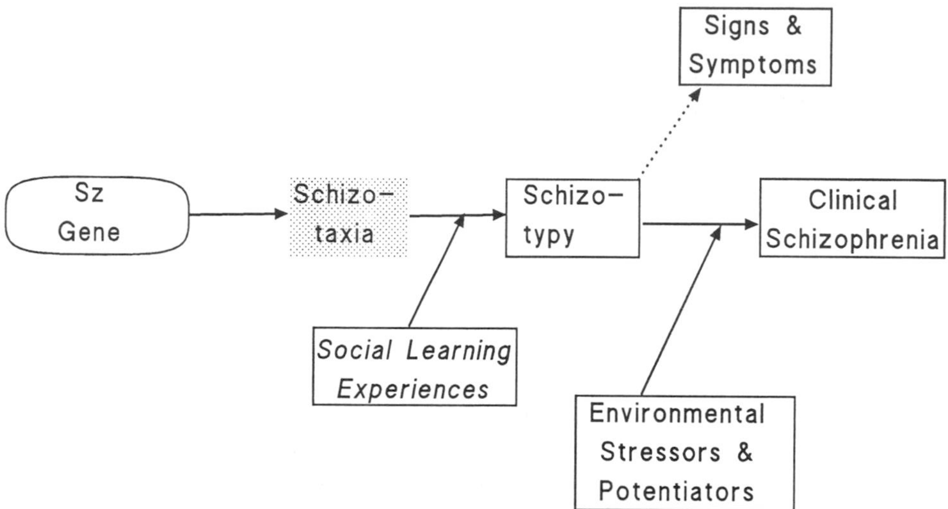

Fig. 15.6. This model is closely related to that advanced by Meehl (1990). A specific gene gives rise to a hypothetical entity called "schizotaxia" (shaded in the model), which, in the presence of certain as yet unknown environmental influences, causes schizotypy, recognizable by specified signs and symptoms as well as through laboratory measures. Although schizotypy is a necessary precondition for clinical schizophrenia, it is not a sufficient cause, since the outbreak of schizophrenia requires both schizotypy and certain environmental stressors as precursors. This model differs from the latent trait model (Figure 15.5). There, schizophrenia and schizotypy are independent of each other, the latent trait being a necessary condition for both.

References

Arboleda, C., & Holzman, P. S. (1985). Thought disorder in children at risk for psychosis. *Archives of General Psychiatry, 42,* 1004–1013.

Asarnow, R. F., Nuechterlein, K. H., & Marder, S. R. (1985). Span of apprehension performance, neuropsychological functioning and indices of psychosis-proneness. *Journal of Nervous and Mental Disease, 171,* 662–669.

Beck, A. T., Ward, C. H., Mendelsohn, M., Mock, J. E., & Erbaugh, J. K. (1961). An inventory for measuring depression. *Archives of General Psychiatry, 4,* 561–571.

Bleuler, E. (1911/1950). *Dementia praecox or the group of schizophrenias* (trans. by H. Zinkin). New York: International Universities Press.

Chapman, L. J., & Chapman, J. P. (1985). Psychosis proneness. In M. Alpert (Ed.), *Controversies in schizophrenia: Changes and constancies* (pp. 157–172). New York: Guilford Press.

Chapman, L. J., & Chapman, J. P. (in press). Psychometric assessment of schizophrenia proneness. In S. Matthysse, D. Levy, F. Benes, & J. Kagan (Eds.), *Psychopathology: The evolving science of mental disorder.* Cambridge: Cambridge University Press.

Chapman, L. J., Chapman, J. P., & Raulin, M. L. (1978). Body-image aberration in schizophrenia. *Journal of Abnormal Psychology, 87,* 399–407.

Cohen, J. (1988). *Statistical power analysis for the behavioral sciences* (2nd ed). Hillsdale, N.J.: Erlbaum.

Coleman, M. J., Carpenter, J. T., Waterneaux, C., Levy, D. L., Shenton, M. E., Perry, J., Medoff, D., Wong, H., Manoach, D., Meyer, P., O'Brien, C., Valentino, C., Robinson, D., Smith, M., Makowski, D., & Holzman, P. S. (1993). The Thought Disorder Index: A reliability study. *Psychological Assessment, The Journal of Consulting and Clinical Psychology, 3,* 346–352.

Cornblatt, B. A., & Erlenmeyer-Kimling, L. (1985). Global attentional deviance as a marker of risk for schizophrenia. *Journal of Abnormal Psychology, 94,* 470–486.

Cronbach, L. J., & Meehl, P. E. (1955). Construct validity in psychological tests. *Psychological Bulletin, 52,* 281–302.

Dixon, J. C. (1963). Depersonalization phenomena in a sample population of college students. *British Journal of Psychiatry, 109,* 371–375.

Edell, W. S. (1987). Role of structure in disordered thinking in borderline and schizophrenic disorders. *Journal of Personality Assessment, 51,* 23–41.

Edell, W. S., & Chapman, L. J. (1979). Anhedonia, perceptual aberration, and the Rorschach. *Journal of Consulting and Clinical Psychology, 47,* 377–384.

Fukushima, J., Fukushima, K., Chiba, T., Tanaka, S., & Yamshita, I. (1988). Disturbances of voluntary control of saccadic eye movements in schizophrenic patients. *Biological Psychiatry, 23,* 670–677.

Fukushima, J., Fukushima, K., Morita, N., & Yamashita, I. (1990a). Further analysis of the control of voluntary saccadic eye movements in schizophrenia patients. *Biological Psychiatry, 28,* 943–958.

Fukushima, J., Morita, N., Fukushima, K., Chiba, T., Tanaka, S., & Yamashita, I. (1990b). Voluntary control of saccadic eye movements in patients with schizophrenic and affective disorders. *Journal of Psychiatric Research, 24,* 9–24.

Funahashi, S., Bruce, C. J., & Goldman-Rakic, P. S. (1991). Neuronal activity related to saccadic eye movements in the monkey's dorsolateral prefrontal cortex. *Journal of Neurophysiology, 65,* 1464–1483.

Goldman-Rakic, P. S. (1991). Prefrontal cortical dysfunction in schizophrenia: The relevance of working memory. In B. J. Carroll & J. E. Barrett (Eds.), *Psychopathology and the brain* (pp. 1–23). New York: Raven Press.

Grinker, R. R., Sr. (1969). An essay on schizophrenia and science. *Archives of General Psychiatry, 20,* 1–24.

Guitton, C., Buchtel, H. A., & Douglas, R. M. (1982). Disturbances of voluntary saccadic eye movement mechanisms following discrete unilateral frontal lobe removals. In G. Lennerstrand, D. S. Zee, & E. Keller (Eds.), *Functional basis of oculomotility disorders* (pp. 497–499). Oxford, U.K.: Pergamon Press.

Guitton, D., Buchtel, H. A., & Douglas, R. M. (1985). Frontal lobe lesions in man cause difficulties in suppressing reflexive glances and in generating goal-directed saccades. *Experimental Brain Research, 58,* 455–472.

Hanson, D. R., Gottesman, I. I., & Meehl, P. E. (1977). Genetic theories and the validation of psychiatric diagnoses: Implications for the study of the children of schizophrenics. *Journal of Abnormal Psychology, 86,* 575–588.

Holzman, P. S. (1982). The search for a biological marker of the functional psychoses. In M. J. Goldstein (Eds.), *Preventive intervention in schizophrenia: Are we ready?* (pp. 19–38). U.S. Government Printing Office.

Holzman, P. S., & Matthysse, S. (1990). The genetics of schizophrenia: A review. *Psychological Science, 1,* 279–286.

Holzman, P. S., Proctor, L. R., Levy, D. L., Yasillo, N. J., Meltzer, H. Y., & Hurt, S. W. (1974). Eye-tracking dysfunctions in schizophrenic patients and their relatives. *Archives of General Psychiatry, 31,* 143–151.

Hurt, S. S., Holzman, P. S., & Davis, J. M. (1983). Thought disorder: The measurement of its changes. *Archives of General Psychiatry, 40,* 1281–1285.

Iacono, W. G., Tuason, V. B., & Johnson, R. A. (1981). Dissociation of smooth pursuit and saccadic eye tracking in remitted schizophrenics. *Archives of General Psychiatry, 38,* 991–996.

Johnston, M. H., & Holzman, P. S. (1979). *Assessing schizophrenic thinking.* San Francisco: Jossey-Bass.

Kendler, K. S., Ochs, A. L., Gorman, A. M., Hewitt, J. K., Ross, D. E., & Mirsky, A. F. (1991). The structure of schizotypy: A pilot multitrait twin study. *Psychiatry Research, 36,* 19–36.

Kraepelin, E. (1896/1919). *Dementia praecox and paraphrenia* (trans. R. M. Barclay). Chicago: Chicago Medical Book.

Levin, S., Holzman, P. S., Rothenberg, S. J., & Lipton, R. B. (1981). Saccadic eye movements in psychotic patients. *Psychiatry Research, 5,* 47–58.

Levin, S., Jones, A., Stark, L., Merrin, E. L., & Holzman, P. S. (1982). Identification of abnormal patterns in eye movements of schizophrenic patients. *Archives of General Psychiatry, 39,* 1125–1130.

Levy, D. L. (in press). Location, location, location: The pathway from behavior to brain locus in schizophrenia. In S. Matthysse, S. Levy, F. Benes, & J. Kagan (Eds.), *Psychopathology: The evolving science of mental disorder,* Cambridge: Cambridge University Press.

Levy, D. L., Holzman, P. S., Matthysse, S., & Mendell, N. R. (1993). Eye tracking and schizophrenia: A critical perspective. *Schizophrenia Bulletin, 19,* 461–536.

Matthysse, S., Holzman, P. S., & Lange, K. (1986). The genetic transmission of schizophrenia: Application of Mendelian latent structure analysis to eye tracking dysfunctions in schizophrenia and affective disorder. *Journal of Psychiatric Research, 20,* 57–65.

Mayer-Gross, W. (1935). On depersonalization. *British Journal of Medical Psychology, 15,* 103–122.

Meehl, P. E. (1962). Schizotaxia, schizotypy, schizophrenia. *American Psychologist, 17,* 827–838.

Meehl, P. E. (1973). MAXCOV-HITMAX: A taxonomic search method for loose genetic syndromes. In P. E. Meehl (Ed.), *Psychodiagnosis: Selected papers* (pp. 200–224). Minneapolis, Minn. University of Minnesota Press.

Meehl, P. E. (1990). Toward an integrated theory of schizotaxia, schizotypy, and schizophrenia. *Journal of Personality Disorders, 4,* 1–99.

Noyes, R., Hoenk, P. R., Kuperman, S., Slymen, D. J. (1977). Depersonalization in accident victims and psychiatric patients. *Journal of Nervous and Mental Diseases, 164,* 401–407.

O'Driscoll, G. A., Strakowski, S., Alpert, N. M., Rauch, S. L., Elliott, D., Levy, D., Matthysse, S., & Holzman, P. S. (1993). Examination of the neural control of eye movements with PET. *Journal of Nuclear Medicine and Technology, 34,* 196.

Park, S., & Holzman, P. S. (1992) Schizophrenics show spatial working memory deficits. *Archives of General Psychiatry, 49,* 975–982.

Park, S., & Holzman, P. S. (1993). Association of working memory deficit and eye tracking dysfunction in schizophrenia: The role of the prefrontal cortex. *Schizophrenia Research, 11,* 55–61.

Park, S., Holzman, P. S., & Levy, D. L. (1993). Spatial working memory deficit in the relatives of schizophrenic patients is associated with their smooth pursuit eye tracking performance. International Congress for Schizophrenia Research, Colorado Springs, CO, 1993. *Schizophrenia Research, 9,* 184.

Patterson, T., Spohn, H. E., Bogia, D. P., & Hayes, K. (1986). Thought disorder in schizophrenia. *Schizophrenia Bulletin, 12,* 460–472.

Pignatti, P. F., & Turco, A. E. (1992). Tracking disease genes by reverse genetics. *Journal of Psychiatric Research, 26,* 287–298.

Rado, S. (1953). Dynamics and classification of disordered behavior. *American Journal of Psychiatry, 110,* 406–416.

Rapaport, D., Gill, M. M., & Schafer, R. (1946/1968). *Diagnostic Psychological Testing* (ed. R. Holt). New York: International Universities Press. (First published in 1946).

Rorschach, H. (1921). *Psychodiagnostics.* (Reprint: New York: Grune & Stratton, 1949).

Sereno, A. B., & Holzman, P. S. (1991). Express and antisaccades in schizophrenic, affective disorder, and normal control subjects. *Society for Neuroscience Abstracts, 17,* 858.

Shenton, M. E., Holzman, P. S., & Solovay, M. (1989). Thought disorder in the relatives of psychotic patients. *Archives of General Psychiatry, 46,* 897–901.

Shenton, M. E., Solovay, M. R., & Holzman, P. S. (1987). Comparative studies of thought disorder: II. Schizoaffective disorder. *Archives of General Psychiatry, 44,* 31–35.

Siever, L. J., Keefe, R., Bernstein, D. P., Coccaro, E. F., Klar, H. M., Zemishlany, Z., Peterson, A. E., Davidson, M., Mahon, T., Horvath, T., & Mohs, R. (1990). Eye tracking impairment in clinically identified patients with schizotypal personality disorder. *American Journal of Psychiatry, 147,* 740–745.

Smeraldi, E., Gambini, O., Bellodi, L., Sacchetti, E., Vita, A., diRossa, M., & Cazzullo, C. L. (1987). Combined measure of smooth pursuit eye movements and ventricle–brain ratio in schizophrenic disorders. *Psychiatry Research, 21,* 293–301.

Solovay, M. R., Shenton, M. E., & Holzman, P. S. (1986). Scoring manual for the Thought Disorder Index, Revised Version. Original version by M. H. Johnston & P. S. Holzman, *Schizophrenia Bulletin, 12,* 483–496.

Solovay, M. R., Shenton, M. E., & Holzman, P. S. (1987). Comparative studies of thought disorder: I. Mania and schizophrenia. *Archives of General Psychiatry, 44,* 13–20.

Spielberger, C. D. (1983). *Manual for the State–Trait Anxiety Inventory.* Palo Alto, Calif.: Consulting Psychologists Press.

Thaker, G. K., Nguyen, J. A., & Tamminga, C. A. (1989). Increased saccadic distractibility in tardive dyskinesia: Functional evidence for subcortical GABA dysfunction. *Biological Psychiatry, 25,* 49–59.

Watkins, J. G., & Stauffacher, J. C. (1952). An index of pathological thinking in the Rorschach. *Journal of Projective Techniques, 16,* 276–286.

Wechsler, D. (1981). *Wechsler Adult Intelligence Scale – Revised (WAIS-R) manual.* New York: The Psychological Corporation.

PART VII
Brain imaging

16

Brain morphology in schizotypal personality as assessed by magnetic resonance imaging

MICHAEL FLAUM and NANCY C. ANDREASEN

Over the past two decades, there have been literally hundreds of studies published in the psychiatric literature on the topic of brain morphology in schizophrenia as assessed by computerized tomography and magnetic resonance imaging (for good overviews, see Gur & Pearlson, 1993; Pearlson & Marsh, 1993; Shelton & Weinberger, 1986). The majority of these reports have employed the strategy of comparing groups of schizophrenics and normal controls in terms of the size of various aspects of brain anatomy. Significant group differences have been demonstrated for many brain regions, most notably, larger ventricular size among the schizophrenics. A host of other studies have explored the relationship between brain morphology and various clinical, neuropsychological, and other neurobiological measures. Although the meaning and implications of these morphological differences have yet to be fully elucidated, there is an emerging sense of confidence within the research community that these neuroimaging findings will provide important clues to the understanding of the etiological and pathophysiological mechanisms underlying schizophrenia.

The primary question that is addressed in this chapter involves the extent to which studies of brain morphology may also serve to provide clues in terms of understanding schizotypal personality. As is evident from this volume, the construct of schizotypy itself remains controversial. Is the distinction between schizotypy and schizophrenia valid? That is, is it really distinct from schizophrenia in terms of its underlying pathophysiology and etiology? Is it merely a milder variant of schizophrenia? Does it share a genetic diathesis with schizophrenia but differ in terms of environmental factors? Is it a different disorder entirely?

To address these questions, a wide variety of approaches have been employed, among them, genetic epidemiological studies, linkage studies, and longitudinal outcome studies, as well as studies of an array of so-called biological markers. Many of these approaches are summarized in this volume. Given the amount of effort and resources that have been devoted to structural neuroimaging research in schizophrenia, it is somewhat surprising how little this technology has thus far been exploited in trying to better understand schizotypy.

In this chapter, we briefly review relevant findings in the schizophrenia–neuroimaging literature, describe those studies that have been done on brain morphology in schizotypy, and discuss how studies of brain morphology may be used to explore alternative models of the relationship between schizotypy and schizophrenia. Examples are provided through preliminary analyses of magnetic resonance imaging (MRI) data that have been collected in our laboratory over the last several years. Alternative strategies, including the study of schizotypal-proneness among normal controls, and its relationship to brain morphology, are also presented. Finally, the limitations of the approach and implications for future research are discussed.

Structural neuroimaging studies of schizophrenia

The effort to understand the basis of mental function and dysfunction by studying brain morphology has not been a recent development. Phrenology, the study of the contours of the skull, was pioneered by Francis Gall in the 1800s based on his theory that the skull's conformation would mirror the underlying brain surface, and prove to be related to specific mental abilities and personality characteristics (Alexander & Selesnick, 1966). Although this theory was never borne out, it did provide a localization model of brain functioning, which was brought into the mainstream by the histological investigations of Brodmann and others. By the turn of the century, advances in microscopy and new staining techniques allowed neuroscientists to perform detailed histopathological evaluations of postmortem brains. Alois Alzheimer was a psychiatrist in Emil Kraepelin's department in Munich, where such studies were being conducted on patients with a variety of mental disorders, most or all of which were presumed to have an "organic" basis. His discovery of the characteristic "plaques and tangles" in the brains of patients who developed progressive dementias later in life led to the recognition of what is now referred to as Alzheimer's disease (Bogerts, 1993). Unfortunately, Alzheimer, Kraepelin, and their contemporaries, using the latest techniques of their day, were unable to elucidate characteristic morphological or histopathological features in patients with dementia praecox. Indeed, their inability to do so partly fueled the enthusiasm for various psychological theories of these disorders, as their negative findings led some to conclude that these patients had "normal" brains.

One clue, however, came from pneumoencephalography (PEG), a neuroradiological technique introduced in 1919. Only eight years later, Jacobi and Winkler used this technique to investigate the brains of 18 individuals with schizophrenia (Jacobi & Winkler, 1927). Their major finding was that of ventricular enlargement. Despite a substantial amount of replication over the subsequent decades, these findings were generally greeted with skepticism, partially owing to two interrelated methodological problems with the technique (Haug, 1962; Huber, 1957). First, the insufflation of air into the ventricular system was thought to cause the appearance of ventricular enlargement in and of itself. Second, as PEG was an invasive technique, most of the studies were uncontrolled, rendering the first limitation even more problematical. Thus, although these studies provided evidence of structural brain abnormalities in schizophrenia, enthusiasm for further exploring the meaning of these findings remained quite limited.

This situation changed rapidly in the 1970s with the introduction of computed tomography (CT). Again, schizophrenia investigators were quick to exploit this new technique, with the first study published only three years after CT was introduced for clinical use (Johnstone, Frith, Crow, Husband, & Kreel, 1976). This study replicated and extended the PEG findings, demonstrating ventricular enlargement as well as evidence of diffuse brain "atrophy" (i.e., widened cortical sulci). Like the PEG findings, these findings were initially greeted with skepticism, as the sample consisted mostly of elderly, chronically institutionalized patients, rendering the results vulnerable to many potentially confounding factors. Over the subsequent decade, however, the ventricular findings in particular were supported by a large number of controlled CT studies, including several based upon samples of young patients who were early in the course of the disorder (reviewed by DeLisi et al., 1991). Indeed, ventricular enlargement in schizophrenia has proven to be a replicable and robust finding. Positive studies (i.e., significantly larger ventricles in patients vs. controls) outnumber negative studies by approximately 3 to 1 (Andreasen, Swayze, Flaum, Yates, Arndt, & McChesney, 1990), and the effect size for comparisons of both lateral and third ventricles between schizophrenics and normal controls has been estimated to be on the order of 0.70, a value considered to be in the "moderate" range (Raz & Raz, 1990). To put this in perspective, such an effect size indicates that the median ventricular size in schizophrenia is approximately equivalent to the 75th percentile for normal controls (Cohen, 1988). Put another way, the average ventricular size in an individual with schizophrenia roughly corresponds to the average ventricular size of normals who are 20 years their senior.

Despite the replicability and robustness of this finding, it is important to recognize that the meaning of ventricular enlargement in schizophrenia has yet to be clearly elucidated. Although a variety of clinical and neurobiological features have been shown to share a significant amount of variance with ventricular size (e.g., poor treatment response, more negative symptoms), ventricular size has not yet proven to be a consistently accurate predictor of any of these characteristics. Further, the finding has been shown to be highly nonspecific, and commonly associated with several other psychiatric and medical conditions such as affective disorders and alcoholism (Jeste, Lohr, & Goodwin, 1988; Swayze, Andersen, Alliger, Ehrhardt, & Yuh, 1990).

Nevertheless, investigators have been able to exploit the finding of ventricular enlargement in addressing a variety of interesting questions about schizophrenia. For example, in an early study by Reveley and colleagues (Reveley, Clifford, Reveley, & Murray, 1982), ventricular size, as assessed by computed tomography (CT), in monozygotic twin pairs discordant for schizophrenia, was used to examine the relative contribution of genetic versus environmental factors to the etiology of schizophrenia. As hypothesized, the ill twins were found to have larger ventricles than their normal co-twins, suggesting something other than genetic factors at play. An unexpected, and highly provocative, finding was that the unaffected co-twins as a group had larger ventricles than did a comparison group of normal twin pairs. Although the sample sizes were small, rendering most of the comparisons nonsignificant statistically, these findings served a heuristic hypothesis-generating function. Specifically, this observation led to the speculation that enlargement of the ventricles – even slight enlargement that would not be considered clinically "abnormal" and could be detected only when compared to an "ideal control" (i.e., an MZ twin) – might be a marker of a genetic predisposition or vulnerability to schizophrenia. The implied corollary to this speculation is that schizophrenia is manifested clinically only when that genetic diathesis is combined with additional environmental factors. While that seems like a lot to speculate from a small amount of data, it is noteworthy that these early CT findings have been subsequently supported by more methodologically sophisticated studies using magnetic resonance imaging (MRI) (Suddath, Christison, Torrey, Casanova, & Weinberger, 1990). Even today, the sample sizes that have been used in these twin paradigms remain too limited to reach definitive conclusions, but they still provide compelling evidence for a "two-hit" (or more properly a "multihit") model of schizophrenia.

MRI has largely supplanted CT over the past decade, because of its superior resolution and because it does not involve any exposure to ionizing radiation. This technique has allowed for a much more detailed investigation of brain morphology, and indeed, a wide variety of morphological abnormalities in addition to ventricular enlargement have now been reported in schizophrenia. These findings, summarized in Table 16.1, suggest that abnormalities may be diffusely distributed throughout the brain.

Our laboratory has recently completed one of the largest MRI studies done to date of this population. Just over 100 individuals with schizophrenia were compared with 90 normal controls, selected to be equivalent to the patient group in terms of age and familial socioeconomic background. In addition to having significantly larger lateral and third ventricles, the patient group was found to have smaller thalamic, hippocampal, and superior temporal gyral volumes than did controls (Flaum et al., in press-b). These findings are summarized in Table 16.2.

To date, none of the findings demonstrating differences in brain tissue volumes (e.g., smaller hippocampi, smaller cerebral size, etc.) have been as consistently reported as has been the case for abnormalities of the ventricular system, and all require further study and replication. At this point, they best serve a hypothesis-generating function and help to steer researchers to specific aspects of the brain in the effort to understand the pathological processes that may underlie the disorder. This is especially the case for those findings that converge with evidence from postmortem studies. Examples include specific cytoarchitectonic abnormalities that have been described in the hippocampi and marked decreases in neuronal density of the thalamus of postmortem brain of schizophrenic individuals (Pakkenberg, 1990; Scheibel & Kovelman, 1981). Other clues may be gleaned from the specificity versus generalized distribution of abnormalities. That is, diffuse abnormalities such as reduced cranial or cerebral size are more suggestive of a generalized developmental disturbance, whereas more focal abnormalities, such as ventricular enlargement in the context of an otherwise normal brain, are more suggestive of a circumscribed event such as an episode of periventricular hemorrhage at or around the time of birth. After decades of skepticism, structural neuroimaging studies have become widely accepted as an integral tool in the investigation of schizophrenia, allowing for large-scale in vivo investigations of these issues.

Neuroimaging studies in schizotypal personality

On the other hand, very few studies of schizotypal personality have employed these techniques. In light of this, those that have been done are worthy of

Table 16.1. *Aspects of brain morphology reported to differentiate groups of schizophrenics versus normal controls with MRI*

Region of interest	Direction (Sz. vs. controls)	Replicability
Lateral ventricles	↑	++++
Third ventricle	↑	+++
Temporal horns	↑	+++
Temporal lobe	↓	++
Hippocampus (± amygdala)	↓	++
Sup. temporal gyrus	↓	+
Basal ganglia (caudate, putamen)	↑	+
Thalamus	↓	+
Cranium	↓	+
Cerebrum	↓	+
Cerebellum	↓	+

careful attention. A brief review of two studies showing ventricular enlargement and greater left versus right frontal horn enlargement in schizotypal patients may be found in Siever (Chapter 12, this volume). In addition, two important imaging studies have thus far been conducted on the sample from the Copenhagen High Risk project. The first of these studies (Schulsinger et al., 1984) examined ventricular size (both lateral and third ventricle) in three groups of individuals, all of whom shared a genetic risk for schizophrenia (i.e., had mothers with schizophrenia). The groups were divided into those individuals who themselves had developed schizophrenia ($n = 7$), those who remained normal ($n = 13$), and a group who were at the time referred to as "borderline schizophrenics" ($n = 11$). This latter group would, by DSM-III through DSM-IV criteria, be most likely defined as having schizotypal personality disorder (SPD). Although the sample sizes were small, and the image analysis techniques were crude by today's standards (planimetric tracing of single CT slices), the findings were intriguing. They noted that the schizophrenics had larger ventricles than the controls, but the borderline (schizotypal) group had the smallest ventricle size of all. This finding was interpreted as consistent with a model in which schizotypy is conceptualized as a condition that shares a genetic diathesis with schizophrenia, but differs in terms of environmental risk factors. It was speculated that ventricular enlargement might reflect a specific environmental insult, such as perinatal anoxia leading to periventricular hemorrhage, and that the genetic diathesis combined with such an environmental insult might result in the later development of schizo-

Table 16.2. *Analysis of covariance testing the effects of diagnosis (schizophrenia vs. control), controlling for stature, age, and gender on regions of interest (ROI) volumes*

Structure (ROI)	*F* values
Third ventricle	11.22***
Lateral ventricles	8.96**
Thalamus	6.82**
Superior temporal gyrus	5.71*
Hippocampus	4.77*
Cerebellum	2.39
Temporal lobes	1.83
Temporal horns	1.42
Caudate nucleus	1.14
Cerebrum	0.29
Cranium	0.26

Note: N = 102 schizophrenics plus 87 normal controls. In controlling for stature, height was used as a covariate for the larger ROIs including cranium, cerebrum, and cerebellum. For all other ROIs, cranial volume was used as the covariate.
$^{*}p < .05$
$^{**}p < .01$
$^{***}p < .001$

phrenia. Again, although that is a lot of speculation from a few data, it provides testable theoretical models and sets the stage for larger studies.

Indeed, subsequent follow-up studies of a much larger sample of this same high-risk group led to an elaboration of this model. Cannon, Mednick, and Parnas (1989) demonstrated that morphological evidence of "multisite neural deficits," as reflected by a decrease in overall brain tissue volume, appeared to be independent of ventricular enlargement. Further, genetic risk was found to be associated the former (i.e., a higher genetic risk predicted more "multisite neural deficits"), whereas ventricular enlargement was significantly associated with a history of obstetrical complications.

Taken together, these two studies lead to specific predictions that can be tested in other data sets. Assuming that ventricular enlargement has largely an environmental origin, the first study leads to the prediction that samples of schizotypes would have ventricular volumes equal to or less than those of normal controls, and significantly less than those of schizophrenics. Assuming that diffuse neural deficits largely reflect genetic risk for schizophrenia, the latter study would lead to the prediction that markers of diffuse neural deficits – that is, decreases in multiple aspects of brain tissue volume –

would occur as commonly among schizotypals as among schizophrenics, and significantly more commonly than among normal controls.

Alternative models of the relationship between schizotypy and schizophrenia can also be tested in a similar fashion. For example, another model of schizotypy is that it is just a milder variant of schizophrenia. If this were the case, then one might expect that schizotypals would tend to lie between normal controls and groups of schizophrenics on any and all potential markers of the disease process. A third model is one that postulates the distinction between schizotypy and schizophrenia to be essentially invalid. That is, schizotypy is the same disorder which, although manifested by a somewhat different pattern of symptoms, is underlain by the same etiological and pathophysiological processes. This latter model would lead to the prediction that schizotypals would be indistinguishable from individuals with schizophrenia on appropriate "disease markers" and that they would differ from normal controls with an effect size similar to that observed between schizophrenics and normals. These models and their associated predictions in terms of brain imaging findings are summarized in Table 16.3.

Preliminary studies from Iowa

We have had the opportunity to begin to examine these models by comparing groups of schizotypes, schizophrenics, and normal controls who had been assessed with MRI in our laboratory. In the process of carrying out the large MRI study mentioned above, approximately 50 subjects who appeared to be within the schizophrenia spectrum, but had diagnoses other than schizophrenia (e.g., schizoaffective disorder, delusional disorder, etc.) were also studied. Included in that group were 10 subjects whose primary DSM-III-R diagnosis was that of schizotypal personality disorder and who has no other Axis I diagnosis. Diagnoses were based upon an extensive medication-free evaluation, multiple sources of information, and a semistructured interview instrument, the Comprehensive Assessment of Symptoms and History (CASH; Andreasen, Flaum, & Arndt, 1992). The schizotypal symptoms for each of these patients had been an essentially lifelong pattern. Further, we were able to follow up all but one of these subjects for at least two years, and follow-up diagnoses remained unchanged.

These 10 subjects were compared to larger groups of individuals who met DSM-III-R criteria for schizophrenia (N = 90), as well as normal controls (N = 60). In an effort to reduce the number of comparisons, we focused only on those regions of interest (ROIs) that had been found to differ significantly between the larger group of schizophrenics and controls (as shown in Table

Table 16.3. *Predictions of how brain morphology among individuals with schizotypal personality disorder (SPD) would be expected to compare to those with schizophrenia (SZ) and normal controls (NC), based on three alternative theoretical models*

	Predictions: Likelihood of:	
Models and their underlying assumptions	Enlarged ventricles	"Multiple neural deficits"
1. SPD and SZ share a common genetic diathesis; but SPD is spared an environmental insult leading to differential pathophysiological processes.	SPD < SZ SPD ≤ NC	SPD = SZ SPD > NC
2. SPD and SZ share common etiopathophysiological processes; but SPD is a milder variant of SZ.	SPD < SZ SPD > NC	SPD < SZ SPD > NC
3. SPD and SZ share common etiopathophysiological processes; the distinction between SZ and SPD is invalid.	SPD = SZ SPD > NC	SPD = SZ SPD > NC

16.2). Thus we were looking at both ventricular measures (both lateral and third ventricle), as well as various measures of brain tissue volume – specifically the thalamic, superior temporal gyral, and hippocampal volumes. We were then able to examine predictions relevant to the ventricular system as well as "multisite neural deficits."

One of the problems inherent in such comparisons has to do with variability in overall body and brain size. That is, a substantial amount of the variance in any subregion of the brain (e.g., hippocampus) is accounted for by overall brain size. Most of the literature on ventricle differences have handled this problem by reporting ventricular brain ratios. Our laboratory has argued against the use of ratio measures and in favor of other methods for accounting for stature (Arndt, Cohen, Alligeh, Swayze, & Andreasen, 1991). As a first attempt to control for differences in overall stature, the comparison groups were selected to be equivalent to the schizotypal group in terms of gender distribution (90% males). In order to account further for variability in stature and head size, cranial volume was entered as a covariate in the analyses. Thus we sought to detect specific aspects of brain abnormality for those aspects of brain morphology that have been implicated in the pathogenesis of schizophrenia. Age was also included as a covariate, as the control group as a whole was older than both patient groups. In order to minimize the effects of outliers, given the small number of schizotypals, the data were transformed to ranks, and nonparametric analyses were carried out.

All subjects underwent MRI with a 1.5-Tesla GE Signa scanner, using identical imaging sequences. Images were obtained in the coronal plane throughout the cranium, with 5-mm slice thickness, and 2.5-mm gaps. Additionally, 3-mm slices with 1.5-mm gaps were obtained throughout the central two-thirds of the brain, in order to improve the resolution for the smaller, subcortical structures. Both proton density and T-2 weighted sequences were used (as the former provides better resolution between gray matter and white matter boundaries, and the latter provides better discrimination between CSF and brain tissue). Immediately after data acquisition, images were transferred to optical disks, and all subsequent image processing was done on a Silicon Graphics work station, using locally developed software (Andreasen et al., 1992a). All 30 sets of images were traced by the same technician, who had extensive experience in structural imaging studies in our lab over the previous eight years. The technician was blind to diagnosis or any clinical or demographic data concerning the subject. Regions of interest (ROIs) were traced on every slide in which they were visualized, and then the pixels within that slice were summed across all slices in which the ROI was traced, yielding volumetric estimates (Arndt, Andreasen, Cizadlo, O'Leary, Swayze, & Cohen, 1994). The volumes of those ROIs, measured separately on the left and right, were summed (e.g., left hippocampus + right hippocampus = hippocampi), as no laterality by diagnostic effects was observed among the larger sample of patients and controls (Flaum et al., in press-b). Reliability was assessed by blindly retracing 21 randomly selected sets of images, and found to be in the excellent range for lateral ventricles (intraclass $r = 0.98$) and third ventricle ($r = 0.86$), good for superior temporal gyri ($r = 0.70$) and hippocampi ($r = 0.64$), and poor for thalamus ($r = 0.35$).

The results of these analyses are shown in Figures 16.1 and 16.2. As expected, the schizophrenic group had significantly larger lateral and third ventricles than did the controls. The mean rank for the schizotypal group was in between the schizophrenics and controls on both measures, but differences were not significant. However, there is a nonsignificant trend for smaller third ventricles in schizotypal compared to schizophrenics ($p = 0.08$, one-tailed).

Figure 16.2 shows the mean ranks across the three groups for volumes of thalamus, superior temporal gyrus, and hippocampus. The schizotypal group did not differ significantly from the controls on any of these measures. Similar to the control group, the schizotypal group showed a significantly greater thalamic volume than did the schizophrenic group. The schizotypal group appeared to lie between the control and schizophrenic group in terms of

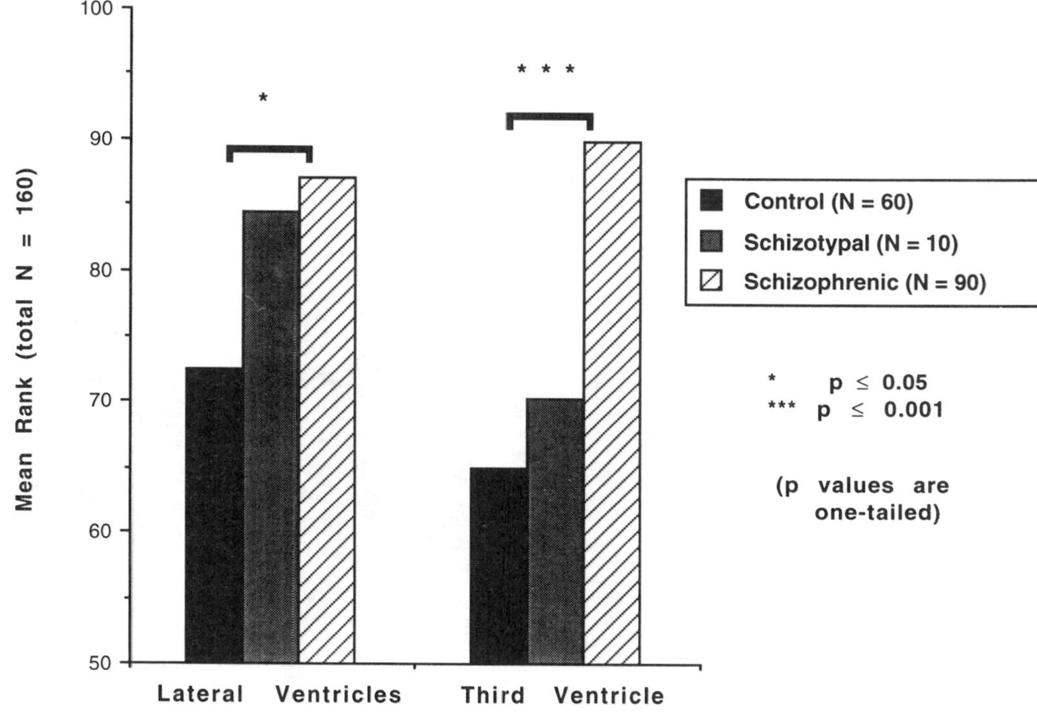

Fig. 16.1. Comparison of lateral and third ventricle volumes across three groups (controls, schizotypals, schizophrenics), based on ranked data, adjusted for age and cranial volume.

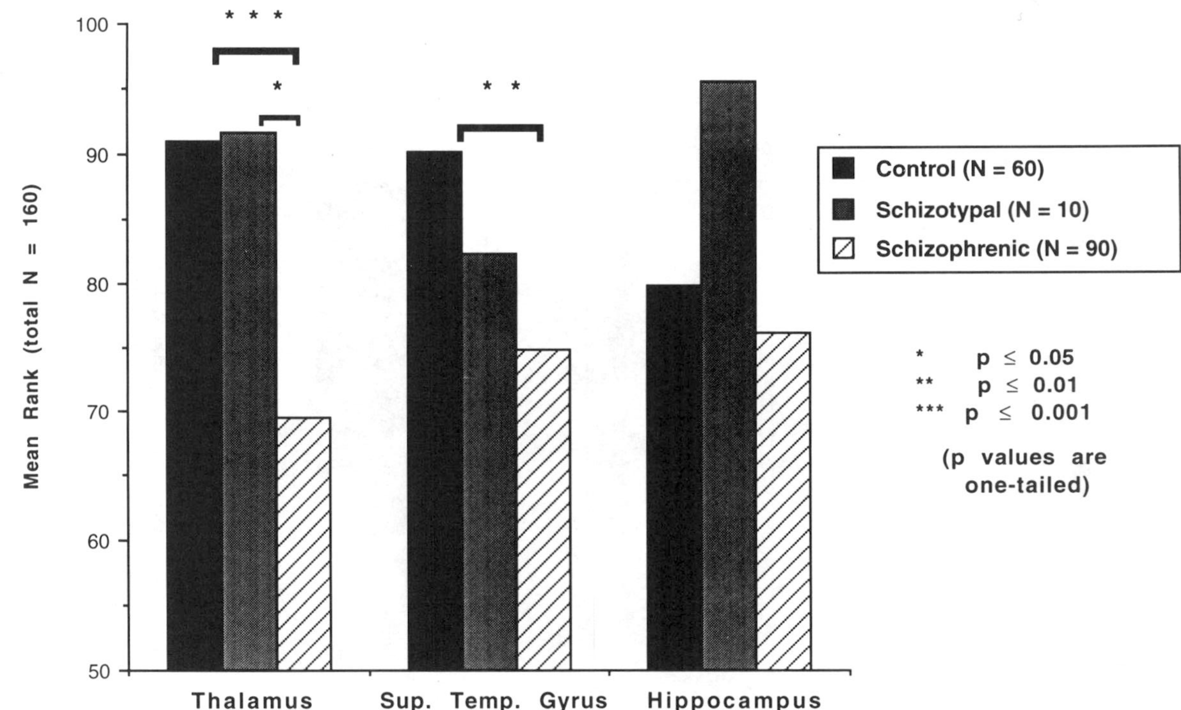

Fig. 16.2. Comparison of thalamic, superior temporal gyral and hippocampal volumes across three groups (controls, schizotypals, schizophrenics), based on ranked data, adjusted for age and cranial volume.

superior temporal gyral volume, and had the largest mean rank for hippocampal volume. However, neither of these comparisons approaches statistical significance.

Although these analyses must be considered quite preliminary in light of the small sample of schizotypals, the degree to which they support or refute the models and predictions described in Table 16.3 can be examined. Model 1 suggests that the schizotypals would more closely resemble the normal controls in terms of ventricle size, and this is partially supported by the finding of no difference for either ventricle measure between schizotypals and controls, but a trend toward smaller third ventricle in schizotypals versus schizophrenics. There is no support, however, for the prediction that measures of tissue volume among the schizotypals would demonstrate a greater resemblance to that of the schizophrenics than to the controls. On the contrary, the schizotypals did not differ from the normals on any of the three tissue measures, but did differ significantly from the schizophrenics on one (thalamus). Therefore, these data provide only very limited support for model 1. The predictions from model 2 are that schizotypals would occupy an intermediate position between schizophrenics and controls on any measure that differentiated the latter two groups. Although the schizotypal group had mean ranks in between the two comparison groups on three of the five measures, the small number of schizotypals preclude any conclusions regarding these predictions. Model 3, which suggests that the distinction between schizotypal personality and schizophrenia is invalid, appears to have the least support from these data. That model would predict that the schizotypals would be indistinguishable from the schizophrenics, and different from the normals. Those differences that were observed were all in the opposite direction; that is, schizotypals differed from schizophrenics but not from normals. Thus these data provide some limited support for the validity of the schizotypal construct. On the whole, however, none of the three models presented in Table 16.3 is strongly supported, as there was no consistent pattern of relationships between the various regions of interest and the diagnostic groups.

This inconsistency in and of itself may tell us something. Should we expect that schizotypals would either resemble or differ from schizophrenics or normals in a consistent manner? Indeed phenomenologically, schizotypals more closely resemble schizophrenics in some respects (e.g., presence of negative symptoms), and normals in others (e.g., absence of positive symptoms). Perhaps brain morphology is more closely tied to specific domains of psychopathology than to any one diagnostic category (Andreasen & Carpenter, 1993).

The primary feature that distinguishes schizotypals from schizophrenics, at least according to DSM-III-R criteria, is the presence of active psychotic symptoms. Thus, it may be that aspects of brain morphology that are related to psychotic symptoms would differ across these diagnostic groups, whereas aspects of brain morphology that are more related to negative symptoms, affective disturbances, cognitive styles, or other indices that are more common to both groups, would be less likely to differ. Rather than comparing brain morphology between diagnosis *x* and comparison group *y*, as has been the case in the vast majority of neuroimaging studies done to date in psychiatry, perhaps we should be looking at the relationship between brain morphology and certain traits or characteristics *within* populations that share certain phenomenological features. That is, a dimensional, rather than categorical, approach may be more powerful in the effort to link clinical manifestations with underlying neurobiological mechanisms.

We have recently employed this type of approach in examining the relationship between brain morphology and symptom patterns and severity among individuals within the broadly defined schizophrenia spectrum. The sample included all of our patients with schizophrenia as well as those with schizoaffective, delusional, psychotic mood and SPD. On the whole, greater symptom severity was found to be correlated with greater ventricular volume and smaller superior temporal and hippocampal volumes. Somewhat surprisingly, it was psychotic symptoms (delusions and hallucinations) that were more predictive of ventricular enlargement than were negative symptoms, whereas negative symptoms were predictive of smaller hippocampal volume. Psychotic symptoms were also significantly predictive of smaller superior temporal gyral volume. Post hoc analyses revealed that this was accounted for almost entirely by hallucinations (rather than delusions), and that it was specific to the left hemisphere. Interestingly, the strength and pattern of the correlations remained stable, even when the pure DSM-III-R schizophrenics were excluded from the analyses. That is, those with schizophrenia-like conditions displayed similar relationships between brain morphology and symptomatology (Flaum, O'Leary, Swayze, Miller, Arndt, & Andreasen, in press-a). This supports the idea that a dimensional rather than categorical approach may be more powerful in the effort to relate neuroanatomical features to clinical/behavior phenomena.

Raine et al. employed such an approach in a study of schizotypal characteristics within a nonclinical population (Raine, Sheard, Reynolds, & Lencz, 1992). Rather than examining a sample of individuals with SPD, they began with a population of normal subjects on whom a variety of measures of schizotypy and psychosis proneness were obtained along with MRI scans.

They found robust negative correlations between several of the schizotypal scale scores and specific MRI measures, most notably left and right prefrontal area. Correlations of similar magnitude were noted between the schizotypal scales and performance on frontal lobe neuropsychological tasks. That is, the smaller the frontal lobes, the higher the schizotypal scores and the poorer the neuropsychological functioning. Thus, in this study, a dimensional, rather than categorical approach was employed with respect to MRI measures, in an effort to relate brain morphology to specific aspects of behavior and neuropsychological performance.

We had the opportunity to begin to explore this approach in a sample of 85 normal controls, all of whom had undergone MRI with the protocol described above. These subjects were also administered tests of psychosis proneness, using scales developed by Chapman and Chapman. Specifically, we used the Physical Anhedonia Scale (61-item version; Chapman & Chapman, 1978) and the Perceptual Aberration Scale (35-item version; Chapman & Chapman, 1976), The Physical Anhedonia Scale reflects negative-like features that may be present in nonclinical populations. All of the items are true–false and include statements such as: "The beauty of the sunset is greatly overrated," and "Sex is OK, but not as much fun as people claim it is." The Perceptual Aberration Scale, on the other hand, assessed more positive-like psychotic proneness, including feelings of depersonalization and derealization. Examples of that scale include "Sometimes I have had feelings that I am united with an object near me," and "At times I have wondered if my body was really my own." Our goal was to determine whether these measures of "psychoses proneness" within normals could be related to those aspects of brain morphology that have been implicated as abnormal among patients with schizophrenic disorders.

The sample included 43 males and 42 females, all of whom were normal volunteers recruited from the community through newspaper advertising. They were screened by a research psychiatrist to rule out any Axis I diagnosis, as well as for a history of schizophrenia in their first-degree relative. Their mean age was 37 years (SD = 16.7). The Chapman scale scores are shown in Table 16.4.

Data analyses consisted of Spearman correlations between each of the Chapman Scale scores and MRI regions of interest. Age was partial in the correlations in order to account for its potentially confounding effect. Cranial volume was also partialed, as in the previous analysis, as we were interested in examining the specific relationships between regions of interest and the psychosis proneness measures, independent of whole brain size or body stature.

Table 16.4. *Chapman scale scores* (N = *85*)

Scale	Mean	S.D.	Range	Potential range
Physical Anhedonia Scale	8.0	5.7	0–24	0–61
Perceptual Aberration Scale	2.3	2.0	0–10	0–35

The results of these correlation analyses are presented in Figure 16.3. Whereas the absolute magnitude of the correlations was relatively small, most were in the expected directions. That is, higher scores on the psychosis proneness scales were associated with larger ventricular sizes, and smaller brain tissue volumes. Interestingly, the only correlation that achieved statistical significance was that between hippocampal volume and the Perceptual Aberration Scale ($r = -0.22$, $p < .05$), indicating reduced hippocampal volume in those with higher perceptual aberration scores.

Clearly, these correlations account for a very small percentage of the overall variance, and only one of many correlations was statistically significant. However, several factors suggest that these findings may be more than just chance findings. First, the range of scores on the psychosis proneness scales was truncated and skewed toward zero as shown in Table 16.4. The reason is that these controls were screened to rule out schizophrenic disorders. Thus, our sample may have consisted of "supernormals," rather than one that would encompass the spectrum of psychosis proneness. The fact that we see any significant correlations at all is therefore somewhat surprising and suggests that in a more generalizable sample, the correlations may be more robust. Second, it is remarkable that it was the hippocampus that proved to be related to psychosis proneness, as, in addition to ventricle size, the hippocampus has been most implicated in both neuroimaging and neuropathological studies of schizophrenia. Finally, with the exception of the thalamic ROI, all correlations were in the expected direction, that is, positive between psychosis proneness and ventricle size, and negative with respect to brain tissue volumes.

While neither of the analyses presented above is in any way conclusive, taken together they provide some support for the idea that brain morphology may be relatable to both phenomenological, as well as etiological factors in schizotypal personality. It is also hoped that they serve to illustrate the types of strategies that may be employed, and limitations that may be encountered, in the use of neuroimaging techniques in this population.

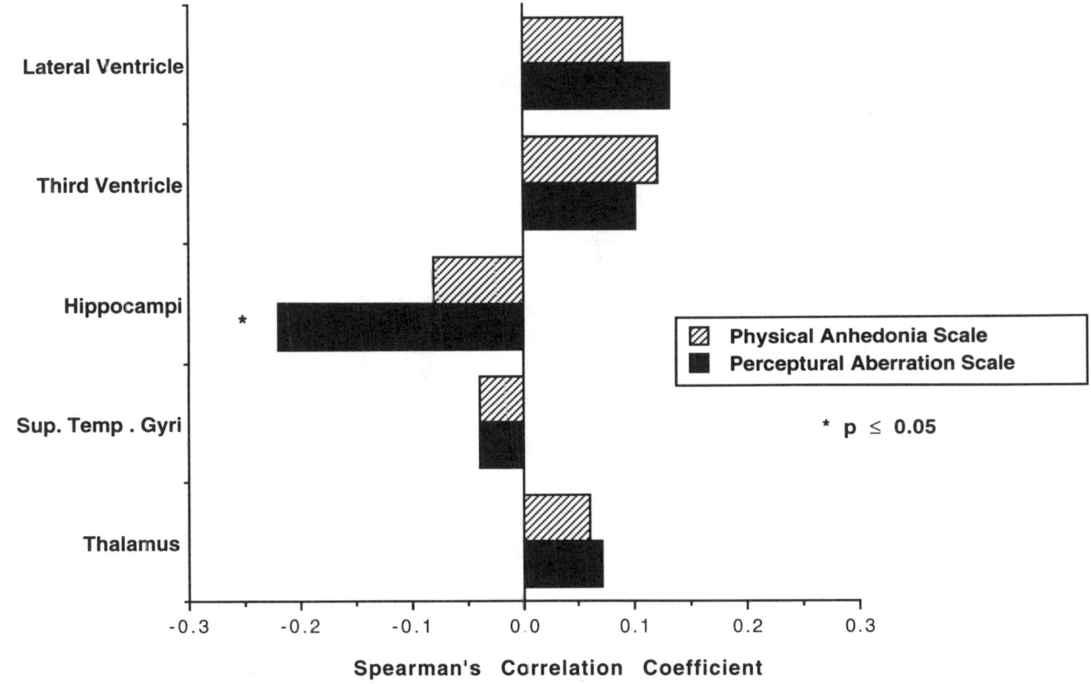

Fig. 16.3. Correlations between Chapman scale scores and region of interest volumes in 85 normal controls.

Methodological considerations

The limited sample size of schizotypals has been repeatedly emphasized because it is a common problem in neuroimaging studies, and one that probably results in the most confusion. Nomograms of power analyses indicate that for group comparisons with a sample size of 10, and a power of .80, the effect size would have to be on the order of 1.3 standard deviations in order to expect to demonstrate a significant difference (Cohen, 1988). The standard deviation for the third and lateral ventricle volumes in these data were on the order of 25–50% of their means, even among the larger normal control group. Thus, the distributions would have to be largely nonoverlapping in order to expect significant differences with samples of this size. In order to detect the expected effect size (0.7), a minimum of 25 subjects per cell would be needed, and this is for the best case scenario in which groups were equivalent on relevant, potentially confounding variables such as stature, age, and so on (Cohen, 1988).

If power analyses indicate the need for larger sample sizes, why is the psychiatric neuroimaging literature replete with studies of ventricular size, as well as other neuroanatomical measures with very small samples? The bottom line is that obtaining adequately large samples is much easier said than done using this approach, and many factors dissuade the investigator from doing so. First of these is the fact that MRI scans are expensive in terms of both cost and person-hours. MRI scans usually cost anywhere from five hundred to eight hundred dollars per subject, and this does not include any of the processing costs. The processing of these images, especially if done manually, can take up to several days for each subject, and requires highly trained personnel, high-speed computers with enormous memory capacity, and methods with established validity.

A second factor that makes it difficult to study large samples has to do with the speed with which technology is progressing. Just as we have all had to accept that our desktop computers will be obsolete before they get dusty, developments in image acquisition and processing techniques often render MRI protocols outmoded by the time the initial reliability and validity work has been completed. Thus if patient flow-through is limited, the investigator faces the choice of either staying with old methods versus changing methods midstream, both of which have serious shortcomings. This problem becomes particularly troubling when dealing with a population such as SPD, in which subject recruitment is inherently more difficult than in disorders, such as schizophrenia, which commonly present for treatment. These types of considerations should serve to caution against the investigator who contemplates doing structural imaging studies as an "add-on" to studies of other measures, unless the available sample population is abundant, resources are plentiful, and flow-through is expected to be rapid. One reasonable solution to this problem involves acceptance of standardized methods that can then be shared across centers in collaborative studies. Other solutions are to follow the model of Raine et al., and focus on schizotypal traits within a more readily available nonclinical population (e.g., students, military groups, etc.).

Finally, these considerations suggest the importance of a priori hypotheses, and the need for replication when interpreting results from brain imaging studies, especially of small samples. We must always keep in mind that brain morphology, as visualized through current imaging modalities, even with the fine-grained resolution of MRI, is still a relatively gross measure, and is only likely to provide subtle clues regarding underlying mechanisms. Just as Alzheimer used the tools of his day to search for these clues, thoughtful neuroscientists today may employ structural neuroimaging for in vivo studies that may further elucidate the underlying causes of a broad array of disorders, including SPD.

Acknowledgments

This research was supported in part by NIMH Grants MH31593 and MH40856; MHCRC Grant MH43271; the Nellie Ball Trust Research Fund, Iowa State Bank & Trust Company, Trustee; and a Research Scientist Award, MH00625.

References

Alexander, F. G., & Selesnick, S. T. (1966). *The history of psychiatry: An evaluation of psychiatric thought and practice from prehistoric times to the present.* New York, Harper & Row.

Andreasen, N. C., & Carpenter, W. T. (1993). Diagnosis and classification of schizophrenia. *Schizophrenia Bulletin, 19,* 199–214.

Andreasen, N. C., Cohen, G., Harris, G., Cizadlo, T., Parkkinen, J., Rezal, K., & Swayze, V. W. (1992a). Image processing for the study of brain structure and function: Problems and programs. *Journal of Neuropsychiatry and Clinical Neuroscience, 4,* 125–133.

Andreasen, N. C., Flaum, M., & Arndt, S. (1992b). The Comprehensive Assessment of Symptoms and History (CASH): An instrument for assessing psychopathology and diagnosis. *Archives of General Psychiatry, 49,* 615–623.

Andreasen, N. C., Swayze, V., Flaum, M., Yates, W. R., Arndt, S., & McChesney, C. (1990). Ventricular enlargement in schizophrenia evaluated with CT scanning: Effects of gender, age, and stage of illness. *Archives of General Psychiatry, 47,* 1054–1059.

Arndt, S., Andreasen, N. C., Cizadlo, T., O'Leary, D. S., Swayze, V. W., & Cohen, G. (1994). Evaluating and validating two methods for estimating brain structure volumes: Tessellation and simple pixel counting. *NeuroImage, 1,* 191–198.

Arndt, S., Cohen, G., Alliger, R. J., Swayze, V. W., & Andreasen, N. C. (1991). Problems with ratios and proportion measures of imaged cerebral structures. *Psychiatry Research: Neuroimaging, 40,* 79–89.

Bogerts, B. (1993). Alois Alzheimer [Essay in: Images in Psychiatry]. *American Journal of Psychiatry, 150,* 1868.

Cannon, T. D., Mednick, S. A., & Parnas, J. (1989). Genetic and perinatal determinants of structural brain deficits in schizophrenia. *Archives of General Psychiatry, 46,* 883–889.

Chapman, L. J., & Chapman, J. P. (1976). Scales for physical and social anhedonia. *Journal of Abnormal Psychology, 85,* 374–382.

Chapman, L. J., & Chapman, J. P. (1978). Body-image aberration in schizophrenia. *Journal of Abnormal Psychology, 87,* 399–407.

Cohen, J. (1988). *Statistical power analysis for the behavioral science.* Hillsdale, N.J.: Lawrence Erlbaum Associates.

DeLisi, L. E., Hoff, A. L., Schwartz, J. E., Shields, D. W., Halthore, S. N., Gupta, S. M., Henn, F. A., & Anand, A. K. (1991). Brain morphology in first-episode schizophrenic-like psychotic patients: A quantitative magnetic resonance imaging study. *Biological Psychiatry, 29,* 159–175.

Flaum, M., O'Leary, D. S., Swayze, V. W., Miller, D. D., Arndt, S., & Andreasen, N. C. (in press-a). Symptom dimensions and brain morphology in schizophrenia and related psychotic disorders. *Journal of Psychiatric Research.*

Flaum, M., Swayze, V. W., O'Leary, D. S., Yun, W. T. C., Ehrhardt, J. C., Arndt, S., Andreasen, N. C. (in press-b). Brain morphology in schizophrenia: Effects of diagnosis, laterality and gender. *American Journal of Psychiatry.*

Gur, R. E., & Pearlson, G. D. (1993). Neuroimaging in schizophrenia research. *Schizophrenia Bulletin, 19,* 337–353.

Haug, J. O. (1962). Pneumoencephalographic studies in mental disease. *Acta Psychiatrica Scandinavica 38* (Suppl. 165), 1–114.

Huber, G. (1957). *Pneumoencephalographische und Psychopathologische Bidler Bei Endogen Psychosen.* Berlin: Springer-Verlag.

Jacobi, W., & Winkler, H. (1927). Encephalographische studien au chronisch schizophrenen. *Arch Psychiatrische Nervenkr, 81,* 299–332.

Jeste, D. V., Lohr, J. B., Goodwin, F. K. (1988). Neuroanatomical studies of major affective disorders: A review and suggestions for further research. *British Journal of Psychiatry, 153,* 444–459.

Johnstone, E. C., Frith, C. D., Crow, T. J., Husband, J., & Kreel, L. (1976). Cerebral ventricular size and cognitive impairment in chronic schizophrenia. *Lancet, 2,* 924–926.

Pakkenberg, B. (1990). Pronounced reduction of total neuron number in mediodorsal thalamic nucleus and nucleus accumbens in schizophrenics. *Archives of General Psychiatry, 47,* 1023–1028.

Pearlson, G. D., & Marsh, L. (1993). Magnetic resonance imaging in psychiatry. *Review of psychiatry* (pp. 347–382). Washington, D.C.: American Psychiatric Press.

Raine, A., Sheard, C., Reynolds, G. P., & Lencz, T. (1992). Pre-frontal structural and functional deficits associated with individual differences in schizotypal personality. *Schizophrenia Research, 7,* 237–247.

Raz, S., & Raz, N. (1990). Structural brain abnormalities in the major psychoses: A quantitative review of the evidence from computerized imaging. *Psychological Bulletin, 108,* 93–108.

Reveley, A. M., Clifford, C. A., Reveley, M. A., & Murray, R. M. (1982). Cerebral ventricular size in twins discordant for schizophrenia. *Lancet, 1,* 540–541.

Scheibel, A. B., & Kovelman, J. A. (1981). Disorientation of the hippocampal pyramidal cell and its processes in the schizophrenic patient. [Letter] *Biological Psychiatry, 16,*101–102.

Schulsinger, F., Parnas, J., Petersen, E. T., Schulsinger, H., Teasdale, T. W., Mednick, S. A., et al. (1984). Cerebral ventricular size in the offspring of schizophrenic mothers. A preliminary study. *Archives of General Psychiatry, 41,* 602–606.

Shelton, R. C., & Weinberger, D. R. (1986). X-ray computerized tomography studies in schizophrenia: A review and synthesis. *Handbook of schizophrenia, Vol. 1: The neurology of schizophrenia* (pp. 207–250). Amsterdam: Elsevier Science.

Suddath, R. L., Christison, G. W., Torrey, E. F., Casanova, M. F., & Weinberger, D. R. (1990). Anatomical abnormalities in the brains of monozygotic twins discordant for schizophrenia. *New England Journal of Medicine, 322* (12), 789–794.

Swayze, V. W., II, Andreasen, N. C., Alliger, R. J., Ehrhardt, J. C., & Yuh, W. T. C. (1990). Structural brain abnormalities in bipolar affective disorder: Ventricular enlargement, and focal signal hyperintensities. *Archives of General Psychiatry, 47,* 1054–1059.

17

The potential of physiological neuroimaging for the study of schizotypy: experiences from applications to schizophrenia

RUBEN C. GUR and RAQUEL E. GUR

With the increased recognition that schizotypy is a legitimate nosological entity that deserves systematic investigation from phenomenological, psychological, and neurobehavioral perspectives, it has become evident that neuroimaging methods should be considered for gaining insight into its pathophysiological substrates. Some pioneering studies using anatomical neuroimaging methods are described in the previous chapter. It is probably fair to suggest at this point that although significant differences in neuroanatomical measures between individuals with schizotypy and healthy controls have been reported, the effects are subtle and the overlap in values is considerable. This should not be surprising, since the same summary would be valid for the (literally) hundreds of such studies in schizophrenia. Thus, the odds are that neuroanatomical abnormalities will explain only some of the behavioral variance associated with schizotypy. While such efforts to establish structural aberrations are prerequisite for interpreting further findings on neural substrates of a behavioral disorder, the hope for larger and more pervasive effects can be turned toward methods for physiological neuroimaging. Behavioral deficits associated with brain disorders can be more extensive than what is attributable to the death of neurons in regions showing anatomical damage. They can be caused by brain cells that are not dead, but are either insufficiently active or too active. Some grave forms of brain dysfunction are caused by abnormalities in regional brain physiological activity. For example, epilepsy has severe behavioral manifestations, and there is evidence for interictal deficits in cognitive and emotional functioning (Dodrill & Wilkus, 1976). However, CT or MRI scans are frequently uninformative or even normal (Gastaut, 1970).

This chapter is intended for investigators of schizotypy who contemplate incorporation of physiological neuroimaging methods, or who wish to have a better appreciation of the potential and limitations of such methods. It will not discuss electroencephalography and will not comment on the new and emerging functional MRI methods, since this would be premature. Thus, the chapter is restricted to isotopic methods. We begin by briefly describing the main methods applied in psychiatric disorders. While this chapter does not provide any technical detail beyond what is necessary to interpret available findings, more comprehensive discussion can be found in several edited volumes (e.g., Phelps, Mazziotta, & Schelbert, 1986; Reivich & Alavi, 1985). Based on our experience in applying some of these techniques in schizophrenia, we then present some of the main issues likely to face the investigator of schizotypy, including resting baseline versus activated measures, quantitative and "subtraction" methods, the choice of behavioral dimensions, and cross-modality integration. These techniques will be illustrated by examples from our work in schizophrenia. We point out some of the complexities not to deter, but to provide much needed perspective for those investigators who think that processing a good sample through a sophisticated device will lead to insight on schizotypy. Such "science ex machina" approaches have not been very productive in schizophrenia and are unlikely to fare better with schizotypy. Our hope is that progress on schizotypy will be expedited by capitalizing on the experience with schizophrenia, and will allow researchers to avoid some of the mistakes made in that regard.

The techniques

Isotopic techniques for imaging neurophysiology make use of the fact that active neurons have metabolic needs for oxygen and glucose, and that cerebral blood flow rates change in response to these needs. Such measures can help identify regions of abnormal physiological activity associated with behavioral deficits. Furthermore, such measures obtained during the performance of cognitive tasks could help delineate brain regions necessary for regulating cognitive processes.

These isotopic techniques for measuring cerebral metabolism and blood flow can be traced to the pioneering method of Kety and Schmidt (1948) for measuring whole-brain metabolism and blood flow. The technique used intracarotid injection of nitrous oxide, and measurement of arterial–venous differences in concentration yielded accurate and reproducible data on brain metabolism and blood flow. However, this technique is limited not only by its restriction to whole-brain values, but also by its invasiveness.

Safe regional measurements were first made possible by the introduction of the xenon-133 (^{133}Xe) clearance techniques for measuring regional cerebral blood flow (rCBF). The highly diffusible ^{133}Xe can be administered as gas mixed in air or in saline. Its clearance from the brain is measurable by stationary scintillation detectors. The rate of clearance enables considerably accurate quantitation of rCBF in the fast-clearing gray matter compartment, as well as calculation of mean flow in gray and white matter. Initial applications used carotid injections (Olesen, Paulson, & Lassen, 1971), which were invasive and only enabled measurements in one hemisphere at a time. In 1975, Obrist and colleagues reported the ^{133}Xe inhalation technique (Obrist et al., 1975), and presented models for quantifying rCBF with this noninvasive procedure. The technique permits simultaneous measurements from both hemispheres, and the number of brain regions that can be measured depends on the number of detectors. Initial studies were performed with up to 16 detectors, 8 over each hemisphere, but there are now commercially available systems with 32 detectors, and more recently a system has been introduced that enables the placement of up to 254 detectors. The quantitative data can be displayed topographically, as is shown in Figure 17.1.

Note that rCBF is typically higher in the front of the brain. This "hyperfrontal" pattern has been observed routinely in normal subjects (Ingvar, 1979). The main limitation of the technique is that it is optimal for measuring rCBF only on the brain surface near the skull, and hence is restricted to the study of cortical brain regions.

Positron emission tomography (PET) has made it possible to measure in vivo biochemical and physiological processes in the human brain, with three-dimensional resolution. Initial work with animals used selectively labeled chemical compounds (radioisotopes) to measure the rate of the biochemical process. This technique has been extended to humans by principles of computed tomography (Reivich et al., 1979), and adapted to use several radionuclides that decay through the emission of positrons. Subjects are administered radionuclides that are unstable because their nuclei have an excess positive charge. The radionuclides are usually given intravenously, and are taken up by tissue. Through the emission of a positron, they get rid of their energy and undergo the process of annihilation where the positrons interact with an electron (negatively charged). The two photons emitted from each annihilation travel in opposite directions, and the energy generated is detected and measured by detector arrays. By computed tomographic principles, the coincidental counts are used to generate images reflecting the regional rate of radionu-

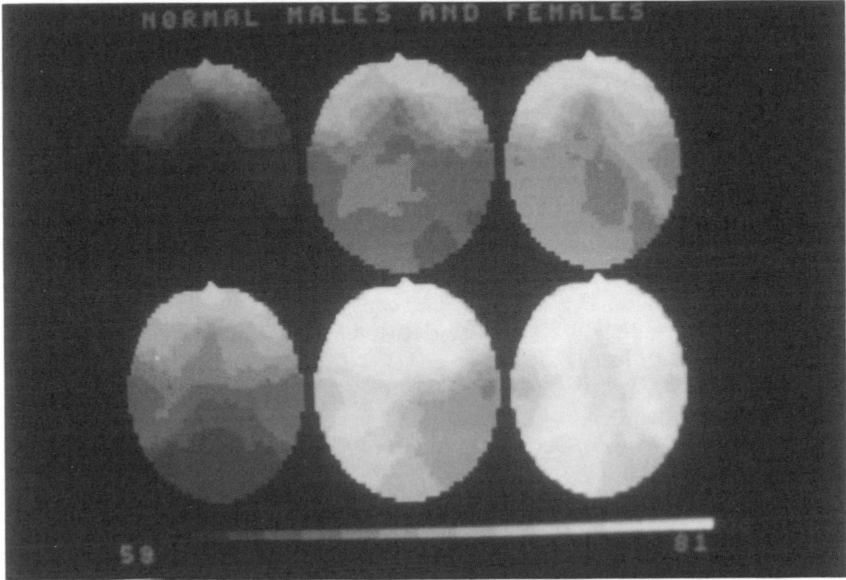

Fig. 17.1. A topographical display of rCBF in a group of normal males (upper row) and females (lower row) during rest (first column), a verbal analogies task (middle column), and a spatial line orientation task (last column). Note the hyperfrontal pattern at rest, the higher CBF in females, and the increased CBF in the left for the verbal and the right for the spatial task. [From R. C. Gur et al. (1991). The impact of neuroimaging on human neuropsychology. In R. G. Lister & H. J. Weingartner (Eds.), *Perspectives on cognitive neuroscience* (p. 422). New York: Oxford University Press. Copyright © 1991 by Oxford University Press. Used by permission.]

clide uptake. This information enables the calculation, depending on the specific radionuclide, of a variety of physiological parameters such as oxygen and glucose metabolism, blood flow, or receptor density of neurotransmitters. In order to relate this physiological information to anatomical ROIs, an atlas of brain anatomy is required. These can be based on computerized images of sliced brains, or on x-ray, CT, or MRI scans. Multiple brain "slices" can be obtained with PET (Figure 17.2).

Another technique for three-dimensional imaging of rCBF is single-photon emission computed tomography (SPECT). The technique uses radionuclides which, unlike positron emitters, do not require the availability of a dedicated cyclotron for their production. However, at present, reliable quantitation of rCBF with available radionuclides that can be safely administered is still very problematic, and much more work is required to allow for its application to systematic neurobehavioral research.

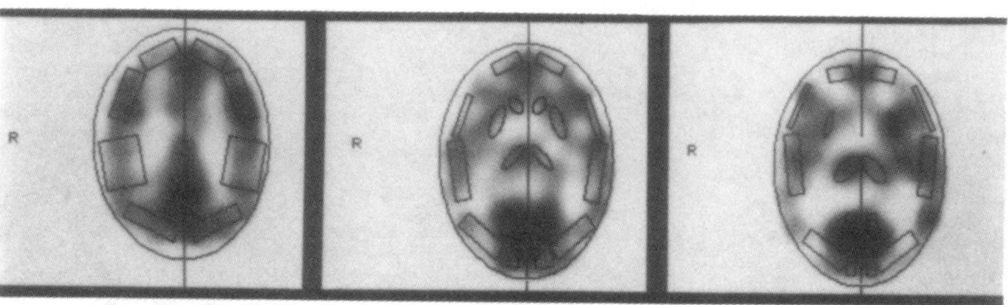

Fig. 17.2. Placement of regions of interest. [From R. E. Gur et al. (1987). Regional brain function in schizophrenia. I. A positron emission tomography study. *Archives of General Psychiatry, 44,* 119–125, p. 121. Copyright © 1987 by the American Medical Association. Used by permission.]

Resting baseline and activated measures

The unique contribution of physiological neuroimaging method is in providing information on the rate of activity of neural systems. This raises the question of measurement conditions: Measures of brain anatomy would not be influenced by the subject's current state of mind – whether the individual is frightened by the procedure or disturbed by conversation among staff members. By contrast, should physiological measures be insensitive to such effects, we would probably lose interest in them as indicators of brain function. Hence, when physiological neuroimaging studies are considered the experimental conditions require careful consideration.

Several investigators have maintained that physiological neuroimaging studies are completely uninformative unless subjects are provided with a task or a uniform stimulation condition. Thus, Buchsbaum et al. (1982, 1984) have used electric shocks and the continuous performance task during measurement of cerebral glucose metabolism with PET. A resting baseline condition, it is argued, is too unstructured, hence unreliable, and would unduly increase intersubject variability.

In contrast, we have argued that a standard resting baseline condition would be invaluable for interpreting activation data and for comparison across studies and research centers. We have described such a condition (Gur et al., 1982) which yields reproducible data (Gur et al., 1983a, 1987a,b; Warach, Gur, Gur, Skolnick, Obrist, & Reivich, 1987, 1992). Furthermore, the variability in the resting values and the regional landscape did not seem random, since it correlated with age (Gur et al., 1987a,b) and gender (Gur et al., 1983a).

With respect to differences in resting baseline activity between patients with schizophrenia and healthy controls, early studies reported reduced overall activity (Mathew et al., 1981, 1982) or reduced activity in frontal regions (the "hypofrontality hypothesis": (Farkas, Wolf, Jaeger, Brodie, Christman, Fowler, 1984; Ingvar & Franzen, 1974). However, other studies of resting CBF and metabolism reported no evidence of resting "hypofrontality" (Buchsbaum et al., 1982, 1984; Shepherd, Gruzelier, Manchanda, & Hirsch, 1983; Weinberger, Berman, & Zec, 1986), and we found normal levels of frontal lobe activity in patients screened for neurological disease or history of events that may alter cerebral metabolism (Gur et al., 1985b, 1987a,b). Differences in resting values between patients and controls were found in laterality indices, suggesting relatively higher left hemispheric values in severely disturbed patients (Gur, Resnick, & Gur, 1989; Shepherd et al., 1983). Furthermore, improvement in clinical status correlated with a shift toward lower left hemispheric relative to right hemispheric metabolism (Figure 17.3). This supports hypotheses derived from behavioral data concerning lateralized abnormalities in schizophrenia (Flor-Henry, 1969; Gruzelier & Venables, 1974), and perhaps the more specific form of the laterality hypothesis, which proposes that schizophrenia is associated with both left hemispheric dysfunction and overactivation of the dysfunctional left hemisphere (R. E. Gur, 1978).

Regardless of one's position in the debate over the value of obtaining resting baseline measures, it became apparent rather early that measures of CBF and metabolism during the performance of cognitive tasks can accentuate differences between patients and controls. For example, in the first study in which we compared medicated patients with schizophrenia to sociodemographically balanced healthy controls, we found no differences in overall or hemispheric CBF using the ^{133}Xe clearance technique, but found distinct abnormalities in the pattern of hemispheric changes induced by verbal (analogies) and spatial (line orientation) tasks. In contrast to controls, who showed greater left hemispheric increase for the verbal and greater right hemispheric increase for the spatial task, patients with schizophrenia had a bilaterally symmetrical activation for the verbal task, thus failing to show left hemispheric dominance for this task, and instead showed greater left than right hemispheric activation for the spatial task (Figure 17.4). Similarly, Weinberger and colleagues found no regional abnormalities in resting CBF of patients with schizophrenia. However, distinct abnormalities were demonstrated in frontal regions during activation with the Wisconsin Card Sorting Test of abstraction and mental flexibility, which is putatively sensitive to frontal lobe damage (Weinberer, Berman, & Zec, 1986).

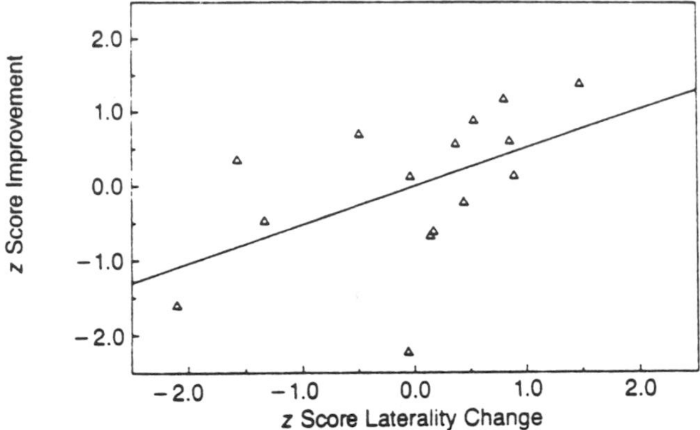

Fig. 17.3. Change in laterality scores from study 1 to study 2 plotted against clinical improvement. Laterality change = study 2 (right–left hemisphere metabolism) – study 1 (right–left hemispheric metabolism). Improvement = (BPRS study 1 – BPRS study 2) / BPRS study 1, where BPRS indicates Brief Psychiatric Rating Scale. Relative right hemispheric increase from study 1 to study 2 is associated with greater improvement [$r(13) = .52$, $p < .05$]. [From R. E. Gur et al. (1987). Regional brain function in schizophrenia. II. Repeated evaluations with positron emission tomography. *Archives of General Psychiatry, 44,* 126–129, p. 128. Copyright © 1987 by the American Medical Association. Used by permission.]

Quantitative and "subtraction" methods

In recognition of the value of activated measurements, an issue that comes immediately to the fore is whether it is important to obtain quantitative parameters of activity. By this we mean the ability to measure with physiological units the rate of blood flow or metabolism. This is an important decision, since quantitation requires the availability of reliable estimates of the isotope arterial concentrations for the input function, which in the case of PET involves arterial catheterization (no reliable methods of CBF quantitation are currently available for SPECT).

A strong argument can be made that the additional effort and risk of quantitative measurements are unnecessary for examining task activation effects since all we are interested in are the task-induced changes in regional landscapes of activity. For this purpose it is sufficient to measure the activity during different task conditions that control for elements of the task, and to subtract the topography of control conditions from that of the condition of interest. The feasibility of this approach was demonstrated elegantly in a series of experiments by Posner, Petersen, Fox, and Raichle (1988) at Washington University, St. Louis. They used rapid bolus injections of oxygen-15–labeled water with PET, where voxel concentration levels were

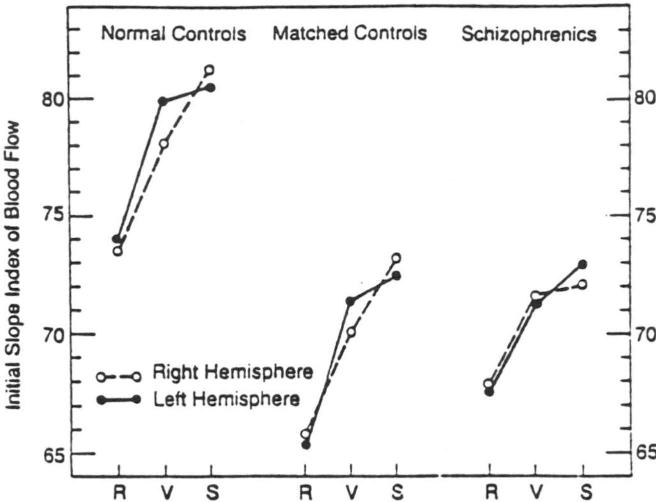

Fig. 17.4. Regional cerebral blood flow in two hemispheres of schizophrenics and matched controls when resting (R), solving verbal analogies (V), and performing spatial tasks (S). Normal control values are from earlier study for comparison with latest matched sample. [From R. E. Gur et al. (1983). Brain function in psychiatric disorders. I. Regional cerebral blood flow in medicated schizophrenics. *Archives of General Psychiatry, 40,* 1250–1254, p. 1253. Copyright © 1983. Used by permission. American Medical Association.]

transformed to proportions of whole-slice and regions were then identified across subjects, using a computerized stereotactic atlas. They showed in healthy subjects how attentional and linguistic subsystems could be isolated by the "subtraction method" (Posner et al., 1988). On the basis of these results, it is fair to conclude that the nonquantitative subtraction method is likely to yield many important insights on brain behavior relations.

However, the subtraction method has several limitations and perhaps may involve some risks. Most importantly, without quantitation it is impossible to tell whether activity in a region of interest has increased, decreased, or stayed the same across conditions. A "hot spot" on the subtraction image refers only to the relative amount of change in the number of counts compared to the other regions. This may address some hypotheses that do not include statements about the relationship between brain activity and mental effort, but will have limited value for linking these constructs. It should be pointed out further that even for hypotheses that are satisfied with statements about relative activation, the subtraction method makes a further questionable assumption of linear relationship between count density and CBF or metabolism.

Lack of quantitation could also lead to error in the interpretation of effects. Recently, Drevets et al. (1992), from the St. Louis group, retracted an earlier report of increased left temporal CBF in anxiety patients during lactate-induced panic attacks. When PET data were cross-registered with MRI based neuroanatomy, it became clear that the "hot spot" was on facial muscles, not brain. Drevets et al. point out that the mistake could have been avoided by anatomical cross-registration, but even without cross-registration a quantitative approach would have revealed that the values are uncharacteristic of brain parenchyma. Cross-registration in its present state when applied to "aggregate brains," as done in the subtraction method, would not safeguard against other artifacts that could be detected by quantitation (e.g., large vessel effects). Thus, while accepting the heuristic value of the subtraction method for identifying neural networks related to behavioral dimensions, we believe it is worthwhile to proceed with caution and use methods that permit quantification in physiological units.

Choice of behavioral dimensions

The selection of particular tasks to be used for activation is ultimately in the hands of the investigator and tailored to test specific hypotheses. However, several considerations could be useful in trying to maximize the yield of such research (Gur, Erwin & Gur, 1992). First and foremost, it is important to begin with well-defined behavioral dimensions, where there is psychometric evidence for convergent and divergent "construct validity" and some neurobehavioral evidence for regional specificity. It is then necessary to find a task that measures this construct and can be adapted for use with neuroimaging. Devising such a task can be rather trivial in some cases, but a challenge in others. When changes in the task are extensive, it would be prudent to find out whether such deviations from standard administration produce changes in the performance and in the task's construct validity.

The ability to obtain performance measures concomitant with the physiological parameters can be helpful in the interpretation of regional effects. For example, in our first experiment with verbal and spatial tasks, we used a Gestalt Completion task for the latter. Whereas the verbal task reliably increased left relative to right hemispheric CBF, the spatial task produced, on the average, bilaterally symmetrical changes. Indeed, of the 36 subjects, all right-handed males, 17 showed greater right and 17 greater left hemispheric increase. The performance data, however, were different between these two groups, with the right hemispheric increase associated with better performance on the spatial task. In general, we found performance data quite essential for evaluating relationships between mental effort and neural activity. For example, in a study of normal young volunteers who were given an easy and a difficult version of a verbal analogies task (within-subject design), we found effects of task difficulty on CBF measured with the ^{133}Xe clearance method. We also found a relationship between the activated CBF and performance, which was mediated by the subjects' anxiety (Gur, Gur, Resnick, Skolnick, Alavi, & Reivich, 1987; Gur, Gur, Skolnick, Resnick, Silver, Chawluk, Muenz, Obrist, & Reivich, 1988).

Beyond the importance of selecting a unitary behavioral dimension and tasks that yield performance measures with established psychometric properties of reliability and validity, task selection can be guided by reference to its relevance to the disorder. In the attempt to understand neural substrates of a psychiatric disorder using the physiological neuroimaging approach, it would make sense to apply tasks for which there is evidence of impairment associated with the disorder. Our initial choice of verbal and spatial tasks was guided by evidence from behavioral measures suggesting dysfunction in cognitive domains associated with the left hemisphere. We have since learned to appreciate Chapman and Chapman's arguments for establishing differential deficit; these can be incorporated into the neuroimaging paradigm by selecting control tasks with comparable psychometric properties. The past decade has also seen the development of efficient and well-standardized neuropsychological testing "batteries." Such batteries provide "neuropsychological profiles" of populations and can be used for establishing areas of differential deficit; the domains can then be selected for further scrutiny by use of activation studies.

Neuropsychological profile

Neuropsychological batteries can be distinguished from standard psychological tests in that they can provide links, based on lesion data, between a profile of behavioral measures and brain topography. A battery developed in our center has shown sensitivity to focal brain lesions (Blonder, Gur, Gur, Saykin, & Hurtig, 1989; Gur, Gur, & Saykin, 1990; Gur, Trivedi, Saykin, & Gur, 1988; Saykin, Gur, Sussmman, & Gur, 1989), and its functional scores could be reliably assigned sensitivity weights for regional brain dysfunction (Gur et al., 1991). When applied to a sample of patients with schizophrenia, it indicated differential deficits in memory processing (Saykin et al., 1991) (Figure 17.5).

To examine the neurophysiological substrate of this memory deficit, we designed a word and face memory task. The target stimuli for the word task were 20 abstract words of 1–3 syllables, selected from Paivio's list (Paivio, Yuille, & Madison, 1968), and matched to 40 distractor words from that list

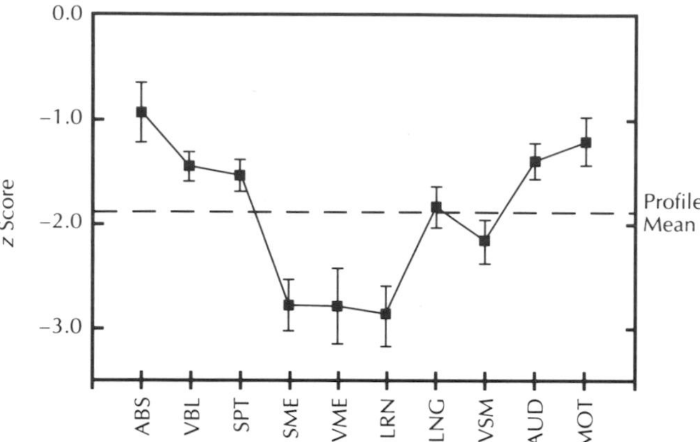

Fig. 17.5. Neuropsychological profile (± SEM) for patients with schizophrenia (*n* = 36) relative to controls (*n* = 36) whose performance is set to zero (± SD). Functions are abstraction (ABS), verbal cognitive (VBI), spatial organization (SPT), semantic memory (SME), visual memory (VME), verbal learning (LRN), language (LNG), visuomotor processing and attention (VSM), auditory processing and attention (AUD), and motor speed and sequencing (MOT). [From A. J. Saykin et al. (1991). Neuropsychological function in schizophrenia: Selective impairment in memory and learning. Archives of General Psychiatry, 48, 618–624, p. 620. Copyright © 1991, American Medical Association.]

for length, abstractness, ratings of imageability, and frequency of use. The corresponding face memory task consisted of straight-angle photographs with neutral expressions. Distractors and targets were matched for ethnicity, gender, and age. When administered to a normative sample, the task produced asymmetrical activation of CBF, measured with the ^{133}Xe clearance method, which was focally restricted to the midtemporal cortex (Gur et al., 1993). The tasks were then applied to a sample of 19 patients with schizophrenia and demographically balanced healthy controls (Gut et al., 1994c). As in earlier studies, patients did not differ from controls in the topographical distribution of resting CBF. However, the pattern of hemispheric activation by the memory tasks was quite different. In contrast to controls who showed the "appropriate" laterality of CBF (L > R verbal, R > L facial) only in the midtemporal region, patients did not show a significantly appropriate effect in this region and instead showed the effects in other regions (Figure 17.6).

Such studies can ideally provide a coherent line of evidence that can further refine current hypotheses on the neural substrates of schizophrenia and schizotypy. As we hope these studies have illustrated, we need to begin with a neurobehavioral hypothesis and then integrate clinical and neuropsychological data with neuroimaging methods. Careful selection of activation tasks can yield a wealth of data that can help direct us in this search.

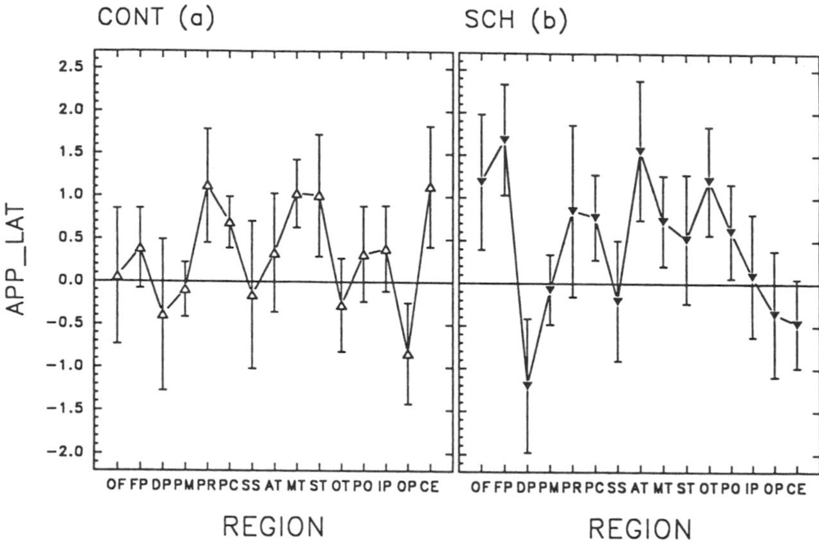

Fig. 17.6. The "appropriate laterality" (APP-LAT) of CBF changes in healthy controls (CONTa) and patients with schizophrenia (b). APP-LAT was defined as Verbal (L-R) + Facial (R-L). Detectors were grouped into 15 regions based on Brodmann areas; orbitofrontal (OF), dorsolateral prefrontal (DP), premotor (PM), frontal pole (FP), precentral (PR), postcentral (PC), somatosensory (SS), anterior temporal (AT), middle temporal (MT), superior temporal (ST), occipitotemporal (OT), parietooccipital (PO), inferior parietal (IP), occipital pole (OP), and cerebellum (CE). Note that controls show a significant elevation of the APP-LAT score above the 0 line only for the target MT region, whereas patients show elevations for the FP, AT, and OT regions but not for the MT region. [Reprinted by permission of Elsevier Science, Inc., from "Cerebral blood flow in schizophrenia: Effects of memory processing on regional activation," by R. E. Gur et al., *Biological Psychiatry, 35* (1), 1994, 3–15. Copyright © 1994 by the Society of Biological Psychiatry.]

Cognition and affect

So far we have restricted the discussion of behavior to cognitive variables, partly because this is the area where most progress has been made. There is reason, however, to believe that perhaps as pertinent to the study of psychiatric disorders, including schizophrenia and schizotypy, is the realm of emotion. This work is more difficult because there are fewer established paradigms and data are meager. Yet there is evidence that application of activation tasks which probe emotional processing may yield unique information on the pathophysiology of schizophrenia.

A simple emotion discrimination task was developed that requires the subject to indicate whether a face is happy, sad, or neutral, and to rate the emotional intensity. The faces were the same as in the memory task except that they expressed happy and sad emotions. The posers were actors and actresses, and expressions were used that could be rated reliably by a normative sample. The task yielded reliable measures of sensitivity and specificity of discriminating happy from neutral and sad from neutral, and was found to be sensitive to gender differences (Erwin et al., 1992). The task also discriminated patients with depression from comparable controls (Gur et al., 1992). When applied to patients with schizophrenia, this task revealed differential impairment relative to an age discrimination task that used the same stimuli (Heimberg et al., 1992). This finding suggests that patients with schizophrenia are impaired in emotional discrimination. We administered the task to a sample of healthy young adults, and found right hemispheric activation for both happy and sad discrimination. However, subtracting happy from sad showed lateralized differences in the frontal region, with happy discrimination associated with relatively greater left hemispheric activation (Gur, Skolnick, & Gur, 1994). The same stimuli were used for standardized mood induction. The effects on mood were robust and reproducible (Schneider et al., 1994), and differential effects were observed on CBF measured with the ^{133}Xe clearance method (Schneider et al., in press) and with PET (Schneider et al., in press). Patients with schizophrenia showed a blunted response to the induction. Thus, it seems that applying emotional probes, in addition to the cognitive probes that are being currently applied, would be of value in patients with schizophrenia and perhaps schizotypal patients.

Cross-modality integration

Throughout this chapter we have attempted to show how hypotheses generated in this area of inquiry can be tested using integration of measures across modalities. This is probably the key for making inroads into our subject matter, yet something that is not easy to do.

Cross-modality integration requires the joint examination of very different types of data, each with its own unreliability and uncertainty. There is need to reduce the data to some parameters that can be interpreted across modalities. Thus, comparing the magnitude of regional task activation with performance may require definition of physiological activation parameters [such as (task – rest per region) ÷ global changes] that could be theoretically linked to performance parameters (such as memory relative to general intellectual abilities). The multitude of data necessarily involved in such integration is also staggering, and utmost care is required to safeguard against excessive Type I error. Sufficiently large samples for exploratory analyses are prohibited by the high costs of the methods, and hence it is particularly important to be guided and driven by hypotheses. On the other hand, the temptation to explore the use of a new technology is natural, and given the novelty of the method, current hypotheses would not lead us very far.

We can divide the data to be integrated into clinical (self- and clinical rating scales, outcome measures, quality of life), neurobehavioral (neuropsychological testing, performance during activation studies), neuroanatomical (volumetric MRI), and neurophysiological. An abnormality at the neuronal level becomes more credible as a potential substrate for the psychiatric disorder if it is correlated with clinical severity. This has motivated our search for neurophysiological correlates of symptom severity (e.g., Gur et al., 1987b, 1989). More recently, we found, using the memory activation paradigm, that clinical, performance, and neurophysiological data can be integrated to link a specific abnormality in the regional neurophysiological response to severity of a cluster of symptoms (Figure 17.7). Thus, as can be seen in Figure 17.7, severity of symptoms of hallucinations and delusions [factor 3 derived from the Scale for the Assessment of Negative Symptoms (SANS) and the Scale for the Assessment of Positive Symptoms (SAPS)] correlated negatively both with the degree of increased CBF for a verbal memory task (left graph), and with performance defined as the "specificity score" (i.e., percentage of items correctly rejected as not belonging to the learning set; middle graph). The notion that the failure to increase activation may relate meaningfully to symptoms and performance is further supported by the positive correlation between CBF increase and performance (left graph). This is obviously a complicated and laborious process, but it is possible to conceive of its success in continuously and systematically refining our hypotheses on brain–behavior relationships.

To illustrate how this paradigm can be applied to the study of schizotypy, we have retrospectively examined our data on CBF in healthy normal subjects in relation to their MMPI scores on the SC scale. As can be seen in Figure 17.8, there were significant correlations between laterality of CBF in subcortical and cortical regions, which differed for baseline compared to measures obtained during activation with the word and face memory tasks. Thus, for baseline CBF, higher SC scores on the MMPI were associated with greater relative left hemispheric activity in the posterior cingulate gyrus, the midfrontal region, and the inferior temporal lobule as well as higher relative right hemispheric activity in the orbital frontal region. The positive correlations are consistent with the hypothesis of left hemispheric overactivation in schizophrenia, and perhaps reflect some continuity with the psychotic dysfunction. By contrast, CBF during performance of the verbal memory task showed a positive correlation with SC only for the hippocampus laterality; that is, higher SC values were associated with relatively higher left hemispheric activity. For thalamus, midfrontal, and inferior frontal regions, these correla-

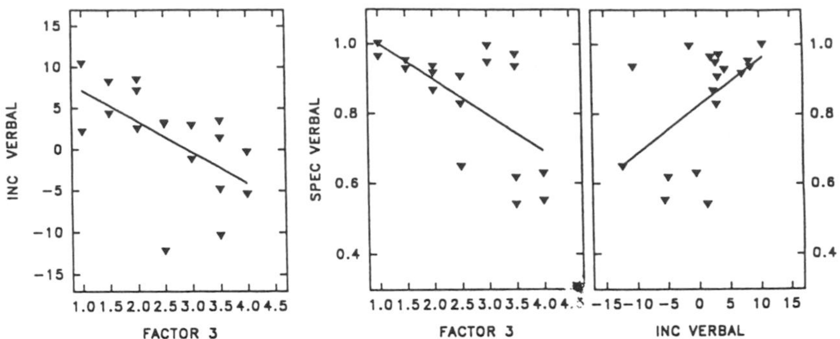

Fig. 17.7. Scatterplots and regression lines depicting correlations between the hallucinations–delusions factor and increase of verbal memory CBF (left graph) as well as verbal memory performance (middle graph), and the scatterplot of verbal CBF increase with verbal memory performance (left graph). CBF increase was defined as verbal-baseline and the performance measure was of specificity (SPEC), defined as percent of items correctly identified as not belonging to the learning set. [Reprinted by permission of Elsevier Science, Inc., from "Cerebral blood flow in schizophrenia: Effects of memory processing on regional activation," by R. E. Gur et al., *Biological Psychiatry, 35* (1), 3–15, 1994. Copyright © 1994 by the Society of Biological Psychiatry.]

tions were negative, suggesting higher SC scores associated with higher relative right hemispheric activation. Thus, while normal subjects will show left hemispheric activation on the verbal task, those with increased SC scores are likely to have less hemispherically appropriate task-related activation in most regions. It seems noteworthy that the midfrontal correlations were opposite for the resting as compared to the activated CBF. We show these data only as an illustration, and caution against their overinterpretation since this is a retrospective and incomplete analysis. However, such studies suggest the utility of the approach and could help pave the way for more systematic research.

Summary

We have tried in this chapter to convey the potential yield of physiological neuroimaging studies in an effort to understand the pathophysiology of neuropsychiatric disorders such as schizophrenia, and believe these considerations apply to the investigation of schizotypy. An impressive array of methods is now available for measuring regional brain physiology, and the application of these methods in other psychiatric disorders has become routine. Whether the results to date can be considered of lasting importance is still debatable. However, with the experience we have gained in "taming" this technology,

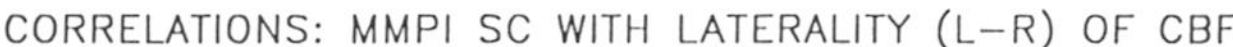

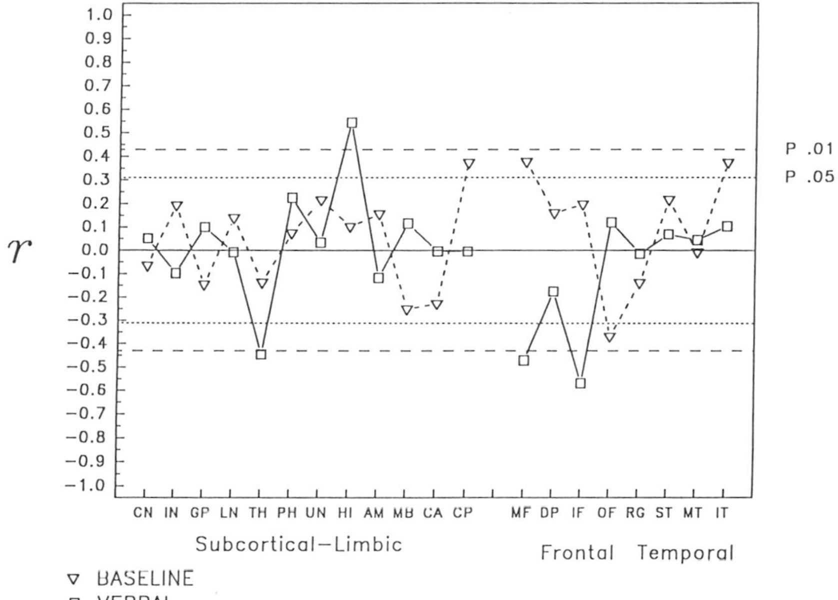

Fig. 17.8. Correlations between the SC score of the MMPI in normal volunteers and the laterality of CBF (defined as L-R) in subcortical-limbic and cortical regions for resting baseline CBF (triangles, dashed line) and CBF during performance of a verbal memory task (squares, solid line). The regions were defined anatomically based on cross-registered MRI scans as follows: caudate nucleus (CN), insula (IN), globus pallidus (GP), lateral lenticular (i.e., putamen) nucleus (LN), thalamus (TH), parahippocampal gyrus (PH), uncus (UN), hippocampus (HI), amygdala (AM), mammillary bodies (MB), anterior cingulate gyrus (CA), posterior cingulate gyrus (CP), midfrontal (MF), dorsolateral prefrontal (DP), inferior frontal (IF), orbital frontal (OF), rectal gyrus (RG), superior temporal (ST), midtemporal (MT), and inferior temporal (IT). Dotted lines were drawn to indicate the .05 level of significance, and the dashed horizontal line shows the .01 significance level.

we should be on our way to making more robust and theoretically heuristic discoveries. This work can be buttressed by the application of well-defined and structured "neurobehavioral probes" that provide psychometrically reliable performance data. Such performance data are particularly helpful in examining correlations with quantitative physiological parameters, and we have tried to argue in favor of such methods as superior to the nonquantitative "subtraction" procedures.

In applying physiological neuroimaging procedures to the study of psychiatric disorders, we have emphasized the need for careful and deliberate choice of activation tasks with respect to the disorder being investigated. In the case of schizophrenia, probes of lateralized functions and, in particular, memory have revealed distinct abnormalities. This may also apply in schizotypy, although we are not aware of comprehensive neuropsychological evaluations that would permit the analysis pointing to differential memory deficits in this population. Should this be demonstrated, it would be intriguing to evaluate schizotypal patients with the kind of memory probes we have applied in schizophrenia.

The most challenging aspect of this work is the integration of neuroimaging data with clinical and neurobehavioral data. This process is still in its infancy in the field of schizophrenia, and is quite difficult to implement, but successful integration will inevitably lead to better understanding of the multifaceted dysfunction characteristic of psychiatric disorders.

Acknowledgments

This work was supported by NIMH Grants MH-43880, MH-48539, MH-00586, MH-42191, and NS-14867.

We thank Helen Mitchell-Sears for her help in preparing this manuscript.

References

Blonder, L. X., Gur, R. E., Gur, R. C., Saykin, A. J., & Hurtig, H. I. (1989). Neuropsychological functioning in hemiparkinsonism. *Brain and Cognition, 9,* 177–190.

Buchsbaum, M. S., Delisi, L. E., Holcomb, H. H., Cappelletti, J., King, A. C., Johnson, J., Hazlett, E., Dowling-Zimmerman, S., Post, R. M., Morihisa, J., Carpenter, W., Cohen, R., Pickar, D., Weinberger, D. R., Margolin, R., & Kessler, R. M. (1984). Anteroposterior gradients in cerebral glucose use in schizophrenia and affective disorder. *Archives of General Psychiatry, 41,* 1159–1166.

Buchsbaum, M. S., Ingvar, D. H., Kessler, R., Waters, R. N., Cappelletti, J., van Kammen, D. P., King, C., Johnson, J. L., Manning, R. G., Flynn, R. W., Mann, L. S., Bunney, W. E., & Sokoloff, L. (1982). Cerebral glucography with positron tomography. *Archives of General Psychiatry, 39,* 251–259.

Dodrill, C. B., & Wilkus, R. J. (1976). Relationships between intelligence and electroencephalographic epileptiform activity in adult epileptics. *Neurology, 26,* 525–531.

Drevets, W. C., Videen, T. O., MacLeod, A. K., Haller, J. W., & Raichle, M. E. (1992). Pet images of blood flow changed during anxiety: Correction. *Science, 256,* 1696.

Erwin, R. J., Gur, R. C., Gur, R. E., Skolnick, B. E., Mawhinney-Hee, M., & Smailis, J. (1992). Facial emotion discrimination: I. Task construction and behavioral findings in normals. *Psychiatry Research, 42,* 231–240.

Farkas, T., Wolf, A. P., Jaeger, J., Brodie, J. D., Christman, D. R., & Fowler, J. S. (1984). Regional brain glucose metabolism in chronic schizophrenia. *Archives of General Psychiatry, 41,* 293–300.

Flor-Henry, P. (1969). Psychosis and temporal lobe epilepsy: A controlled investigation. *Epilepsia, 10,* 363–395.

Gastaut, H. (1970). Clinical and electroencephalographic classification of epileptic seizure. *Epilepsia, 11,* 102–113.

Gruzelier, J. H., & Venables, P. H. (1974). Bimodality and lateral asymmetry of skin conductance orienting activity in schizophrenics: Replication and evidence of lateral asymmetry in patients with depression and disorders of personality. *Biological Psychiatry, 8,* 55–73.

Gur, R. C., Erwin, R. J., & Gur, R. E. (1992). Neurobehavioral probes for physiologic neuroimaging studies. *Archives of General Psychiatry, 49,* 409–414.

Gur, R. C., Erwin, B. J., Gur, R. E., Zwil, A. S., Heimberg, C., & Kraemer, H. C. (1992). Facial emotion discrimination. II. Behavioral findings in depression. *Psychiatry Research, 42,* 241–251.

Gur, R. C., Gur, R. E., Obrist, W. D., Hungerbuhler, J. P., Younkin, D., Rosen, A. D., Skolnick, B. E., & Reivich, M. (1982). Sex and handedness differences in cerebral blood flow during rest and cognitive activity. *Science, 217,* 659–661.

Gur, R. C., Gur, R. E., Resnick, S. M., Skolnick, B. B., Alavi, A., & Reivich, M. (1987). The effect of anxiety on cortical cerebral blood flow and metabolism. *Journal of Cerebral Blood Flow and Metabolism, 7,* 173–177.

Gur, R. C., Gur, R. E., Skolnick, B. E., Resnick, S. M., Silver, F. L., Clawluk, J. B., Muenz, L., Obrist, W. D., & Reivich, M. (1988). Effects of task difficulty on regional cerebral blood flow: Relationships with anxiety and performance. *Psychophysiology, 25,* 392–399.

Gur, R. C. (1991). The impact of neuroimaging on human neuropsychology. In R. G. Lister & H. J. Wingartner (Eds.), *Perspective on cognitive neuroscience.* New York: Oxford University Press.

Gur, R. C., Gur, R. E., Rosen, A. D., Warach, S., Alavi, A., Greenberg, J., & Reivich, M. (1983b). A cognitive–motor network demonstrated by positron emission tomography. *Neuropsychologia, 21,* 601–606.

Gur, R. C., Jaggi, J. L., Ragland, J. D., Resnick, S. M., Shtasel, D., Muenz, L., & Gur, R. E. (1993). Effects of memory processing on regional brain activation: Cerebral blood flow in normal subjects. *International Journal of Neuroscience, 72,* 31–44.

Gur, R. C., Ragland, J. D., Resnick, S. M., Skolnick, B. E., Jaggi, J., Muenz, L., & Gur, R. E. (1994a). Lateralized increases in cerebral blood flow during performance of verbal and spatial tasks: Relationship with performance level. *Brain and Cognition, 24,* 244–258.

Gur, R. C., Saykin, A. J., Blonder, L. X., & Gur, R. E. (1988b). "Behavioral imaging": II. Application of the quantitative algorithm to hypothesis testing in a population of hemiparkinsonian patients. *Neuropsychiatry, Neuropsychology and Behavioral Neurology, 1,* 87–96.

Gur, R. C., Skolnick, B. E., & Gur, R. E. (1994b). Effects of emotional discrimination tasks on cerbral blood flow: Regional activation and its relation to performance. *Brain and Cognition, 25,* 271–286.

Gur, R. C., Trivedi, S. S., Saykin, A. J., & Gur, R. E. (1988a). "Behavioral imaging" – a procedure for analysis and display of neuropsychological test scores: I. Construction of algorithm and initial clinical evaluation. *Neuropsychiatry, Neuropsychology and Behavioral Neurology, 1,* 53–60.

Gur, R. C., Trivedi, S. S., Saykin, A. J., Resnick, S. M., Malamut, B. L., & Gur, R. E. (1985a). Behavioral imaging. *Journal of Clinical and Experimental Neuropsychology, 7,* 633.

Gur, R. E. (1978). Left hemisphere dysfunction and left hemisphere overactivation in schizophrenia. *Journal of Abnormal Psychology, 87,* 226–238.

Gur, R. E., Gur, R. C., & Saykin, A. J. (1990). Neurobehavioral studies in schizophrenia: Implications for regional brain dysfunction. *Schizophrenia Bulletin, 16,* 445–451.

Gur, R. E., Gur, R. C., Skolnick, B. E., Caroff, S., Obrist, W. D., Resnick, S., & Reivich, M. (1985b). Brain function in psychiatric disorders: III. Regional cerebral blood flow in unmedicated schizophrenics. *Archives of General Psychiatry, 42,* 329–334.

Gur, R. E., Jaggi, J. L., Shtasel, D. L., Ragland, J. D., & Gur, R. C. (1994c). Cerebral blood flow in schizophrenia: Effects of memory processing on regional activation. *Biological Psychiatry, 35,* 3–15.

Gur, R. E., Mozley, P. D., Resnick, S. M., Shtasel, D., Kohn, M., Zimmerman, R., Herman, G., Atlas, S., Grossman, R., Erwin, R., & Gur, R. C. (1991). Magnetic resonance imaging in schizophrenia-I. Volumetric analysis of brain and cerebrospinal fluid. *Archives of General Psychiatry, 48,* 407–412.

Gur, R. E., Resnick, S. M., Alavi, A., Gur, R. C., Caroff, S., Dann, R., Silver, F. L., Saykin, A. J., Chawluk, J. B., Kushner, M., & Reivich, M. (1987a). Regional brain function in schizophrenia: I. A positron emission tomography study. *Archives of General Psychiatry, 44,* 119–125.

Gur, R. E., Resnick, S. M., & Gur, R. C. (1989). Laterality and frontality of cerebral blood flow and metabolism in schizophrenia: Relationship to symptom specificity. *Psychiatry Research, 27,* 325–334.

Gur, R. E., Resnick, S. M., Gur, R. C., Alavi, A., Caroff, S., Kushner, M., & Reivich, M. (1987b). Regional brain function in schizophrenia: II. Repeated evaluation with positron emission tomography. *Archives of General Psychiatry, 44,* 126–129.

Gur, R. E., Skolnick, B. E., Gur, R. C., Caroff, S., Rieger, W., Obrist, W. D., Younkin, D., & Reivich, M. (1983a). Brain function in psychiatric disorders: I. Regional cerebral flow in medicated schizophrenics. *Archives of General Psychiatry, 40,* 1250–1254.

Heimberg, C., Gur, R. E., Erwin, R. J., Shtasel, D. L., & Gur, R. C. (1992). Facial emotion discrimination: III. Behavioral findings in schizophrenia. *Psychiatry Research, 42,* 253–265.

Ingvar, D. H. (1979). "Hyperfrontal" distribution of the cerebral matter flow in resting wakefulness: On the functional anatomy of the conscious state. *Acta Neurologica Scandinavica, 60,* 12–25.

Ingvar, D. H., & Franzen, G. (1974). Distribution of cerebral activity in chronic schizophrenia. *Lancet, 2,* 1484–1486.

Kety, S. S., & Schmidt, C. F. (1948). The nitrous oxide method for the quantitative determination of cerebral blood flow in man: Theory, procedure and normal values. *Journal of Clinical Investigation, 27,* 476–483.

Mathew, R. J., Duncan, G. C., Weinman, M. L., & Barr, D. L. (1982). Regional cerebral blood flow in schizophrenia. *Archives of General Psychiatry, 39,* 1121–1124.

Mathew, R. J., Meyer, J. S., Francis, D. J., Schoolar, J. C., Weinman, M., & Mortel, K. F. (1981). Regional cerebral blood flow in schizophrenia: A preliminary report. *American Journal of Psychiatry, 138,* 112–113.

Obrist, W. D., Thompson, H. K., Wang, H. S., & Wilkinson, W. E. (1975). Regional cerebral blood flow estimated by ^{133}Xenon inhalation. *Stroke, 6,* 245–256.

Olesen, J., Paulson, O. B., & Lassen, N. A. (1971). Regional cerebral blood flow in man determined by the initial slope of the clearance of intra-arterially injected ^{133}Xe. *Stroke, 2,* 519–540.

Paivio, A., Yuille, J. C., & Madison, S. A. (1968). Concreteness, imagery, and meaningfulness values for 925 nouns. *Journal of Experimental Psychology* (Monogr. Suppl.), *76* (No. 1, 1–25).

Phelps, M., Mazziotta, J. C., & Schelbert, H. R. (Eds.). (1986). *Positron emission tomography and autoradiography: Principles and applications for the brain and heart.* New York: Raven Press.

Posner, M. I., Petersen, S. E., Fox, P. T., & Raichle, M. E. (1988). Localization of cognitive operations in the human brain. *Science, 240,* 1627–1631.

Reivich, M., & Alavi, A. (Eds.). (1985). *Positron emission tomography.* New York: A. R. Liss.

Reivich, M., Kuhl, D., Wolf, A. P., Greenberg, J., Phelps, M., Ido, T., Casella, V., Fowler, J., Hoffman, E., Alavi, A., Som, P., & Sokoloff, L. (1979). The 18-*F*-fluorodeoxyglucose method for the measurement of local cerebral glucose utilization in man. *Circulation Research, 44,* 127–137.

Saykin, A. J., Gur, R. C., Sussman, N. M., & Gur, R. E. (1989). Memory deficits before and after temporal lobectomy: Effect of laterality and age of onset. *Brain and Cognition, 9,* 191–200.

Schneider, F., Gur, R. C., Gur, R. E., Harper-Mozley, L., Smith, R. J., Mozley, P. D., Censits, D. M., & Alavi, A. (1995). Mood effects on cerebral blood flow correlate with emotional self-rating: A PET H_2 ^{15}O study. *Psychiatry Research,* in press.

Schneider, F., Gur, R. C., Gur, R. E., & Muenz, L. (1994). Standardized mood induction with happy and sad facial expressions. *Psychiatry Research, 51,* 19–31.

Schneider, F., Gur, R. C., Jaggi, J. L., & Gur, R. E. (1994). Differential effects of mood on cortical cerebral blood flow: A ^{133}Xenon clearance study. *Psychiatry Research,* in press.

Sheppard, G., Gruzelier, J., Manchanda, R., & Hirsch, S. R. (1983). 15-0 positron emission tomographic scanning in predominantly never treated acute schizophrenic patients. *Lancet, 2,* 1448–1452.

Warach, A., Gur, R. C., Gur, R. E., Skolnick, B. E., Obrist, W. D., & Reivich, M. (1987). The reproducibility of the Xe-133 inhalation technique in resting studies: Task order and sex related effects in healthy young adults. *Journal of Cerebral Blood Flow and Metabolism, 7,* 702–708.

Warach, S., Gur, R. C., Gur, R. E., Skolnick, B. E., Obrist, W. D., & Reivich, M. (1992). Decreases in frontal and parietal lobe regional cerebral blood flow related to habituation. *Journal of Cerebral Blood Flow and Metabolism, 12,* 546–553.

Weinberger, D. R., Berman, K. F., & Zec, R. F. (1986). Physiologic dysfunction of dorsolateral prefrontal cortex in schizophrenia: I. Regional cerebral blood flow evidence. *Archives of General Psychiatry, 43,* 114–125.

PART VIII
Conclusion

18

Schizotypal personality: synthesis and future directions

TODD LENCZ and ADRIAN RAINE

What is schizotypy?

The purpose of this final chapter is to attempt a broad survey of current scientific inquiry into schizotypal personality and provide directions for future research. As will be seen, some of these directions represent the consensus of the contributors to this volume, whereas others reflect areas of sharp disagreement or divergence of perspectives. In the course of examining the specific contributions of the chapters in this volume to our understanding of schizotypy, it is important to bear in mind the critical conceptual issues that emerged from the proceedings of the conference. Perhaps the central question can be simply stated: What is schizotypy? This question is not as straightforward as it seems. Indeed, after 100 years of schizophrenia research, there are still lively debates on the definition of that term; research on schizotypy is in its infancy relative to its parent field, schizophrenia. Only in the last 15 years has the full force of modern clinical science been brought to bear on the nature of schizotypy, despite the fact that the origins of the concept can be traced back to Bleuler (see Ingraham, Chapter 2, this volume).

Two additional questions emerge in parallel to the first: (1) Why do we study schizotypal personality? and (2) How should we approach studying it? This chapter attempts to synthesize some answers to these questions, based on the work presented in the 17 preceding chapters. Given the early stage of the science, however, more questions will be raised than answered. Consequently, this chapter attempts to provide conceptual and methodological directions for future research that might address these questions.

Examination of the chapters in this volume, or even a random survey of the literature on schizotypy, will reveal that various researchers define schizotypy differently; consequently, they utilize a variety of instruments to tap these traits. In order to compare the findings across studies, one must be familiar with the varying definitions applied to the construct called schizotypy. Generally speaking, there are four different approaches one might take to begin to define schizotypal personality: consensual, historical, theoretical, and empirical. Before embarking on this review, we should note that these four approaches are separable only in theory; in the actual published record, they are intertwined, as we show below. The four-part division used here calls the reader's attention to certain critical components in the evaluation of the schizotypy construct.

Consensual definition

The consensual definition of schizotypy can be found in the DSM-III-R (APA, 1987), and is relatively unchanged in the DSM-IV (APA, 1994). The DSM defines schizotypy as an Axis II personality disorder, which means that the symptoms must be present by early adulthood and must be enduring and persistent across situations and circumstances. Because of the categorical nature of the DSM, schizotypal personality disorder (SPD) is automatically viewed as a dichotomous entity, so that each patient either is or is not schizotypal. In addition, the category has a prototypic symptom structure, meaning that any given patient need only have five of the nine criteria to receive the diagnosis. Thus, there can exist, for example, two individuals with the diagnosis of SPD who only have one trait in common.

The advantages of utilizing this definition are familiar from debates concerning the merits of DSM itself (e.g., Millon, 1991). Specifically, the criteria are readily accessible to all in the field, are relatively well-operationalized, and have established interrater reliability. In addition, studies using DSM-based assessments of SPD have the advantage of sampling a wide range of symptoms thought to be related to factors of cognitive aberrations, interpersonal deficits, and disorganized behavior (Raine, Reynolds, Lencz, Scerbo, Triphon, & Kim, 1994). Recently, several well-tested and comprehensive instruments have been developed to assess the nine DSM-III-R symptoms, including clinical interview manuals such as the Personality Disorders Examination (Loranger, Susman, Oldham, & Russakof, 1987) and the Structured Clinical Interview for the DSM-III-R (Spitzer, Williams, & Gibbon, 1987), as well as one self-report measure, the Schizotypal Personality Questionnaire (Raine, 1991). Finally, the use of DSM-based assessment protocols allows for a coherent method of assessing psychotic and affective (Axis I) symptoms that may confound the diagnosis of schizotypy (Siever, Kalus, & Keefe, 1993).

The disadvantages of the DSM system primarily stem from the manner in which the criteria were selected. As noted in Loring Ingraham's contribution to this volume, the original items selected for SPD in the DSM-III were based on the results of a single study: the Danish adoption study of Kety et al. (1975). The selection of the original symptoms of SPD for DSM-III (Spitzer, Endicott, & Gibbon, 1979) were subject to limitations in the original design of the Danish study as well as to the assumptions made by Spitzer et al.

Origins of DSM classification

Although the Danish adoption study was comprehensive in nature and of seminal importance, its limitations have been detailed by Kendler (1985). Specifically, Kety and his colleagues changed their working definition of schizotypy (which they called latent or borderline schizophrenia) between the first and second phases of the study. In the first (Copenhagen) phase of the study, Kety et al. (1975) examined hospital records of relatives of schizophrenic subjects and controls. The criteria examined for latent schizophrenia included predominantly "positive" symptoms such as thought disorder, odd speech, and cognitive slippage, although some items for social and interpersonal impairments were also included. Kety (1985) has indicated that this bias derived from the fact that, at least in the first phase of the study, he was diagnosing schizotypy only in those adoptees with severe enough pathology to be hospitalized. Positive symptoms are simply more noticeable and are more likely to result in hospitalization. In the second phase of the study, the first-degree relatives of the schizophrenic probands were studied by use of interviews. In this phase, Kety used DSM-II criteria for latent schizophrenia, which was drawn from Bleuler's account; he therefore discovered more of the negative symptoms that Bleuler had identified.

When Spitzer et al. (1979) were developing the SPD criteria, they selected the eight criteria that most effectively (in terms of sensitivity and specificity) picked out the subjects in Kety's study who had received a diagnosis of borderline or latent schizophrenia. However, they made this determination irrespective of whether such subjects were relatives of schizophrenics. The implicit assumption was that schizotypy was not essentially linked to schizophrenia; that is, Spitzer and his colleagues assumed that there would be no significant difference between SPD in the biological relatives of schizophrenics compared to the general population. As will be seen below, this may have impacted the criteria they selected, which lean more heavily toward the positive symptoms.

Gunderson, Siever, and Spaulding (1983) reanalyzed the Danish adoption data and gave diagnoses of DSM-III SPD and borderline personality disorder

(BPD) to the index adoptees and their relatives who had originally been diagnosed with borderline (or latent) schizophrenia. These researchers found SPD diagnoses to be much more common among the relatives with borderline schizophrenia as opposed to the index cases; on the other hand, most (9 out of 10) of the index cases who had originally received a diagnosis of borderline schizophrenia were diagnosed by Gunderson et al. as BPD. They also kept a tally of non–DSM-III symptoms of both the positive and negative variety. Using discriminant function analysis, these researchers found that a set of six criteria, five of which were social–interpersonal deficits, best identified those schizotypals who were biological relatives of schizophrenics (as opposed to the index cases). Conversely, they found that psychotic-like symptoms, such as illusions and magical thinking, were actually more effective in identifying subjects with BPD.

Historical definitions

The discrepancy in results between the studies of Spitzer et al. (1979) and Gunderson et al. (1983) mirrors an historical division spanning 80 years between two competing methods of examining and identifying schizotypal symptomatology. On the one hand, many early descriptive psychiatrists (e.g., Bleuler, Kretschmer, and Kallman) identified a syndrome in the relatives of schizophrenics involving social withdrawal and other "negative" symptoms, but not involving psychosis. Other psychiatrists (Zilboorg, Hoch, and Polatin) noticed transient or subclinical psychotic experiences ("positive" symptoms) in patients who were not necessarily related to schizophrenics. These symptoms were linked to schizophrenia by their surface similarity of type.

The details of this distinction can be found elsewhere (see Ingraham, Chapter 2, this volume; Kendler, 1985); however, it is important to note here that this division has not been resolved. It is still not clear whether these descriptive psychiatrists were identifying two syndromes or two variations of the same syndrome, or simply emphasizing two aspects of a single syndrome. Thaker and colleagues (Thaker, Moran, Cassady, Ross, & Adani, 1993) have presented some recent evidence to suggest that schizotypals who had a family history positive for schizophrenia had a greater incidence of social–interpersonal symptoms compared to schizotypals without schizophrenic relatives. They further found that the former group were characterized by significantly more eye tracking abnormalities. Condray and Steinhauer (1992), on the other hand, found no difference between schizotypals with and without schizophrenic relatives on the Continuous Performance Test, a measure of sustained attention; both groups were impaired relative to controls. Unfortunately, these two studies nearly exhaust the literature in this area. A major direction for future research will be to compare schizotypals from the general population to those who have schizophrenic relatives on measures of symptomatology as well as on biological variables.

Theoretical considerations

The definitions of schizotypy offered by the DSM and the early descriptive psychiatrists are, to a large extent, explicitly atheoretical. However, much of the research on schizotypy reviewed in this book derives from two seminal theoretical models: the categorical and the dimensional.

The categorical model, originated and developed by Meehl (1962, 1990), is discussed at length by Lenzenweger and Korfine (Chapter 7, this volume) as well as by Tyrka, Haslam, and Cannon (Chapter 8, this volume). According to this model, schizotypy is a discrete diagnostic entity (taxon) that shares the same genetic basis as schizophrenia. Moreover, this genetic basis is hypothesized to involve a single, isolable locus. The possible existence of other genetic determinants that may influence the degree of expression of the gene in behaviors is not excluded; these genes are termed "polygenic potentiators" by Meehl. The essential elements of this perspective are (1) its focus on schizotypy as a dichotomous trait that one either has or does not have, (2) the hypothesis that the basis of this trait can be isolated in a genetically determined "integrative neural defect," and (3) the notion that this genetic basis is also the genetic basis for schizophrenia. Thus, this perspective links schizotypy and schizophrenia on a spectrum of disorder while underscoring the gulf between these stages and "normality." The Chapmans' scales of psychosis proneness were constructed with elements of this model in mind (Chapman, Chapman, & Kwapil, Chapter 5, this volume).

The second model stands in seeming contradiction to the first. This model, derived from the influential personality theories of Hans Eysenck (1960), holds that schizotypy is simply near the extreme end of a continuum of normal personality processes. According to this model, there is no fundamental discontinuity among normality, schizotypy, and schizophrenia; all differences are of degree, not of kind.

Claridge and Beech (Chapter 9, this volume) endorse a similar, though less radical, view. They agree with Eysenck that research should begin with normal personality processes rather than defect states. However, they do not require absolute continuity at the extreme end of the spectrum (see Figure 9.1 in Claridge & Beech's chapter); psychotic and other disordered symptoms can emerge discontinuously owing to environmental stressors and other predisposing factors. Although this model explicitly eschews using schizophrenia genetic theory as a starting point, it seems not inconsistent with the multifactorial polygenic model of schizophrenia as articulated by Gottesman and Shields (1982) and Fowles (1992). The polygenic model, in contrast to Meehl's view, holds that there is no single gene primarily responsible for vulnerability to schizophrenia; what is required is that a threshold number from a pool of possible "vulnerability" genes must be reached for an individual to be at risk for schizophrenia.

Evaluation

The only direct empirical method developed specifically to test the taxonicity of schizotypy is statistical modeling, using Meehl's MAXCOV-HITMAX procedure (Meehl, 1973). Several studies using this method have provided empirical support for the categorical model (see Lenzenweger & Korfine, Chapter 7; Tyrka et al., Chapter 8, this volume). Although these data are strong and consistent in their support of a categorical model, they are not yet conclusive.

Lenzenweger and Korfine's studies analyze the Chapman's Perceptual Aberration Scale (PAS), which is designed to tap unusual symptoms of body image distortion that would be endorsed only by those with a strong degree of pathology (Chapman et al., Chapter 5, this volume). It is possible that the nature of the scale influenced the results. Lenzenweger and Korfine note that the base-rate estimates provided by the MAXCOV-HITMAX procedure should not be influenced by the item endorsement frequency. However, the possibility that results are determined by the nature of the scale is supported by a MAXCOV-HITMAX study by Earleywine, Dawson, and Hazlett (1994). These researchers replicated the finding that the PAS is taxonic (categorical) in nature. However, they also found that scores on the Chapmans' Magical Ideation (MI) scale, which is not skewed toward highly unusual items, are distributed continuously. It should also be noted that the MI scale is perhaps a better predictor of subsequent psychosis (Chapman et al., Chapter 5, this volume). In addition, although the two studies presented by Lenzenweger and Korfine (Chapter 7, this volume) show convergent results, they leave a significant discrepancy concerning the base rate of the taxon (10% in their first study vs. 5% in their second).

Similarly, the MAXCOV study by Tyrka et al. presents several strongly convergent findings supporting the categorical model of schizotypy. However, generalizability of the findings is again limited, in this case by the nature of the sample. These researchers found a high base rate of schizotaxia (averaging about 50%) in their high-risk sample of offspring of schizophrenics. However, a question is raised by the relatively high rate (15–20%) of schizotaxia in the low-risk sample composed of children of nonschizophrenics. This study needs to be supplemented by another, using similar items in a general population; as noted above, it remains an open question whether schizotypy in relatives of schizophrenics has the same etiology as that found in the general population.

The report of Tyrka et al. raises a second question to be pursued by future research: What is the stability of this taxon over time? According to Meehl's theory, this genetically based taxon should be highly stable over time, with any detected shifts primarily due to measurement error. It is theoretically possible that fluctuations in the polygenic potentiators or environmental conditions could affect expression of schizotypal signs and symptoms. However, according to Meehl's theory, such fluctuations would need to be large in magnitude to cause someone to not appear schizotypal, since schizotaxia is manifested in schizotypy "on all actually existing reinforcement regimes" (Meehl, 1990, p. 35). Although Tyrka et al. found that the overall base rates for membership in the schizotypal taxon were relatively consistent across time, they also reported that individual subjects were not always consistent over time. This points to the need for more in-depth longitudinal analysis of how these symptoms evolve in relation to life stress, developmental milestones, and so on. The need for more longitudinal research to examine the relative stability or lability of schizotypal symptoms is addressed again in a later section.

A final piece of empirical evidence affecting evaluation of these theories comes from a recent family study by Torgersen and colleagues (Torgersen, Onstad, Skre, Edvardsen, & Kringlen, 1993). This study reported that schizotypal personality disorder was present in only 20% of monozygotic (MZ) twins of schizophrenics. This datum disconfirms a strong version of Meehl's hypothesis, which would predict that all MZ twins of schizophrenics would carry the schizotaxia gene and therefore would be schizotypal. Still it is possible that these twins still carry the gene, but do not express it in the form of observable schizotypal symptoms.

While the differences between the categorical and dimensional approaches to schizotypy should not be overlooked, it is possible to take some steps toward reconciling these models. It may be that some schizotypal traits (such as body image distortions) are categorical in nature, whereas other traits, such as those positive symptoms tapped by Claridge's STA or the Chapmans' MI, are distributed normally throughout the population. This possibility is not inconsistent with Meehl's general theory, insofar as he posits that some schizotypal features, such as anhedonia, are not part of the core schizotypal syndrome and are not taxonic in nature. Such symptoms, according to Meehl, are manifestations of polygenic potentiators, not reflecting the hypothesized single schizogene. With respect to such symptoms, the two theories are not in disagreement.

The two theories diverge, however, on the issue of whether there is a single "core" schizotypal deficit that is taxonic in nature. Given the heterogeneity of schizotypy alluded to in the historical overview above, it is possible that a monolithic theory will not suffice to explain all the phenomena labeled as "schizotypy." Perhaps both theories are correct in describing certain subpopulations of schizotypals, marked by differing constellations of symptoms. Heterogeneity of schizotypy is supported by the common research finding of high variance within schizotypal samples on biological measures (cf. Dawson et al., Chapter 11, this volume; Holzman et al., Chapter 15, this volume). It will be important for future researchers to discover how many of those identified as schizotypals are what Meehl would term "phenocopies," lacking the hypothesized core genetic neural defect. If this number is nonnegligible, against Meehl's predictions, then we must grapple with the question of how to classify such cases. Such a decision would require data on the relation between this form of schizotypy and other variables, such as neuropsychological performance and subsequent development of psychosis.

Other empirical approaches

We have already discussed two empirical approaches to schizotypy: MAXCOV-HITMAX and the Danish adoption study. In addition to these, there is a large body of empirical research that examines the validity of individual traits or symptoms hypothesized to be part of the schizotypy construct. This research falls into two basic types: clinical studies of comparative diagnostic efficiency, and laboratory studies of biological markers and other "external" variables.

Clinical studies

In the last 10 years, clinical research on SPD has been focused primarily on two goals. First, researchers have examined the discriminant validity of SPD items with respect to BPD. Second, studies have examined the relative diagnostic efficiency of the various criteria in hospital settings.

The literature

Perhaps the central question of the clinical literature on schizotypal personality is the issue of overlap with borderline personality disorder (BPD). In a representative study, Widiger, Frances, Warner, and Bluhm (1986) examined the rates of SPD and BPD symptoms in 83 nonpsychotic hospital inpatients. SPD and BPD were found to have a high rate of overlap; 24 patients had BPD only, 29 had SPD only, and 29 received both diagnoses. Other studies have found rates of overlap as high as 58% (Serper et al., 1993). This phenomenon is common to most of the Axis II disorders (Widiger, Frances, Spitzer, & Williams, 1988), and raises the question of the placement of schizotypy on Axis II. Some argue that this rate of overlap supports a dimensional view of schizotypy and of the personality disorders in general (e.g., Widiger, Trull, Hurt, Clarkin, & Frances, 1987). Others suggest that item selection in DSM-III was flawed, thus blurring distinctions between SPD and BPD. For example, George and Soloff (1986) point to the exclusion of transient psychotic-like episodes from the DSM criteria for BPD; this exclusion was intended to decrease the overlap between the two categories (Spitzer et al., 1979). George and Soloff (1986) believe that this move had the unintended, paradoxical effect of increasing the overlap of the two categories. They suggest that this occurred because many BPD patients (67% in their sample) experience such episodes, which are then classified as perceptual aberrations under SPD criteria. Yet another suggestion, posited by Serper et al. (1993), is that patients with combined SPD and BPD represent a distinct diagnostic category of severely impaired patients. In their study, these overlap subjects had significantly more impairment on MMPI scales 8 (Schizophrenia), 1 (Hypochondriasis), and 7 (Psychasthenia) compared to pure SPD or pure BPD patients, even though the overlap group did not meet more SPD criteria than the pure SPD group or more BPD criteria than the pure BPD group.

In a separate study, Widiger, Frances, and Trull (1987a) examined the base rates, positive predictive power (PPP), and negative predictive power (NPP) of the various symptoms to compare their diagnostic relevance and efficiency in the clinical setting. They concluded that in clinical settings, the cognitive–perceptual symptoms were more significant in diagnosing SPD than the social–interpersonal symptoms. Social–interpersonal deficits, such as no close friends, were very common across all diagnoses, and therefore were not specifically pathognomic for SPD.

Evaluation

At one level, these studies of clinical populations are effective insofar as they identify and answer a well-defined research question: What is the distribution of and relationship among the various symptoms in a given setting or population? For example, these studies have consistently shown a pattern of the relative prevalence and overlap of SPD and BPD diagnoses across clinical settings. However, it may be difficult to utilize psychometric statistical techniques such as PPP and NPP to draw broader inferences concerning the relative importance of the items and the overall meaning or definition of the diagnostic entities. As Widiger et al. (1987a) admit, these psychometric techniques were originally designed to examine the effectiveness of various self-contained indicators (e.g., test scores or questionnaire items) for tapping a previously (and externally) defined criterion. Widiger et al. (1987a) use these techniques to examine the effectiveness of SPD criteria in diagnosing SPD itself, which is entirely defined by those same criteria. While classificatory science necessarily involves a circular bootstrapping process, the circle of reasoning in the Widiger et al. (1987a) study may be a bit too tightly closed in on itself.

This circularity exists because there is no external validation, such as other scales or biological markers. It should be noted that such validation does not need to be seeking an ontological definition of a "disease entity." Widiger et al. appear correct when they say that diagnostic efficacy is dependent upon the setting and purposes of the differential diagnosis. Validation can be defined entirely contextually. Future studies can expand on these findings by specifying the relevant features of their respective settings. In an inpatient facility, for example, the external variables might include response to treatment, discharge decisions, and other clinically relevant dependent measures.

This philosophical difficulty in identifying the "true" nature of a disorder, and the need for contextual clarity, are underscored by the attempts of many researchers to increase the differentiation between SPD and BPD. For example, in a recent review of the clinical/diagnostic literature, Kotsaftis and Neale (1993) indicated that traitlike constricted affect was the symptom that best differentiates SPD from BPD, insofar as BPD is typically marked by extremes of affect and affective lability. (When present in borderline patients, flat affect tends to be related to depressive episodes, and is therefore state-dependent.) They suggest that this symptom be made a necessary (but not sufficient) condition for the diagnosis of SPD to be assigned. This suggestion appears to make sense clinically, and it would certainly serve the goal of decreasing the rate of overlap between the two disorders. Such differentiation may serve important clinical goals, such as planning treatment strategies, and this possibility should be tested with clinical trials. However, it does not necessarily answer the question of "true" schizotypy; it may instead create an artificial division that blinds us to a "true" overlap between the disorders, which may be based in similar neurochemical or psychosocial pathogenic processes. In an attempt to "carve nature at the joints," we must avoid the temptation to invent artificial joints at which to carve.

Despite these weaknesses, one strength of the clinical approach that has potential for further development is in the more general issue of comorbidity. These studies are particularly enlightening when they go outside the constructs themselves to examine other scales or symptoms that co-occur with SPD or BPD differentially. For example, Rosenberger and Miller (1989) reported a higher rate of drug abuse and affective disorder in BPD subjects compared to the SPD subjects. Serper et al. (1993), in addition to the MMPI findings discussed above, determined that high hostility, as measured by the Buss–Durkee Hostility Inventory, may be a critical indicator separating BPD patients from schizotypals. Further studies are needed that utilize these external variables, ranging from hostility to substance use to depressive symptomatology. In addition, demographic factors such as gender and ethnicity also need to be examined across settings. Such studies can give us a better picture of whom the mental health service tends to encounter under the label "schizotypal."

Biological studies

Given the biological revolution in the schizophrenia literature over the last 25 years, it is not surprising that most of the research on SPD has explored the biological properties of schizotypy. Consequently, the majority of the contributions to this volume are biological or inspired by the biopsychosocial paradigm. These chapters are too richly packed to be summarized here; in this section, we highlight the key issues addressed and approaches employed.

Genetics studies

The first major biological approach to the definition of schizotypy comes from genetics studies. Researchers in this tradition attempt to identify and isolate schizotypy by examining which symptoms have increased prevalence in the first-degree relatives of schizophrenics. This effort attempts to identify empirically which traits are phenotypic manifestations of the "core" schizophrenic deficit(s). As reviewed by Ingraham (Chapter 2, this volume), most (but not quite all) studies of the relatives of schizophrenics have confirmed the increased prevalence of schizotypy, variously defined. Further, several of these studies have converged on the so-called negative symptoms, or social–interpersonal deficits, as being the critical items contributing to the results.

Two lingering questions must be addressed by future family, twin, and adoption studies, however. The first concerns the specificity of these findings, given the increased prevalence of social difficulties and schizotypy in some familial studies of affective disorders. A recent study addressing this issue (Torgersen et al., 1993) indicates that excessive social anxiety, in particular, may have the highest sensitivity and specificity for identifying relatives of schizophrenics as compared to relatives of depressed probands. An additional problem comes from the lack of strong evidence finding an increased rate of schizophrenia in the relatives of schizotypals. Some have interpreted this as a strike against the genetic theory of schizotypy or that the data support the multifactorial theory over the single-locus or mixed model (Ritsner, Karas, & Ginath, 1992). Because of the low base-rate nature of schizophrenia, however, more studies are needed and the data pooled together to be sure that the weakness of these findings is not spurious.

Machon et al. (Chapter 3, this volume) take a novel approach to validating schizotypy in relation to schizophrenia. These researchers compared the prevalence of schizotypal symptomatology in several birth cohorts of schizophrenics. One cohort had been exposed to a severe influenza virus in the second trimester of gestation, while the remaining cohorts served as controls for trimester of exposure and season of birth. Traitlike suspiciousness and paranoia were found to be significantly elevated in the second-trimester-exposed cohort, even after positive schizophrenic symptoms and delusions had been factored out. Further, those rated as chronically suspicious and exposed in the second trimester had a notably higher incidence of schizophrenia. The authors suggest that these results indicate that chronic suspiciousness, as distinguished from discrete paranoid delusions, represent the symptomatic expression of the "core" neurodevelopmental disruption that underlies the risk for schizophrenia. As the authors note, this hypothesis must now be tested by expanding the research base to include nonschizophrenics exposed to the virus at the critical period. Generalizability from this study, however, is uncertain; it is unclear whether virus-exposed schizophrenics are representative of schizophrenics in general or represent a distinct subgroup.

Biological markers

The remainder of biological research into the nature of schizotypy works from the assumption that there is some genetic link to schizophrenia. Much of it follows on the heels of biological investigations into schizophrenia, which have sought biological markers of the presumed neuronal pathophysiology of schizophrenia. Since such research is etiological in nature, the goal is to identify stable traits that are not merely the by-products of the disease or state-dependent indices of current symptomatology, but rather are present irrespective of the waxing and waning of symptoms.

Much biological research in schizotypy seeks to provide validation for these markers by investigating subjects who putatively carry the genetically based deficit but who lack outright psychosis. Thus, schizotypal research is an important window onto schizophrenia, for such research overcomes the well-known confounds and obstacles of schizophrenia research. These include the difficulties of maintaining and assessing motivation and task-focus in actively symptomatic patients. In addition, the effects on dependent measures of neuroleptic medication and institutionalization (often long-term), which serve as a confound in studies of schizophrenics, are generally not an issue for schizotypal subjects. Furthermore, replication in schizotypals of deficits found in schizophrenics lends additional support to the hypothesis that such deficits are genetically based etiological factors and not simply by-products of the disease state.

In this volume, six chapters focus primarily on examining a variety of putative markers at three different "levels" of psychobiological analysis: (1) biological indicators such as homovanillic acid levels in the blood; (2) psychophysiological responses such as startle eye-blink modification, eye movements, and electrodermal responding; and (3) neuropsychological performance on tasks of memory, attention, and executive functions, as well as lateralized brain asymmetries (see, in this volume, Siever, Chapter 12; Dawson et al., Chapter 11; Holzman et al., Chapter 15; Raine et al., Chapter 10; Lencz et al., Chapter 13; Gruzelier, Chapter 14, respectively). Each of these research areas has a long history of investigation in schizophrenic subjects, and the studies presented in these chapters take the research one step further, with very promising results. In many cases, the results are so rich, that it is more difficult than expected to identify the "core" deficit.

For example, Raine et al. (Chapter 10), in their review of the literature on skin conductance orienting responses and schizotypy, demonstrated that previously published studies have provided evidence of three disparate relationships: (1) decreased responsivity related to "negative" symptoms (e.g., anhedonia); (2) decreased responsivity related to presence of "positive" schizotypal symptoms (e.g., perceptual aberrations); and (3) increased responding related to "positive" features of schizotypy. The new results reported by Raine et al. suggest a fourth possibility: that schizotypals are marked by an abnormal pattern of responding in which orienting increases, rather than habituates, over the first three trials. Raine et al. suggested that one cause of this discrepancy may be the difference in scales used to identify schizotypy. For example, the new results were the first in the area to utilize DSM-III-R diagnosed schizotypals, as opposed to subjects scoring high on self-report measures. However, even studies using the same scales achieved discrepant results. Perhaps the most significant aspect of the new study reported by Raine et al. is that it examined a different dependent measure – pattern of habituation – rather than an aggregate level of responding. This study therefore added the dimension of time, and revealed that schizotypals show a different pattern of changes over time in response to a stimulus as compared to controls.

Similar to Raine et al. in their literature review, Lencz et al. (in Chapter 13) found a variety of deficits reported in published studies of neuropsychological performance in schizotypals. Given the original purpose of such studies, the wide array of positive results almost constitutes an embarrassment of riches. It has been extremely important to the validation of the very concept of schizotypy (as the schizophrenia phenotype) to confirm that populations defined as schizotypal or psychosis prone share similar neurocognitive deficits to schizophrenics and their first-degree relatives. The number of studies reporting such deficits lends strong support to the general notion that schizotypy and schizophrenia share a similar neurocognitive, and presumably genetic, basis. In addition, each study provides specific external validation to the particular schizotypal symptoms under examination, which have ranged from positive, cognitive–perceptual symptoms to more negative, social–interpersonal deficits. However, the attempt at specification of the "core" deficit has been limited by the sheer volume of positive findings. As noted by Lencz et al., studies on schizophrenics have tended to show across-the-board deficits on tasks that exceed a threshold of difficulty (e.g., Spaulding, Garbin, & Dras, 1989), and the identification of differential deficits is rather difficult (Chapman & Chapman, 1973). Schizotypals, who show much more limited functional impairment compared to schizophrenics, have been expected to show circumscribed cognitive deficits as well.

Dawson et al. (Chapter 11) report a carefully designed study in an attempt to specify the affected components of information processing in schizotypals. These researchers sought to determine whether the deficit in information processing involves automatic, preconscious processing immediately after stimulus exposure; the alternate hypothesis posited that the key deficit involved consciously controlled attentional mechanisms. In order to compare these hypotheses, they designed two experimental protocols involving the modification of the startle eye-blink response by presentation of stimuli prior to the blink-eliciting stimulus. Subjects scoring high on the Chapmans' scales of psychosis proneness showed significantly less prepulse modification when instructed to attend to the prepulse. Dawson et al. concluded that the deficit, therefore, lay in controlled (active) processing. But these authors cite another study (Cadenhead, Geyer, & Braff, 1993), which found deficits in schizotypals in a passive (automatic processing) paradigm. However, these studies are difficult to compare because they utilized different methodology as well as employed different subject selection strategies; Cadenhead et al. examined DSM-diagnosed schizotypals. Further research is needed to control for these factors.

One final interesting question to emerge from the results discussed by Dawson et al. is the issue of specificity. One of the prerequisites for a biological marker for a disorder is that the deficit be specific to members of that group. By definition, a marker is supposed to mark members of one diagnostic group to the exclusion of others. However, Dawson et al. note that startle eye-blink modification is not specific to the schizophrenia spectrum. Still, this research avenue can be useful, insofar as the other disorders (e.g., Huntington's disease) with this indicator have more well-known neuropathology. An examination of these areas of overlap with other disorders may help us to map the affected neurocircuitry underlying schizophrenia and schizotypy.

Another specific theory attempting to map the neurocircuitry hypothesizes that the core of both schizotypy and schizophrenia are frontal lobe deficits, whereas schizophrenics have additional impairments in limbic circuitry (Walker & Gale, Chapter 4). Some support for this model is provided by studies showing that schizotypals have increased perseverative errors on the Wisconsin Card Sorting Task (WCST) and increased errors on the Continuous Performance Test (reviewed in Lencz et al., Chapter 13), as well as increased prevalence of deficits in delayed response memory (Holzman et al., Chapter 15). All of these tasks have been shown to be sensitive to frontal damage in studies of brain-lesioned patients as well as functional neuroimaging studies. However, schizotypals have also been shown to have poorer verbal memory (Lencz et al.; Gruzelier, Chapters 13 and 14) and decreased latent inhibition (Claridge & Beech; Lencz et al., Chapters 9 and 13), which have been linked to temporal and limbic deficits (Lencz et al., 1992; Venables, 1992).

What makes model testing so difficult at this juncture is that almost all published studies to date look at only one dependent measure or several tests of the same construct (e.g., frontal deficits). At the same time, it is not always clear if two measures purporting to tap the same construct are in fact the same. For example, Lencz et al. (Chapter 13) cite studies in which two measures of frontal deficits (Stroop interference and negative priming) are significantly correlated with each other, but only one is significantly correlated with schizotypy.

Consequently, multitrait, multimethod studies are needed in order to tease out differential deficits. For example, a study testing the hypothesis of Walker and Gale (Chapter 4) would require that schizotypals be tested both with a few frontal tasks such as the Wisconsin Card Sort and with tests that have been empirically validated as tapping temporolimbic functioning. One such task is the Wechsler Memory Scale logical memory section (prose passages); the percent retention index has been shown to be strongly correlated with hippocampal pathology (Lencz et al., 1992; Sass et al., 1992). As noted above, several tests tapping each proposed deficit would be ideal for honing in on the core processes.

This dissociation of deficits can be attempted at this time only retrospectively by reviewing the literature from several different labs. For example, Lencz et al. (Chapter 13) reviewed the literature on tasks of cerebral hemispheric asymmetries in schizotypy. By examining the pattern of deficits across studies, the review indicated that an abnormality in the process of interhemispheric transfer of information provided a better fit to the total pool of data compared to theories of unilateral hemispheric over- or underactivation.

The difficulty of comparing results across different studies, however, comes from differences in subject selection. Studies of schizotypy differ in their subject selection along at least three dimensions, which tend to confound comparison of results. The first is the population from which the schizotypal subjects are drawn, ranging from severely dysfunctional inpatients to relatives of schizophrenics to volunteers from the general population to college undergraduates. These different types of subjects are likely to present with different symptom severity, and the meaning of various diagnostic criteria may well be dissimilar. For example, magical thinking in an undergraduate may be as benign as an overly uncritical belief in the dormitory ouija board, while an inpatient rated as having magical beliefs may be verging on psychotic delusions.

Secondly, studies vary as to which instruments are used to rate schizotypal symptoms. Some utilize clinical interviews of DSM-III-R items, but most employ self-report questionnaires which tend to tap only one set of schizotypal traits, such as the cognitive–perceptual distortions tapped by the STA or the Perceptual Aberrations scale. Finally, studies differ in their statistical approach: Some examine group differences between diagnosed schizotypals or high scorers on scales and "normal" controls, whereas others employ correlational techniques, examining the relationship between schizotypy and biological variables across a full spectrum of unselected subjects. This distinction is not merely statistical; it has theoretical implications relating to the categorical and dimensional models described above. Selection of subjects and methods may artificially skew the results toward one interpretation or the other, or may blind researchers to possible results available from the other method. In the future, researchers should explicitly address competing models and definitions of schizotypy by comparing the results across several subject pools and methodologies.

An intriguing empirical example of this need comes from two studies recently conducted by Raine and colleagues (Benishay, Raine, & Lencz, 1994; Raine, Lencz, Scerbo, Reynolds, Redmon, Brodish, Bird, Kim, & Triphon, 1991). These studies examined the relationship between schizotypy and perseverative errors on the WCST. Both studies utilized undergraduate volunteers, who were initially screened with the SPQ and then administered items from the schizotypal section of the SCID diagnostic interview. The difference was that the first study was based on the categorical model, whereas the second employed the dimensional approach. In the first study (Raine et al., 1991), 14 subjects who were diagnosed with DSM-III-R schizotypal personality disorder were compared to 32 subjects who were not schizotypal and had scored in the bottom 10% of all students on the SPQ. There were no significant differences between the groups on perseverative errors or any other measure derived from the WCST.

In the second study (Benishay, Raine, & Lencz, 1994), correlational analyses were used to compare WCST performance and schizotypal scores from the SCID. This design permitted separate analyses for each of three symptom factors: cognitive–perceptual abnormalities, social–interpersonal deficits, and disorganized behavior. Social–interpersonal symptoms were significantly correlated with perseverative errors (Spearman's rho = 0.28; $p = 0.04$).

Interestingly, this latter study had fewer subjects ($n = 39$) as compared to the first. Therefore, statistical power was not a likely explanation for the difference in findings. Importantly, none of the subjects in the latter study met DSM criteria for the diagnosis of SPD. Nevertheless, a significant effect of schizotypy was found. Thus, the comparison lends support to the dimensional model of schizotypy; as noted by Gangestad and Snyder (1985), if a true underlying dimensionality exists, a group difference design will lose potential variance and impede the discovery of significant results. (Conversely, if a true taxon exists, use of a correlational design will increase error variance, thereby decreasing the possibility of a significant finding.)

Biological studies and factor analysis

This comparison of studies also draws our attention to the emerging evidence that schizotypy is not a monolithic construct, but rather composed of several factors. The three factors mentioned above have been replicated in a variety of studies reviewed by Venables (Chapter 6); this factor structure is also confirmed by the new data reported by Gruzelier (Chapter 14). The new data reported by Venables also alert us to the possibility that there may be additional factors, such as anhedonia, that are not part of the DSM criteria that were the basis of the factor analysis of Raine et al. (1994). As Venables notes, however, factor analysis can be very sensitive to the items selected for inclusion, and does not necessarily confirm that any particular items are an essential part of the hypothesized construct. Other forms of validation are needed for each hypothesized factor.

Venables's chapter also illustrates how the three-factor model of schizotypy bears many similarities to recent studies demonstrating three factors underlying schizophrenia. This similarity implies that schizotypal researchers must take into account the issues that have emerged concerning the factors of schizophrenia. For example, future studies of biological markers must be very clear about which symptoms are under consideration, and should look for dissociations between symptom clusters. Two different types of symptoms may have different, or even opposite, neurocognitive correlates. For example, the new data reported by Gruzelier (Chapter 14) indicate that a left hemisphere bias is found in subjects scoring high on measures of disorganized schizotypal symptoms (odd speech and behavior), whereas subjects scoring high on a scale of social–interpersonal deficits were marked by a right hemisphere processing bias.

A second implication concerns the etiologic relationship between these factors. One possibility, suggested by the historical division noted earlier in this chapter, is that there are two or more different disorders that have been, at various times, labeled schizotypy. Thus, there may be "schizotypies," just as some have suggested that there are several schizophrenias (e.g., Heinrichs, 1993). Another possibility is that these represent multiple etiopathophysiologies which interact to produce the observable pathology of schizotypal personality disorder. Such a theory would be consonant with an integration of the categorical and dimensional viewpoints discussed above. It may be that the individual traits of schizotypy are normally distributed throughout the population, but combine synergistically to produce a full-blown clinical disorder. An analogy to this synergistic process is the action potential of a neuronal membrane; membrane potentials vary "dimensionally" within a certain range, but then quickly spike to a different range (an action potential) when a critical threshold is reached, owing to positive feedback loops.

Siever (Chapter 12) suggests that cognitive aberrations and interpersonal deficits represent separable clinical syndromes with separable pathophysiologies. He reports his research demonstrating that hypodopaminergia in the frontal cortex is related to deficit-like, social–interpersonal symptoms, whereas hyperdopaminergia in the limbic/subcortical region is found in patients with psychotic-like symptoms. In a number of cases, the upregulation of subcortical dopamine metabolism may be a secondary reaction to frontal reductions in dopamine. If and when these two symptoms interact with an individual predisposition toward sensitivity to dopamine, the result is the pattern of symptoms observed in schizophrenia.

Thus, at least three models can be specified to describe the relationship among factors of schizotypal personality: (1) They may be completely separate entities thrown together by historical accident; (2) they may be separate dimensional traits which interact to form a categorical clinical syndrome; or (3) they may be separable but related syndromes which combine to produce schizophrenia. It is also possible that some symptoms are more important than others; that is, some may represent "core" features that are necessary but not sufficient for the disorder, whereas others are more nonspecific vulnerability factors. Zubin (1985) went so far as to suggest that premorbid personality variables are independent factors that interact with the vulnerability for schizophrenia but are not constitutive of that vulnerability; they do not represent a "core" to schizophrenia. Of course, this begs the question of whether or not there is a categorical "core" to the disorder, and what the meaning of the word "core" is here. Meehl (1990) would say that the core is that part which shares the same major gene as schizophrenia. Another, more clinical, framework might suggest that the core symptoms are those that are most specific to the disorder, or respond to a specific treatment. It is also possible that the prototypic nosological system of DSM best describes the situation: There is no single core.

Future research needs to test these hypotheses at both the clinical/phenomenological level and the physiological/neurocognitive level. Longitudinal studies are needed to examine the evolution of the clinical presentation of schizotypal symptoms. For example, does the presence of cognitive and perceptual aberrations in childhood result in difficulties in interacting with others? Are social–interpersonal deficits secondary to cognitive deficits, or vice versa? Or is there no systematic relationship between the two over time? Similarly, researchers should examine whether there are systematic relationships at the biological level, such as the dopaminergic mechanism that Siever (Chapter 12) proposes that links negative and positive symptoms.

Pleiotropy and the interpretation of marker studies

A possible confound to interpreting factor structure and biological marker studies is the pleiotropy hypothesis suggested by Holzman et al. (Chapter 15).

This theory states that while there may be a single major gene underlying both schizophrenia and schizotypal personality, the gene may take on a variety of different phenotypic manifestations. These researchers make the analogy to neurofibromatosis, which leads to the distinctive tumorous lesions only in a minority of those who carry the gene; most gene carriers can show a variety of lesser symptoms. This theory poses a problem for researchers investigating biological correlates of schizotypy, insofar as individuals possessing the gene may show schizotypal symptoms, or eye tracking deficits, or neurocognitive deficits, or any combination of the above. Thus, the biological markers, although linked genetically to schizotypal traits, may appear separate from those traits in a given research subject or pool of subjects. This hypothesis can be extended by further breaking down the schizotypal clinical symptoms into subsyndromes, which may be disparate manifestations of the same genotype. This heterogeneity of expression may account for the high degree of variance reported in the studies of Holzman et al. (Chapter 15), as well as Dawson et al. (Chapter 11). On the other hand, the strong convergence of findings pointing toward frontal lobe deficits does not support this theory. Still, this possibility can be taken into account in designing studies in at least three possible ways: (1) Studies should be designed to test the same subjects on a variety of different markers, with the prediction that partially overlapping subsets of schizotypals will show physiological abnormalities; (2) relatively large sample sizes should be employed in the expectation of modest yet robust findings; (3) statistical tests of variance or dispersion of subjects should be performed to test the hypothesis that the schizotypal group shows a broader range of scores. It should be noted that the above suggestions assume a group difference approach, as this theory is a refinement of the categorical approach of Meehl.

Longitudinal pathways

A final consideration that may confound the interpretation of findings in biological studies is one that has been underexamined in the literature, namely temporal issues of stability and long-term development of schizotypy. Since schizotypal personality is widely viewed as a stable, lifelong mode of personality organization, a tacit assumption of the literature is that schizotypal features and correlates do not change much over time. In this volume, however, Gruzelier (Chapter 14) has demonstrated that the short-term effects of test anxiety can have an effect on the relationship between schizotypal symptom factors and their correlates in cerebral hemispheric activity. Specifically, he reported that test anxiety reversed the normal asymmetry in which left hemisphere processes are dominant. This mimicked the relationship between social–interpersonal deficits and hemispheric asymmetry, and abolished the significant relationship between disorganized symptoms and left hemisphere dominance.

Siever, Kalus, and Keefe (1993) also call attention to the role of affective lability in the expression of schizotypal symptoms. These investigators note that borderline patients can show schizotypal-like symptoms of cognitive distortions under conditions of high stress or affective lability. They emphasize the need to assess symptomatology over time to ensure that reported symptoms are traitlike and not simply state-dependent. As with the Gruzelier findings, this point also underscores the importance for future biological researchers to confirm their results using retesting of the same subjects.

One potentially complicating factor, however, is the inherent instability of some schizotypal characteristics, such as perceptual distortions and ideas of reference. While theoretically traitlike and occurring repeatedly over the lifespan, they can wax and wane over time, depending on conditions of stress and other factors. Indeed, some researchers have suggested that instability and cognitive lability and dysregulation are an intrinsic component of the schizotypal syndrome (Claridge, 1993, personal communication). If this is true, then retesting schizotypal subjects may not prove to be an effective means of identifying brain–behavior relationships. Rather, some test of dispersion or change over time would be needed. The new results reported by Raine et al. (Chapter 10), provide a good example of how an examination of change over time can shed new light on previous studies with conflicting results. This finding highlights the importance of the word "process" in the oft-used phrase "information processing."

While the aforementioned researchers emphasized short-term fluctuations in state, long-term developmental issues are also of interest in schizotypy. As noted earlier, research should be conducted to examine the dynamic interaction of symptoms and brain deficits over time, to address whether some symptoms are primary whereas others are secondary or compensatory. To name just one possible example, it could be hypothesized that unusual speech and behavior are the "core" symptoms, leading to difficulty in social situations, interpersonal anxiety, and a retreat into fantasy, paranoia, and ideas of reference. Alternately, plausible scenarios could be constructed with any permutation of this sequence. To test these competing scenarios, researchers must track these symptom features longitudinally from childhood to early adulthood. Walker and Gale (Chapter 4) provide some hypotheses concerning the motoric abnormalities that might be expected in schizotypal children. Future longitudinal research can test their neurodevelopmental hypothesis at both physiological and behavioral levels.

Relationship to schizophrenia

Discussion of longitudinal development inevitably leads to a consideration of the longitudinal relationship between schizotypy and schizophrenia. One of the major goals of schizotypal research is to identify individuals at risk for schizophrenia and understand the mechanism of psychotic breakdown. Unfortunately, the field has not had sufficient time to conduct many longitudinal studies required to examine this hypothesis. Chapman, Chapman, and Kwapil (Chapter 5) report that the Chapman scale of Magical Ideation is predictive of later psychosis. Contrary to predictions, however, this effect was not specific for schizophrenic psychosis, nor did it hold for the other scales of putative psychosis proneness. Given the low base-rate nature of schizophrenia, follow-up data are needed on many more subjects in order to judge the validity of the hypothesis.

Even if schizotypals do not become schizophrenic, much can be learned from longitudinal research. Specifically, research is needed to examine those cognitive and physiological measures on which schizotypals do not show deficits or abnormalities. Such measures may serve as protective factors – that is, specific strengths of a schizotypal that maintain a stable, compensated personality structure. For example, one hypothesized protective factor is IQ (Venables, 1989). It has been suggested that schizotypals with a high IQ are able to process and mediate the cognitive dysregulation, directing it toward creativity rather than psychosis.

The challenges to this area of research are twofold. First, they must identify robust effects, so that nonsignificant findings due to lack of experimental power are not overinterpreted as protective factors. Second, the assumptions underlying the notion of protective factors must be tested. The critical assumption is that schizotypy and schizophrenia share the same genetic basis (single or multiple genes), and that schizophrenics have some extra factor(s) that push(es) them into psychosis. While many researchers would agree with this model, other models have been proposed. For example, Holzman's pleiotropy model posits that all manifestations of the essential genotype, from eye movement abnormalities to schizotypy to schizophrenia, are equipotential rather than cumulative. That is, one person may have eye movement impairments and schizotypy, whereas another may have schizotypy and memory deficits, and so on. Walker and Gale (Chapter 4) suggest that there may be some forms of schizotypy that are "terminal," that is, they are the end point of a pathophysiological process that is unrelated to schizophrenic etiology. This "terminal SPD" is similar to the model of phenocopies described by Meehl (1990). For these models, the assumptions underlying the search for protective factors do not hold.

As noted above, most of the literature on neurocognitive studies of schizotypy have looked for deficits in schizotypals analogous to those in schizophrenics to support the hypothesis that such deficits are genetically linked and not the result of psychosis, medication, or institutionalization. From this perspective, the lack of deficits in schizotypals may be interpreted as a potential protective factor. However, it is possible that schizotypals may show neurocognitive performance that reveals neither deficits nor protective factors. In two contributions to this volume (Claridge & Beech; Lencz et al., Chapters 9 and 13), data are presented which suggest that schizotypy may be related to *superior* performance on certain tasks of priming, incidental learning, and cerebral hemispheric processing. These authors do not suggest that these data reflect protective factors in the schizotypals. Rather, they interpret them as revealing an underlying dimension of neurophysiological organization that results in an inverted-U pattern of performance.

By this model, neurocognitive performance factors such as cognitive disinhibition may increase as one moves along a spectrum from normality through schizotypy to schizophrenia. In schizotypals, cognitive disinhibition may have relatively benign effects, actually improving performance on tasks of incidental learning and producing nonpsychotic cognitive–perceptual symptoms. As this disinhibition increases in schizophrenics, its effects become malignant, resulting in cognitive overload, poor performance on tests, and psychotic symptomatology.

Other methodological issues

We have seen how the assumptions made about the relationship between schizotypy and schizophrenia can have effects on research design and interpretation of results. Two other methodological issues can be extrapolated from the schizophrenia literature and should be applied to schizotypy research: sex differences and comorbidity with substance abuse. Neuroimaging studies, which have increased exponentially in the schizophrenia literature, will also be discussed as an important future direction for schizotypy research.

Schizophrenia research has revealed that females and males may demonstrate differences in the rate, transmission, and expression of schizophrenia (e.g., Goldstein, Tsuang, & Faraone, 1989). Females tend to show less genetic transmission of schizophrenia, and a more acute onset with fewer premorbid symptoms compared to male schizophrenics. This hypothesis is supported by Claridge and Hewitt's (1987) finding of a decreased heritability for schizotypy in females as compared to males. It may be that in males, the schizotypy construct reveals root antecedents of the schizophrenic syndrome(s), whereas for females, high schizotypy may be caused by social/environmental factors that are not reflected in neurocognitive studies. Further research, comparing male and female schizotypals both with and without schizophrenic relatives, is required to examine this hypothesis. From this analysis, it would be predicted that female schizotypals would have fewer schizophrenic relatives, but those who did would show performance abnormalities similar to those of male schizotypals. In any event, researchers cannot assume that male and female schizotypals will have the same biological correlates, and research reviewed by Lencz et al. (Chatper 13) indicates that males are more likely to show significant abnormalities.

Researchers should also bear in mind that schizotypal symptoms may have different pathognomonic significance for the two sexes insofar as females in the general population tend to show relatively higher levels of self-report cognitive–perceptual aberrations, whereas males show higher levels of social–interpersonal deficits (Raine, 1992). Thus, a female SPD patient with high levels of social–interpersonal symptomatology may have a higher degree of pathology than a male with the same degree of symptomatology, and vice versa.

Biological research into schizophrenia has also had to grapple with the fact that schizophrenics have an increased incidence of some forms of substance abuse (Mueser et al., 1990). Recent evidence collected in our lab indicates that this is also true of schizotypals drawn from a general community sample. In our current work, we are examining subjects from temporary employment agencies, using the SPQ as a screening instrument. Those scoring in the top and bottom percentiles of SPQ scores receive a full DSM-III-R clinical interview using the SCID. We have found that 81% of those scoring above the cutoff score on the SPQ receive a diagnosis of SPD. However, approximately 50% of these diagnosed schizotypals meet DSM-III-R criteria for past or present substance dependence. This provides a potential confound to studies examining neuropsychological and psychophysiological performance. One approach is to eliminate subjects with significant substance abuse. However, such an approach may sacrifice ecological validity, insofar as half of schizotypals would be excluded; the resulting subject pool may not be a representative sample of schizotypals. Drug use may play a significant etiological role for many schizotypals; for example, cocaine or amphetamine use may increase sensitivity to dopamine, thereby increasing positive symptoms. On the other hand, the inclusion of substance-abusing subjects obscures the etiological source of biological deficits. An alternative approach is to covary this factor out by use of statistical techniques; however, this approach may also sacrifice validity (Lord, 1969). Future studies are needed to confirm the increased prevalence of substance abuse disorders associated with schizotypal personality; if prevalence is as high as 50%, then marker studies should divide schizotypal samples into two groups and compare them with abuse-positive and -negative controls.

Finally, neuroimaging is a rapidly growing field that will prove extremely useful in identifying brain structure–function relationships in schizotypals (Flaum & Andreasen, Chapter 16; Gur & Gur, Chapter 17). A search of the MEDLINE periodical database for the years 1991–3 reveals 219 articles on schizophrenia and brain imaging, as compared to one study (Raine, Sheard, Reynolds, & Lencz, 1992) found under the key words "schizotypal personality" and "brain imaging." Raine et al. (1929) found negative correlations between schizotypy, as measured by the STA (primarily positive symptoms), and frontal lobe size. Future MRI studies are needed to replicate and extend these findings to important brain regions such as the hippocampus and corpus callosum. Functional imaging (such as positron emission tomography and fats MRI), can identify which areas of the brain are activated during task performance. The combination of structural and functional brain imaging available with the fast MRI technique (Alper, 1993) will allow future researchers to map affected cortical pathways involved with task performance in marker studies. Undoubtedly, imaging studies will proliferate in schizotypal research over the next 10 years.

Conclusions

A survey of the state of schizotypal research today reveals a surprising diversity of conceptualizations of the disorder and methodological approaches for studying it. The field is still very young, with some promising research avenues having only one or two published studies available for consideration. Current controversies in the parent discipline, schizophrenia, spill over into schizotypal research, opening up such difficult issues as heterogeneity and factor structure.

Given the complexity of the issues concerning the nature of schizotypy and the limited information we have accumulated to date, there is no singular answer to the question, What is schizotypy? Rather, we should consider that the term "schizotypal personality" denotes an open concept (Pap, 1953). An open concept is a "black box" that is known only through its relation to other, more operationalized concepts in a nomological network. The goal of research is to slowly encroach on the boundaries of the black box to reduce the proportion of the unknown to the known. In the specific case of schizotypy, operationalized elements of the nomological network include, for example, the oft-demonstrated relationship between decreased negative priming and Claridge's STA. The underlying construct that is being tapped, however, still remains open to debate and further research.

Currently, the boundaries of the concept are large enough to accommodate research approaching the box from different angles and using different research paradigms: for example, those applying a psychiatric, categorical diagnostic approach as opposed to those utilizing dimensional, psychometric means of identifying schizotypy. It is possible that this process will reveal that there are several discriminable phenomena that have all been labeled "schizotypy," owing to some substantial overlap or by historical accident. Indeed, this possibility already has some support, given (1) the historical dichotomy noted previously, (2) the multiplicity and divergence of findings from a variety of studies, and (3) the current evidence concerning the heterogeneity of schizophrenia (e.g., Heinrichs, 1993).

The most important purpose of exploring this open concept is not to lead to a final, definitive answer to the question, What is schizotypy? Rather, the primary goals of this research are defined by the particular instrumental ends of the research team/community. For example, some researchers may seek as their primary goal the discovery of genetic markers for schizophrenia. These researchers would examine schizotypy in a different context than researchers in a clinical setting examining efficacy of drug treatment for schizotypal personality disorder. Researchers in the former category would need to examine differences between schizotypals with and without schizophrenic relatives; the latter might be dealing with a much more severe disorder and be concerned with overlap with borderline personality disorder. Thus, the context of the researcher changes the nomological network that surrounds the open concept of schizotypy. As Millon (1991, p. 245, referring also to Schwartz, 1991) notes:

> In the desire to discover the essential order of nature, one is concerned with but a few of the infinite number of elements that may be chosen, and one's choices are narrowed only to those aspects of nature that may best answer the questions that are posed. The concepts and categories that scientists construct are only optional tools to guide the observation and interpretation of the natural world; different concepts and categories may be formulated as alternatives to understanding the same subject of inquiry.

This quote calls our attention to the constructive element in any formulation of the definition of a psychopathology; researchers and clinicians, guided by their own interests as well as the data, construct the boundaries of a disorder in order to answer the questions that are most relevant to them.

Given the essential role of contructivism in the investigation of psychopathology, researchers must be very clear as to the assumptions and contextual needs that are driving their research. Researchers of schizotypal personality, in particular, must justify their use of the particular definition they employ. As shown above, the use of correlational approaches to biological markers can lead to different results as compared to studies with the group difference approach. Interpretation of results in any given study is limited to the particular methodology and measures employed; generalization to an overarching concept of "schizotypy" cannot be made without further experimentation.

This chapter has shown how interpretation of results across studies can be confounded by the use of different instruments. The generalizability of results of future studies of schizotypal personality would be aided by the casting of a wide net. Where possible, researchers should utilize the multitrait, multimethod design (Campbell & Fiske, 1959) to test the convergence of different constructions of schizotypy. In addition, we would recommend adding the elements of "multisubject, multianalysis" design, entailing comparison of results on subjects from different sources (relatives of schizophrenics, hospitals, undergraduates), as well as of different statistical approaches (correlational, group differences, tests of dispersion). Future schizotypal researchers may find it fruitful to utilize an unconventional mixed design, in which three groups of subjects are selected: (1) a group of diagnosed schizotypals, (2) a control group without schizotypal symptoms, and (3) a randomly selected group with varying degrees of symptomatology. The first two groups can be utilized for group differences comparisons, while the third group can be the source of correlational analyses.

A final goal for future schizotypal research is the development of etiological models. To date, most researchers have tacitly subsumed the etiology of schizotypy under the etiology of schizophrenia. These assumptions have been based primarily on the classic diathesis–stress model, in which a relatively static vulnerability interacts with discrete stressors to produce schizophrenia. This model has immensely added to our knowledge of schizophrenia, and research into schizotypy can help clarify and articulate the link. A number of contributors to this volume have suggested possibilities at the genetic level (Holzman et al., Chapter 15), the neurodevelopmental level (Machon et al., Chapter 3), the neurobiological level (Siever; Walker & Gale, Chapters 12 and 4), and the phenomonological level (Claridge & Beech, Chapter 9).

In pursuing etiological models, future schizotypal research may benefit from theoretical advances made in biosocial research of other disorders. The traditional diathesis–stress model is an *interactional* model in which the elements are conceived as being relatively discrete and static. Current developments in other personality disorders point toward biosocial *transactional* models, in which genetics and environment reciprocally determine each other dynamically over time (Scarr & McCartney, 1983). In such a model, the child's genetically determined temperament is seen as eliciting a particular type of parenting environment, which in turn reinforces some elements of that temperament and punishes others, and so on. The individual is seen as an active creator of his or her environment, which in turn shapes the subsequent choices of the individual. According to the transactional model, the accretion of these choices over the course of time constitutes the individual's personality. Future research using a longitudinal biosocial approach will help shed light on these transactional etiological processes in schizotypal personality.

Acknowledgments

Research described in this chapter was supported by a National Institute of Mental Health (NIMH) Shared Instrumentation Grant by BRSG S07 RR07012-21 awarded by the Biomedical Research Support Group. In addition, the first author was supported by NIMH Grant MH10463-01.

The authors are grateful to Deana S. Benishay for her helpful comments.

References

Alper, J. (1993). Echo-planar MRI: Learning to read minds. *Science, 261,* 556.

American Psychiatric Association (1987). *Diagnostic and statistical manual of mental disorders,* 3rd edition, revised. Washington, D.C.: APA Press.

American Psychiatric Association (1994). *Diagnostic and statistical manual of mental disorders,* 4th edition, revised. Washington, D.C.: APA Press.

Benishay, D. S., Raine, A., & Lencz, T. (1994). Dissociations between neuropsychological impairments and factors of schizotypy. Manuscript in preparation.

Cadenhead, K. S., Geyer, M. A., & Braff, D. L. (1993). Impaired startle prepulse inhibition and habituation in patients with schizotypal personality disorder. *American Journal of Psychiatry, 150*(12), 1862–1867.

Campbell, D. T., & Fiske, D. W. (1959). Convergent and discriminant validation by the multitrait–multimethod matrix. *Psychological Bulletin, 56,* 81–105.

Chapman, L. J., & Chapman, J. P. (1973). Problems in the measurement of cognitive deficits. *Psychological Bulletin, 79,* 380–385.

Condray, R., & Steinhauer, S. R. (1992). Schizotypal personality disorder in individuals with and without schizophrenic relatives: Similarities and contrasts in neurocognitive and clinical functioning. *Schizophrenia Research, 7,* 33–41.

Claridge, G., & Hewitt, J. K. (1987). A biometrical study of schizotypy in a normal population. *Personality and Individual Differences, 8,* 303–312.

Earleywine, M., Dawson, M. E., & Hazlett, E. (1994). A MAXCOV-HITMAX study of the Chapmans' scales of psychosis-proneness. (Unpublished manuscript).

Eysenck, H. J. (1960). Classification and the problem of diagnosis. In H. J. Eysenck (Ed.), *Handbook of abnormal psychology.* London: Pitman.

Fowles, D. C. (1992). Schizophrenia: Diathesis–stress revisited. *Annual Review of Psychology, 43,* 303–336.

Gangestad, S., & Snyder, M. (1985). "To carve nature at its joints": On the existence of discrete classes of personality. *Psychological Review, 92,* 317–349.

Goldstein, J. M., Tsuang, M. T., & Faraone, S. V. (1989). Gender and schizophrenia: Understanding the heterogeneity of the illness. *Psychiatry Research, 27,* 243–253.

Gottesman, I. I., & Shields, J. (1982). *Schizophrenia, the epigenetic puzzle.* New York: Cambridge University Press.

Gunderson, J. G., Siever, L. J., & Spaulding, E. (1983). The search for a schizotype: Crossing the border again. *Archives of General Psychiatry, 40,* 15–22.

Heinrichs, R. W. (1993). Schizophrenia and the brain. Conditions for a neuropsychology of madness. *American Psychologist, 48*(3), 221–233.

Kendler, K. S. (1985). Diagnostic approaches to schizotypal personality disorder: A historical perspective. *Schizophrenia Bulletin, 11,* 538–553.

Kety, S. S. (1985). Schizotypal personality disorder: An operational definition of Bleuler's latent schizophrenia. *Schizophrenia Bulletin, 11,* 590–594.

Kety, S. S., Rosenthal, D., Wender, P. H., Schulsinger, F., & Jacobsen, B. (1975). Mental illness in the biological and adoptive families of adopted individuals who have become schizophrenic: A preliminary report based on psychiatric interviews. In R. R. Fieve, D. Rosenthal, & H. Brill (Eds.), *Genetic research in psychiatry* (pp. 147–165). Baltimore: Johns Hopkins University Press.

Kotsaftis, A., & Neale, J. M. (1993). Schizotypal personality disorder I: The clinical syndrome. *Clinical Psychology Review, 13,* 451–472.

Lencz, T., McCarthy, G., Bronen, R. A., Scott, T. M., Inserni, J. A., Sass, K. J., Novelly, R. A., Kim, J. H., & Spencer, D. D. (1992). Quantitative magnetic resonance imaging in temporal lobe epilepsy: Relationship to neuropathology and neuropsychological function. *Annals of Neurology, 31,* 629–637.

Loranger, A. W., Susman, V. L., Oldham, J. M., & Russakof, L. M. (1987). The Personality Disorder Examination: A preliminary report. *Journal of Personality Disorders, 1,* 1–13.

Lord, F. M. (1969). Statistical adjustments when comparing pre-existing groups. *Psychological Bulletin, 72,* 336–337.

Meehl, P. E. (1962). Schizotaxia, schizotypy, schizophrenia. *American Psychologist, 17,* 827–838

Meehl, P. E. (1973). MAXCOV-HITMAX: A taxonomic search method for loose genetic syndromes. In P. E. Meehl (Ed.), *Psychodiagnosis: Selected papers.* Minneapolis, Minn.: University of Minnesota.

Meehl, P. E. (1990). Toward an integrated theory of schizotaxia, schizotypy, and schizophrenia. *Journal of Personality Disorders, 4,* 1–99.

Millon, T. (1991). Classification of psychopathology: Rationale, alternatives, and standards. *Journal of Abnormal Psychology, 100,* 245–261.

Mueser, K. T., Yarnold, P. R., Levinson, D. F., Singh, H., Bellack, A. S., Kee, K., Morrison, R. L., & Yadalam, K. G. (1990). Prevalence of substance abuse in schizophrenia: Demographic and clinical correlates. *Schizophrenia Bulletin, 16,* 31–56.

Pap, A. (1953). Reduction-sentences and open concepts. *Methods, 5,* 3–30.

Raine, A. (1991). The SPQ: A scale for the assessment of schizotypal personality based on DSM-III-R criteria. *Schizophrenia Bulletin, 17,* 555–564.

Raine, A. (1992). Sex differences in schizotypal personality in a nonclinical population. *Journal of Abnormal Psychology, 101,* 361–364.

Raine, A., Lencz, T., Scerbo, A., Reynolds, C., Redmon, M., Brodish, S., Bird, L.,

Kim, D., & Triphon, N. (1991). Schizotypal personality: Factor structure, sex differences, psychiatric differences, handedness, genetics, psychophysiology, and neurophysiology. Poster presented at 1991 meeting of the Society for Research in Psychopathology. Cambridge, Mass.

Raine, A., Reynolds, C., Lencz, T., Scerbo, A., Triphon, N., & Kim, D. (1994). Cognitive–perceptual, interpersonal, and disorganized features of schizotypal personality. *Schizophrenia Bulletin, 20,* 191–201.

Raine, A., Sheard, C., Reynolds, G. P., & Lencz, T. (1992). Pre-frontal structural and functional deficits associated with individual differences in schizotypal personality. *Schizophrenia Research, 7,* 237–247.

Ritsner, M., Karas, S., & Ginath, Y. (1992). Relatedness of schizotypal personality to schizophrenic disorders: Multifactorial threshold model. *Journal of Psychiatric Research, 27,* 27–38.

Rosenberger, P. H., & Miller, G. A. (1989). Comparing borderline definitions: DSM-III borderline and schizotypal personality disorders. *Journal of Abnormal Psychology, 98,* 161–169.

Sass, K. J., Sass, A., Westerveld, M., Lencz, T., Novelly, R. A., Kim, J. H., & Spencer, D. D. (1992). Specificity in the correlation of verbal memory and hippocampal neuron loss: Dissociation of memory, language, and verbal intellectual ability. *Journal of Clinical and Experimental Neuropsychology, 14,* 662–672.

Scarr, S., & McCartney, K. (1983). How people make their own environments: A theory of genotype–environment effects. *Child Development, 54,* 424–435.

Schwartz, M. A. (1991). The nature and classification of the personality disorders: A re-examination of basic premises. *Journal of Personality Disorders, 5,* 25–30.

Serper, M. R., Bernstein, D. P., Maurer, G., Harvey, P. D., Horvath, T., Klar, H., Coccaro, E. F., & Siever, L. J. (1993). Psychological test profiles of patients with borderline and schizotypal personality disorders: Implications for DSM-IV. *Journal of Personality Disorders, 7,* 144–154.

Siever, L. J., Kalus, O. F., & Keefe, R. S. (1993). The boundaries of schizophrenia. *Psychiatric Clinics of North America, 16,* 217–244.

Spaulding, W., Garbin, C. P., & Dras, S. R. (1989). Cognitive abnormalities in schizophrenic patients and schizotypal college students. *Journal of Nervous and Mental Disease, 177,* 717–728.

Spitzer, R. L., Endicott, J., & Gibbon, M. (1979). Crossing the border into borderline personality and borderline schizophrenia. *Archives of General Psychiatry, 36,* 17–24.

Spitzer, R. L., Williams, J. B., & Gibbon, M. (1987). *Structured clinical interview for DSM-III-R personality disorders (SCID-II).* New York: New York State Psychiatric Institute, Biometrics Research.

Thaker, G., Moran, M., Cassady, S., Ross, D., & Adani, H. (1993). Eye movements in schizophrenia spectrum personality disorders: Familial vs. non-familial samples. (Abstract) *Schizophrenia Research, 9,* 168–169.

Torgersen, S., Onstad, S., Skre, I., Edvardsen, J., & Kringlen, E. (1993). "True" schizotypal personality disorder: A study of co-twins and relatives of schizophrenic probands. *American Journal of Psychiatry, 150,* 1661–1667.

Venables, P. H. (1989). The Emmanual Miller lecture 1987: Childhood markers for adult disorders. *Journal of Child Psychology and Psychiatry and Allied Disciplines, 30,* 347–364.

Venables, P. H. (1992). Hippocampal function and schizophrenia: Experimental psychological evidence. *Annals of the New York Academy of Sciences, 658,* 111–127.

Widiger, T. A., Frances, A., Spitzer, R. L., & Williams, J. B. (1988). The DSM-III-R personality disorders: An overview. *American Journal of Psychiatry, 145,* 786–795.

Widiger, T. A., Frances, A., & Trull, T. J. (1987a). A psychometric analysis of the social–interpersonal and cognitive–perceptual items for the schizotypal personality disorder. *Archives of General Psychiatry, 44,* 741–745.

Widiger, T. A., Frances, A., Warner, L., & Bluhm, C. (1986). Diagnostic criteria for the borderline and schizotypal personality disorders. *Journal of Abnormal Psychology, 95,* 43–51.

Widiger, T. A., Trull, T. J., Hurt, S. W., Clarkin, J. F., & Frances, A. (1987b). A multidimensional scaling of the DSM-III personality disorders. *Archives of General Psychiatry, 44,* 557–563.

Zubin, J. (1985). Negative symptoms: Are they indigenous to schizophrenia? *Schizophrenia Bulletin, 11,* 461–470.

PART IX
Appendix

Semistructured interviews for the measurement of schizotypal personality

DEANA S. BENISHAY and TODD LENCZ

It has been 15 years since the introduction of schizotypal personality disorder (SPD) as an official diagnostic entity in DSM-III (APA, 1980). In that time, a number of semistructured clinical interviews have been developed to assess for SPD. These interviews serve to complement the self-report instruments reviewed by Chapman et al. (Chapter 5, this volume); the clinical interview schedules, while significantly more time consuming, were designed in order to obtain more detailed and potentially more accurate information than self-report instruments. Specifically, the use of clinical interviews attempts to overcome false negatives related to a lack of self-awareness or defensiveness, as well as false positives due to misunderstanding on the part of subjects of the requirement that symptoms be longstanding.

In addition to these purposes, the observations of the interviewer can be used to rate directly the presence of schizotypal signs, which are supposed to be evident to an outside observer, as opposed to symptoms, which are problems reported by the subject. The three observable schizotypal signs listed in DSM-III-R (APA, 1987) include constricted or inappropriate affect, odd speech, and odd appearance or behavior. It should be noted that the ratings of the other six SPD symptoms in clinical interviews are based on "self-report," although this term is usually applied to paper-and-pencil questionnaires (Loranger, 1992). However, clinical interview measures allow the diagnostician to follow up on the subject's self-report, and to assess whether the subject properly understands the question – for example, by asking for concrete details or anecdotes. In this way, clinical interview measures have the potential to increase greatly the validity of clinical diagnosis.

The purpose of this appendix is to review briefly the interview schedules that include an assessment of SPD. We focus specifically on the research literature, reporting the reliability and internal validity of these instruments. We do not describe results pertaining to "external" validating variables such as biological correlates or neuropsychological deficits; the relation of these variables to interview-diagnosed schizotypy is described in Parts V, VI, and VII of this volume.

Before proceeding with the review, a few general points should be considered. First, there are two types of reliability that may be reported: test–retest and same-interview reliability methods (Grove, Andreasen, McDonald-Scott, Ketter, & Shapiro, 1981). In the test–retest method, the same subject is interviewed by two different experimenters on separate occasions, whereas in the same-interview method, the subject is interviewed by one experimenter while another either sits silently and observes, or observes tapes later on. The latter form of reliability is a scientifically more rigorous one, insofar as it involves two independent tests of the same phenomenon (the patient's clinical state). Additionally, the test–retest method contains more sources of error (Zimmerman, 1994). Specifically, in addition to differing in their diagnostic rating of the subjects' responses, the raters in a test–retest design may vary in the way in which they ask questions. Further, the subject's clinical state may change from one testing session to the other. Hypothetically, a time lag should not substantially alter the subject's presentation with respect to personality disorders, which are supposed to be composed of stable, lifelong traits. However, there is growing evidence that a person's mood can substantially affect his or her recall of previous life events (Kihlstrom, 1989). Therefore, studies of test–retest reliability are subject to the potential confound of change in clinical state, such as remission of depression, especially since most of the studies reported below were conducted on patient populations (Loranger et al., 1991).

Interpretation of the validity results must be tempered by an awareness of two possible sources of error other than the assessment instrument being tested. First, most studies compare interview results to self-report measures such as the Millon Clinical Multiaxial Inventory (MCMI) as a test of concurrent validity. However, the validity of such measures themselves is open to question; specifically, the MCMI is considered to have the tendency of overdiagnosing personality disorders (Loranger, 1992; Zimmerman, 1994). Second, since the clinical interviews are based on DSM-III and DSM-III-R criteria, the maximum validity (as well as reliability) of these instruments is bounded by the quality of the DSM criteria. These criteria range from relatively narrowly defined symptoms, such as no close friends or confidants, to somewhat more vaguely worded signs and symptoms requiring significant interpretation and/or operationalization. For example, individual raters may differ on what constitutes "excessive" social anxiety or "odd" appearance. By the same token, the relatively high reliability and validity figures reported in some studies demonstrate that this task is not impossible.

Finally, in considering the studies reported below or in developing future research, the researcher should determine the reason for using the structured interview. The major difference between the interview schedules below is that some test for all personality disorders, whereas others test for SPD only. If the study is conducted in a clinical setting, or if an examination of comorbidity is desired, then it is important to use a diagnostic instrument that tests for all personality disorders, such as the Structured Clinical Interview for DSM-III Personality Disorders (SIDP), the Structured Clinical Interview for DSM-III-R personality disorders (SCID), or the Personality Disorder Examination (PDE). However, if the goal of research is simply to identify a schizotypal sample or to examine the schizotypal symptomatology in a very detailed way, then the Schedule for Schizotypal Personalities (SSP) or the Structured Interview for Schizotypy (SIS) may be more appropriate. In the review below, scales measuring all PDs will be discussed first, as there is more research on these instruments; scales specially designed for SPD only will be reviewed at the end.

Structured clinical interview for DSM-III personality disorders (SIDP)

The SIDP (Pfohl, Stangl, & Zimmerman, 1983) was the first semistructured interview schedule developed to test and improve DSM-III Axis II validity and reliability. The SIDP-R is the revised edition for DSM-III-R (Pfohl, Blum, Zimmerman, & Stangl, 1989). Both versions of this interview have been tested for reliability and validity, as well as presence and comorbidity of Axis II disorders. Each of these structured interviews consists of 160 items, a scoring manual, and takes 60–90 minutes to administer to the subject if an Axis I diagnosis has already been made. Additionally, there is a 30-minute informant interview. Each interview is arranged in 16 sections, around major domains of personality such as "level of social interaction." During the interview, the diagnostician records the subject's open-ended responses. At the end of each section, the relevant criteria of each personality disorder are scored according to level of severity on a 0–2 scale. This format was designed to reduce redundancy due to overlap of criteria across more than one disorder. Scores are assigned only to symptoms from the DSM; no general scores are assigned. A score of 1 means that the variable is present, and a 2 means that it is severe. No published data on norms are available.

The authors specify several features of the instrument designed to increase accuracy. First, the questions specifically ask the subject to describe their "usual" behavior, outside of the presence of any acute psychopathology. Second, the interview also includes a section in which an informant is contacted to verify the accuracy of the reports; when the subject and informant conflict, the interviewer must decide the relative veracity of each respondent based on clarity and specificity of responses. Finally, the interviewer is directed to determine if the subject's personality has substantially changed, and to score the predominant personality of the past five years if there have been significant alterations.

Reliability

Stangl, Pfohl, Zimmerman, Bowers, and Corenthal (1985) tested the reliability of the SIDP on a sample made up mostly of inpatients (n = 131). About half of the subjects (n = 63) were rated by a second interviewer, usually as silent observer of the same interview. They reported interrater reliability (kappa) for presence or absence of a personality disorder at .71 ($p < .001$). Interrater reliability for SPD was somewhat lower (coefficient kappa = .62, $p < .001$ for SPD). This kappa is "barely acceptable" according to Stangl et al. (1985). The diagnostic frequency of SPD in this sample was 9% (12 subjects).

Nazikian, Rudd, Edwards, and Jackson (1990) also found a comparable reliability using a same-interview design in a small sample of patients (n = 10). In addition to comparing diagnostic outcome, which was too limited to quantify, these researchers utilized a dimensional index of the number of items scored for each patient and reported a significant correlation (Pearson's r) of .70 ($p < .05$) for schizotypal items. Jackson, Gazis, Rudd, and Edwards (1991) also utilized categorical and dimensional comparisons of joint-interview reliability; for SPD, reliabilities were .67 (kappa) and .59 (r), respectively. In a subsample (n = 104) selected for joint interview from a larger study of 808 relatives of psychiatric patients, Zimmerman and Coryell (1990) reported a coefficient kappa of 1.0 for SPD using the SIDP. However, it should be noted that the overall base rate of SPD in the larger sample was 3%, so the reported kappa is based on perhaps only three cases (the specific number is not reported).

One study of joint-interview reliability (Hogg, Jackson, Rudd, & Edwards, 1990) reported a much lower correlation (r = .399) between dimensional scores of SPD in a sample of 40 recent-onset schizophrenics. In this study, SPD had one of the lowest interrater reliabilities of all the personality disorders. Given the strong relationship between schizophrenia and SPD, this datum is unsettling in terms of validity of the instrument for this disorder.

In contrast to these relatively positive results for concurrent reliability, a study of six-month test–retest reliability by van den Brink et al. (1986, cited in Reich, 1989) found a kappa of .14 for SPD. This very low number might in fact be inflated, insofar as near misses were counted as agreements. Similarly, Pfohl et al. (1987) reported kappa of .22 for SPD in 36 depressed inpatients reassessed after 6–12 months.

Validity

The validity of the SIDP has also been tested in a number of studies, usually in terms of concurrent/convergent validity with self-report questionnaires. These studies have almost always found very low concordance between the SIDP and self-report instruments such as the MCMI (Millon, 1983), the MCMI-II (Millon, 1987), and the Personality Disorders Questionnaire (PDQ; Hyler & Reider, 1984). For example, several studies comparing the SIDP with the MCMI (Hogg et al., 1990; Gazis, Rudd, & Edwards, 1991; Miller, Streiner, & Parkinson, 1992; Nazikian et al., 1990) found diagnostic concordance for SPD to be zero or close to zero (maximum kappa = .34). Dimensional comparisons were similarly low (maximum r = .394). These results cannot be easily ascribed to a difference in thresholds, as the evidence on false positives and negatives is mixed. In a number of these studies, the MCMI tended to diagnose more personality disorders in general, whereas the SIDP tended to result in more diagnoses of SPD specifically.

A recent study comparing the MCMI-II with SIDP in a sample of 21 bipolar patients found that each scale identified only one patient with SPD, but the two scales identified different patients (Turley, Bates, Edwards, & Jackson, 1992). Differences in the SIDP and the MCMI do not necessarily invalidate the SIDP, insofar as the MCMI was developed prior to the DSM-III and does not utilize the same conceptual basis (Widiger, Williams, Spitzer, & Francis, 1985). However, similarly low concordance rates were found in studies of the PDQ (Zimmerman & Coryell, 1990) and personality disorder scales derived from the MMPI (Miller et al., 1992), both of which were specifically designed in accordance with DSM-III. In these studies, the low concordance was found for SPD specifically, which tended to be detected less frequently by the SIDP as compared to the self-report scales, as well as for PDs in general.

Revision for DSM-III-R

As noted above, Pfohl and colleagues have released a revised version of the SIDP in accordance with the revisions in DSM-III-R (Pfohl et al., 1989). Blashfield, Blum, and Pfohl (1992) compared kappas for agreement between the SIDP and SIDP-R in a sample of 72 inpatients. While the concordance (kappa) for any personality disorder was moderate (.569), the concordance for SPD was the lowest of all (–.25). The number of subjects diagnosed with SPD decreased from 8 to 2. The authors attribute this marked shift to two factors: (1) the increased number of symptoms needed for threshold in DSM-III-R (5 of 9 symptoms, as opposed to 4 of 8); (2) the deletion from DSM-III-R of the most frequently endorsed symptom, "hypersensitivity to criticism."

Advantages and disadvantages

The SIDP/SIDP-R has several notable features that may serve as advantages or disadvantages, depending on the purposes for which it is to be used. The scale is comprehensive, providing assessments for all the DSM personality disorders. This is useful in studies examining comorbidity, but the scale does not provide detailed information on schizotypal symptomatology outside of the nine DSM-III-R criteria. Questions are grouped by topic, rather than by disorder, which the authors suggest helps to avoid clinician bias and the halo effect; however, it may also limit the use of valid clinical judgment and intuition. One structural feature of the SIDP and SIDP-R that is almost certainly an advantage is that it provides for the collection of data from an informant, in order to corroborate the reports of the subject. However, the use and effects on diagnosis of informant data have not been examined in detail empirically.

One final advantage of the SIDP/SIDP-R is that it has been widely used in the research literature, and has acceptable reliability. This allows for comparability across laboratories for research utilizing this instrument. However, as noted above, the long-term test–retest reliability and validity in comparison to other instruments are so far unsubstantiated by the data.

Structured clinical interview for DSM-III-R personality disorders (SCID-II)

The SCID-II (Spitzer, Williams, & Gibbon, 1987; Spitzer, Williams, Gibbon, & First, 1990) is designed to evaluate 11 DSM-III-R PD diagnoses, as well as the proposed category of self-defeating PD. It consists of 160 items, each representing one of the DSM diagnostic criteria for a symptom. Each item is rated on a 1–3 scale: inadequate information (rated "?"), not present (rated 1), subthreshold (2), or present (3). When the number of criteria for a PD is met, a diagnosis is made. In these respects, the SCID-II is structurally similar to the SIDP. One structural difference is that the SCID-II package includes a questionnaire containing all of the symptoms presented in a self-report format; this feature is designed to save time by allowing the interviewer to follow up only on questions that are answered "yes" by self-report, or in diagnostic categories that appear to be close to threshold.

Reliability

Studies reporting joint-interview reliability for the SCID-II tend to show good concordance for the instrument as a whole as well as for SPD in particular. Fogelson et al. (Fogelson, Nuechterlein, Asarnow, Subotnik, & Talovic, 1991), studying 45-first-degree relatives of psychotic patients, reported intraclass correlation coefficients (ICCs) ranging from .60 to .84, with SPD = .73, although the number of cases of SPD was limited (n = 2). Arntz and associates (van Beijsterveldt, Hoekstra, Hofman, Eussen, & Sallaerts, 1992) found similar same-interview reliability in an item-by-item analysis of a Dutch version. For SPD items, reliability ran from .74 to .97 for the six symptoms, while the three signs (odd speech, odd appearance or behavior, and inappropriate/constricted affect) had much lower reliability (.42, .49, and 0.0, respectively). Kappa for SPD diagnosis was an acceptable .65, and kappa for the total instrument was .80. On the other hand, a study by Renneberg and colleagues (Renneberg, Champless, Dowdall, Fauerbach, & Gracely, 1992), while not providing results for each disorder, reported that PDs in the odd cluster (SPD, schizoid PD, and paranoid PD) had the lowest concordance of all (kappa = .45).

Validity

Studies of the validity of SCID-II diagnoses for SPD have demonstrated mixed results and point to key sources of variability. Renneberg et al. (1992) reported low correspondence (kappa = .19) between the MCMI-II and the SCID-II for the odd cluster. This figure improved substantially (.44–.52) when the cutoff threshold was increased on the MCMI-II, thereby reducing the number of positive diagnoses. Hyler and colleagues (Hyler, Skodol, Kellman, Oldham, & Rosnick, 1990) found a similar concordance (.48) for SPD between the PDQ-Revised and SCID-II in a sample of 87 applicants to inpatient treatment almost all of whom had severe Axis II pathology. In a separate study of less severely disturbed applicants for outpatient treatment (Hyler, Skodol, Oldham, Kellman, & Doidge, 1992), the kappa for SPD was –.03.

These results indicate first that the diagnostic outcome of a given self-report measure can change drastically with a small change in cutoff scores; by the same token, the subjective threshold used by an interviewer can have significant effects on the outcome. Second, studies of reliability and validity are quite sensitive to the population being studied, possibly because the kappa statistic is dependent on the number of total patients given the diagnosis, and is very sensitive to disagreement if the base rate for a disorder is low. Additionally, the strength of the pathology in a severely disturbed sample may artificially inflate agreement.

One study examined the predictive validity of the SCID-II by comparing diagnoses to those given after "longitudinal expert evaluation using all data" (Skodol, Rosnick, Kellman, Oldham, & Hyler, 1988). This evaluation was made on 20 inpatients after an average hospitalization of 30.8 weeks. These researchers found that the SCID-II had a diagnostic power (percentage accuracy) of .90.

Advantages and disadvantages

The SCID-II has the advantages of being comprehensive and specifically tailored to DSM-III-R by the authors of that manual. The SCID-II can be utilized conveniently in conjunction with the SCID-P (Spitzer et al., 1987), which tests for Axis I pathology. In addition, the SCID-II has the potential of being faster to administer because of the preinterview questionnaire. However, the questionnaire may reduce the validity of the instrument, given the reported discrepancies between self-report and interview diagnoses.

Two sources of potential biasing on the SCID-II have been posited. First, it has been suggested that because the questions on the SCID-II are very direct, subjects may be more likely to deny them (Renneberg et al., 1992). Widiger and Frances (1987) propose that the organization of questions by syndrome may cause a halo effect, but it is also possible that this effect may represent legitimate clinical judgment.

Personality Disorders Exam (PDE)

The PDE (Loranger, Susman, Oldham, & Russakoff, 1987; Loranger et al., 1985) is an interview assessing for all personality disorders in DSM-III-R, has 328 items, and takes approximately 90 minutes to administer. The interview is organized around five headings: work, self, interpersonal relations, affect, and impulse control. Like the SIDP and SCID-II, each item is scored on a 3-point scale: not present or clinically significant, present below threshold, clinically significant; the interviewer can also indicate if not enough information is available. Diagnoses for each personality disorder can be made either based on a psychometrically determined cutoff score or by an experienced clinician; dimensional scores are also available. The PDE utilizes a diagnostic window of five years in order to define the concept of "longstanding." The PDE is being translated by the WHO into other languages to be used in WHO research (Loranger et al., 1994).

Reliability

In their initial report, Loranger et al. (1987) demonstrated that same-interview interrater reliability was very high for SPD rated dimensionally (ICC = .98) and categorically (kappa = .80); all other PDs evaluated also had higher scores than reported for other instruments. O'Boyle and Self (1990) reported high ICCs (.89–1.0) for dimensional scores for all PDs. The lowest reported kappa for SPD is an acceptable .62 (Standage & Ladha, 1988). The international version of the PDE (IPDE; Loranger et al., 1994) also shows strong same-interview reliability for dimensional scores and number of criteria met (.87/.82 for SPD).

Results for temporal stability are less strong. Loranger et al. (1994) reported good six-month stability for the IPDE when measured by the same interviewer (ICC = .81/.69 for SPD). O'Boyle and Self (1990) reported no significant change in dimensional scores for SPD in 17 depressed patients in remission at two-month follow-up. However, a study by Stuart, Simons, Thase, and Pilkonis (1992) found the opposite results in a sample of depressed patients who had been rated by the PDE as positive for one or more PDs. Nine of the 10 who were successfully treated for depression no longer were diagnosed with PDs at the completion of treatment (12 weeks). Similarly, Ames-Frankel et al. (1992) reported a 0.0 kappa for the SPD diagnosis at a 6-week interval for 30 bulimic outpatients.

Validity

Soldz, Budman, Demby, and Merry (1993) examined the diagnostic agreement between the MCMI-II and the PDE on 97 mental health outpatients, and found that the self-report measure identified far more personality disorders, including SPD. Concordance between the two measures was low (for any PD, kappa = .23; for SPD, kappa = –.02). Hyler et al. (1990, 1992) compared the PDE to the PDQ-R and found the same pattern as they had found for the SCID-II: for the severely disturbed inpatients, concordance for SPD was moderate (.54), whereas for outpatient applicants, kappa = 0.0.

Hyler et al. (1990, 1992) also compared the PDE with the SCID-II in both samples, with results similar to those for the PDQ (SPD kappa = .44 for the inpatients, 0.0 for the outpatients). O'Boyle and Self (1990) found low concordance for depressed inpatients between PDE and SCID-II (kappa = .08 for the odd cluster as a whole). Oldham and colleagues (Oldham, Skodol, Kellman, Hyler, Rosnick, & Davies, 1992) found a striking similarity of prevalence rates of SPD as measured by the SCID-II and PDE, but kappa was moderate at best for SPD (between .30 and .59). This study also demonstrated that despite the similarities in prevalence for SPD, the patterns of comorbidity were markedly different; in general, the PDE showed a greater degree of comorbidity for schizotypy, despite the fact that the PDE showed lower overall prevalence of PDs compared to the SCID-II. This finding indicates that the evaluation of the prevalence of schizotypy on these instruments may be anomalous relative to the ratings of the other disorders.

Advantages and disadvantages

One strength of the PDE is its broad coverage of so many items, allowing for the generation of a personality profile, similar to the MMPI profile. However, it is also potentially more time-consuming than the SCID-II. Requiring further investigation are the substantial discrepancies between the PDE and the SCID-II; these may be due to differences in probes, the different arrangement of the items (by disorder vs. by content area), or a different threshold. Future studies are needed in which external variables (such as biological markers) are differentially correlated with scales from the SCID-II and PDE.

Personality Assessment Schedule (PAS)

The PAS (Tyler & Alexander, 1979) was created by British researchers in relation to ICD criteria for personality disorders. The scale contains 24 items covering a range of characteristics, each of which is rated on a 9-point scale.

The unique feature of the PAS is that the interview is conducted separately with both a patient and a close informant, and the information given by the informant is given more weight in final scoring and assessment. The scale also contains a cluster-analytic algorithm to generate categorical diagnoses in five categories: normal, sociopathic, passive-dependent, anankastic (obsessional), or schizoid. While the questions cover topics relevant to schizotypy, a new algorithm would need to be generated to allow for diagnosis of SPD.

Reliability

Despite the fact that the PAS was developed in Britain, Tyrer et al. (1984) demonstrated moderate-to-good cross-national reliability for the scale in a joint-interview study of American and British interviewers (ICCs = .66–.94 for informants and .51–.91 for subjects on the 24 personality variables). Concordance for presence or absence of a PD was strong (kappa = .6 to .8). Tyrer, Strauss, and Cicchetti (1983) found that test–retest reliability at 2.9 years was inconsistent across items (ICCs = –.09 to .73 for the 24 scales). The authors reported data indicating that much of this inconsistency may be due to changes in clinical state in a subgroup of the patients.

Schedule for interviewing borderlines (SIB)/schedule for schizotypal personalities (SSP)

The SIB (Baron & Gruen, 1980; Baron, Asnis, & Gruen, 1981) contains 70 items, and measures both SPD (Schedule for Schizotypal Personalities, SSP), as well as borderline personality disorder (Schedule for Borderline Personalities). The interview takes 1–2 hours to administer, and has 10 subscales of 1–8 items each. The subscales represent each of the eight DSM-III SPD criteria as well as two additional symptoms – depersonalization/derealization and transient delusions or hallucinations.

Each of the 10 subscales can be evaluated by a variety of scoring methods. First, each item on the subscale is rated on a 1–4 scale. The subscale is rated categorically (statement score), and two dimensional scores are also available: a scaled score, representing the sum of the scale scores of the items, and a summary rating of severity (scale of 1–4). Age of onset is also recorded, but there is no minimum or maximum limit set. While the item content was originally drawn primarily from the DSM-III criteria, the SSP was the first to be originally field-tested on first-degree relatives of schizophrenic patients. Also, because of the limited scope of the SSP compared to schedules for all PDs, this scale contains many more probes and alternate phrasings for questions relating to SPD. It is possible that this may result in the relative overestimation of the prevalence of SPD, insofar as it casts a wider net, and each symptom subscale has a low threshold, requiring only one response scored as mild or above to be counted as present.

Reliability

Baron et al. (1981) evaluated the joint-interview interrater reliability of the scale scores for each of the 10 subscales; ICCs were very good, ranging from .95 to .97. Similarly, ICCs for six-month test–retest reliability ranged from .61 to .91. Concordance for the diagnosis of SPD was also good (kappa = .88). The joint-interview reliability figures were replicated in a larger study of schizophrenics' relatives (ICCs = .68–.99; kappa = .92; Baron, Gruen, Rainer, Kane, Asnis, & Lord, 1985). Other studies (Goldberg, Schulz, Schulz, Resnick, Hamer, & Friedel, 1986; Jacobsberg, Hymowitz, Barasch, & Frances, 1986; Perry, O'Connell, & Drake, 1984) found similarly positive results (all ICCs and kappas > .64). Perry et al. (1984) also found high six-month test–retest reliability for the scale scores (ICCs = .57–.91); however, the statement scores (present/absent decisions for each criterion) were not as reliable (ICCs = .09 to 1.0). Still, retest reliability for the SPD diagnosis was a strong 0.84.

Validity

Two studies have examined the validity of the SSP in comparison to concurrent expert clinicians' judgment (Baron et al., 1985; Perry et al., 1984). Perry et al. (1984) found that all of the SSP scales had moderate to good sensitivity (50–88%) and specificity (64–100%) in discriminating SPD case, identified through clinical consensus, from controls. Baron et al. (1985) validated the instrument by showing that it could identify greater prevalence of SPD in relatives of schizophrenics as compared to relatives of matched controls. No studies have been reported that compare the SSP to other self-report or interview measures of schizotypy.

Advantages and disadvantages

The SSP provides more detailed information on SPD than the scales discussed above and achieves high (concurrent) reliability; however, it does not allow for determination of comorbidity with other Axis II disorders. One important feature is that the self-report measures of the schizotypal signs has been validated against clinicians' observation (Perry et al., 1984). The SSP also has demonstrated strength specifically in the population it was designed on – that is, relatives of schizophrenics, who constitute an important research group.

The Structured Interview of Schizotypy (SIS)

The SIS (Kendler, Lieberman, & Walsh, 1989) was the only scale developed specifically as a research tool for those studying schizotypy and schizophrenia. According to its authors, it was not designed for clinical use insofar as it (1) includes a much broader range of potentially relevant items beyond those in DSM definition of SPD, but does not assess for all PDs; and (2) generates dimensional data, rather than a categorical diagnosis. There are numerous items for each symptom, and "skip-outs" are provided to eliminate the need to assess further in an area where the subject gives negative responses. In addition, the authors sought to improve upon previous instruments by adding (1) closed response format (e.g., "often," "sometimes," "rarely," "never") allowing for quicker assessment of more items; (2) comprehensive assessment of schizotypal signs (giving the interviewer specific guideposts for rating these signs); (3) questions phrased in nondeviant ways; and (4) contextual assessments of the meaning of items (e.g., ideas of reference may be justified in someone with a severe facial disfigurement). Finally, the SIS provides coverage of childhood and adolescent personality features; most questions are asked about the subjects' functioning in the last three years.

Reliability and validity

In initial pilot studies, joint-interview reliabilities were high for symptoms (ICCs > .67, except for the symptom "impulsivity"). However, inconsistent reliabilities were obtained for the signs (ICCs = 0.0 to .65). Kendler et al. (1989) note that many of the low reliabilities may have been artifacts due to low variance in the sample; reliabilities reported for a larger pilot sample were substantially better than those for the initial pilot (ICCs = .56 to .80). As with the SSP studies, validity was assessed by demonstrating that a number of predicted subscales (corresponding to the DSM-III-R criteria for SPD) have significantly higher ratings in relatives of schizophrenics as compared to relatives of controls. More studies are needed to assess the advantages of using this instrument over the SSP, and to validate the potential benefits posited by the authors.

Concluding comments

One finding that was prevalent across instruments was that the self-report questionnaires reported a greater prevalence of personality disorders in general than did the semistructured interviews. This may be for several reasons: (1) State factors may affect self-report measures more than interviews (Renneberg et al., 1992); (2) the interview asks when the symptoms have occurred, and explicitly requires long-term duration; (3) some of the interview questions may seem deviant, and make subject underreport symptoms for fear of the interviewer's judgment. Future studies are needed in order to understand the impact on outcome, treatment, and other correlates of self-report versus interview-diagnosed PDs. Many of the scales showed good joint-interview interrater reliability, but few have examined different interviewer reliability. Future studies also need to closely examine long-term test–retest reliability, which does not appear to be strong for these instruments and may be strongly impacted by changes in clinical state. This issue cuts to the core of our understanding of personality disorders as lifelong traits. If we are unable accurately to assess lifetime stability of these traits, than the accuracy of our diagnostic system for Axis II can be called into question.

References

Ames-Frankel, J., Devlin, M. J., Walsh, B. T., Strasser, T. J., Sadik, C., Oldham, J. M., & Roose, S. P. (1992). Personality disorder diagnoses in patients with bulimia nervosa: Clinical correlates and changes with treatment. *Journal of Clinical Psychiatry, 53,* 90–96.

American Psychiatric Association (1980). *Diagnostic and statistical manual of mental disorders,* 3rd edition. Washington D.C.: American Psychiatric Association.

American Psychiatric Association (1987). *Diagnostic and statistical manual of mental disorders,* 3rd edition, revised. Washington D.C.: American Psychiatric Association.

Arntz, A., van Beijsterveldt, B., Hoekstra, R., Hofman, A., Eussen, M., & Sallaerts, S. (1992). The interrater reliability of a Dutch version of the Structured Clinical Interview for DSM-III-R Personality Disorders. *Acta Psychiatrica Scandinavica, 85,* 394–400.

Baron, M., Asnis, L., & Gruen, R. (1981). The Schedule for Schizotypal Personalities (SSP): A diagnostic interview for schizotypal features. *Psychiatry Research, 4,* 213–228.

Baron, M., & Gruen, R. (1980). *The Schedule for Interviewing Borderlines* (*SIB*). New York: N.Y. State Psychiatric Institute.

Baron, M., Gruen, R., Rainer, J. D., Kane, J., Asnis, L., & Lord, S. (1985). A family study of schizophrenic and normal control probands: Implications for the spectrum concept of schizophrenia. *American Journal of Psychiatry, 142*(4), 447–455.

Blashfield, R., Blum, N., & Pfohl, B. (1992). The effects of changing Axis II diagnostic criteria. *Comprehensive Psychiatry, 33*(4), 245–252.

Fogelson, D. L., Nuechterlein, K. H., Asarnow, R. F., Subotnik, K. L., & Talovic, S. A. (1991). Interrater reliability of the Structured Clinical Interview for DSM-III-R, Axis II: Schizophrenia spectrum and affective spectrum disorders. *Psychiatry Research, 39,* 55–63.

Goldberg, S. C., Schulz, S. C., Schulz, P. M., Resnick, R. J., Hamer, R. M., & Friedel,

R. O. (1986). Borderline and schizotypal personality disorders treated with low-dose thiothixene vs placebo. *Archives of General Psychiatry, 43,* 680–686.

Grove, W. M., Andreasen, N. C., McDonald-Scott, P., Keller, M B., & Shapiro, W. (1981). Reliability studies of psychiatric diagnoses. *Archives of General Psychiatry, 38,* 408–413.

Hogg, B., Jackson, H. J., Rudd, R. P., & Edwards, J. (1990). Diagnosing personality disorders in recent-onset schizophrenia. *Journal of Nervous and Mental Disease, 178*(3), 194–199.

Hyler, S. E., & Reider, C. (1984). *Personality Diagnostic Questionnaire Revised (PDQR),* New York, N.Y.: New York State Psychiatric Institute.

Hyler, S. E., Skodol, A. E., Kellman, H. D., Oldham, J. M., & Rosnick, L. (1990). Validity of the Personality Diagnostic Questionnaire – Revised: Comparison with two structured interviews. *American Journal of Psychiatry, 147,* 1043–1048.

Hyler, S. E., Skodol, A. E., Oldham, J. M., Kellman, H. D., & Doidge, N. (1992). Validity of the Personality Diagnostic Questionnaire – Revised: A replication in an outpatient sample. *Comprehensive Psychiatry, 33*(2), 73–77.

Jackson, H. J., Gazis, J., Rudd, R. P., & Edwards, J. (1991). Concordance between two personality disorder instruments with psychiatric inpatients. *Comprehensive Psychiatry, 32*(3), 252–260.

Jacobsberg, L. B., Hymowitz, P., Barasch, A., & Frances, A. J. (1986). Symptoms of schizotypal personality disorder. *American Journal of Psychiatry, 143*(10), 1222–1227.

Kendler, K. S., Lieberman, J. A., & Walsh, D. (1989). The Structured Interview for Schizotypy (SIS): A preliminary report. *Schizophrenia Bulletin, 15*(4), 559–571.

Kihlstrom, J. F. (1989). On what does mood-dependent memory depend? *Journal of Social Behavior and Personality, 4,* 23–32.

Loranger, A. W. (1992). Are current self-report and interview measures adequate for epidemiological studies of personality disorders? *Journal of Personality Disorders, 6*(4), 313–325.

Loranger, A. W., Lenzenweger, M. F., Gattner, A. F., Susman, V. L. (1991). Trait–state artifacts and the diagnosis of personality disorders. *Archives of General Psychiatry, 48*(8), 720–728.

Loranger, A. W., Sartorius, N., Andreoli, A., Berger, P., Buchheim, P., Channabasavanna, S. M., Coid, B., Kahl, A., Diekstra, R. F. W., Ferguson, B., Jacobsberg, L. B., Mombour, W., Pull, C., Ono, Y., & Regier, D. A. (1994). The International Personality Disorder Examination. *Archives of General Psychiatry, 51,* 215–224.

Loranger, A. W., Susman, V. L., Oldham, J. M., & Russakoff, L. M. (1985). *Personality Disorder Examination (PDE): A Structured Interview for DSM-III-R Personality Disorders.* White Plains, N.Y.: New York Hospital–Cornell Medical Center, Westchester Division.

Loranger, A. W., Susman, V. L., Oldham, J. M., & Russakoff, L. M. (1987). The Personality Disorder Examination: A preliminary report. *Journal of Personality Disorders, 1*(1), 1–13.

Miller, H. R., Streiner, D. L., & Parkinson, A. (1992). Maximum likelihood estimates of the ability of the MMPI and MCMI personality disorder scales and the SIDP to identify personality disorders. *Journal of Personality Assessment, 59*(1), 1–13.

Millon, T. (1983). *Millon Clinical Multiaxial Inventory,* 3rd edition. (MCMI). Minneapolis, Minn.: National Computer Systems.

Millon, T. (1987). *Manual for the Millon Clinical Multiaxial Inventory – II.* Minneapolis, Minn.: National Computer Systems.

Nazikian, H., Rudd, R. P., Edwards, J., & Jackson, H. J. (1990). Personality disorder assessment for psychiatric inpatients. *Australian and New Zealand Journal of Psychiatry, 24,* 37–46.

O'Boyle, M., & Self, D. (1990). A comparison of two interviews for DSM-III-R personality disorders. *Psychiatry Research, 32,* 85–92.

Oldham, J. M., Skodol, A. E., Kellman, H. D., Hyler, S. E., Rosnick, L., & Davies, M. (1992). Diagnosis of DSM-III-R personality disorders by two structured interviews: Patterns of comorbidity. *American Journal of Psychiatry, 149,* 213–220.

Perry, J. C., O'Connell, M. E., & Drake, R. (1984). An assessment of the Schedule for Schizotypal Personalities and the DSM-III criteria for diagnosing schizotypal personality disorder. *Journal of Nervous and Mental Disease, 172*(11), 674–680.

Pfohl, B., Blum, N., Zimmerman, M., & Stangl, D. (1989). *Structured Clinical Interview for DSM-III Personality Disorders, Revised* (SIDP-R). Iowa City, Ia.: University of Iowa Hospitals and Clinics.

Pfohl, B., Coryell, W., Zimmerman, M., & Stangl, D. (1987). Prognostic validity of self-report and interview measures of personality disorder in depressed inpatients. *Journal of Clinical Psychiatry, 48*(12), 468–472.

Pfohl, B., Stangl, D., & Zimmerman, M. (1983). *Structured Interview for DSM-III Personality Disorders* (SIDP). Iowa City, Ia.: University of Iowa Hospitals and Clinics.

Reich, J. H. (1989). Update of instruments to measure DSM-III and DSM-III-R personality disorders. *Journal of Nervous and Mental Disease, 177*(6), 366–370.

Renneberg, B., Champless, D. L., Dowdall, D. J., Fauerbach, J. A., & Gracely, E. J. (1992). The Structured Clinical Interview for DSM-III-R, Axis II and the Millon Clinical Multiaxial Inventory: A concurrent validity study of personality disorders among anxious outpatients. *Journal of Personality Disorders, 6*(2), 117–124.

Skodol, A. E., Rosnick, L., Kellman, D., Oldham, J. M., & Hyler, S. E. (1988). *American Journal of Psychiatry, 145*(1), 1297–1299.

Soldz, S., Budman, S., Demby, A., & Merry, J. (1993). Diagnostic agreement between the Personality Disorder Examination and the MCMI-II. *Journal of Personality Assessment, 60*(3), 486–499.

Spitzer, R. L., Williams, J. B. W., & Gibbon, M. (1987). *Structured Interview for DSM-III-R (SCID).* New York: New York State Psychiatric Institute, Biometrics Research.

Spitzer, R. L., Williams, J. B. W., Gibbon, M., & First, M. B. (1990). *Structured Interview for DSM-III-R Personality Disorders (SCID-II, version 1.0).* Washington D.C.: American Psychiatric Press.

Standage, K., & Ladha, N. (1988). An examination of the reliability of the Personality Disorder Examination and a comparison with other methods of identifying personality disorders in a clinical sample. *Journal of Personality Disorders, 2,* 267–271.

Stangl, D., Pfohl, B., Zimmerman, M., Bowers, W., & Corenthal, C. (1985). A Structured Interview for the DSM-III Personality Disorders. *Archives of General Psychiatry, 42,* 591–596.

Stuart, S., Simons, A. D., Thase, M. E., & Pilkonis, P. (1992). Are personality assessments valid in acute major depression? *Journal of Affective Disorders, 24,* 281–290.

Turley, B., Bates, G. W., Edwards, J., & Jackson, H. J. (1992). MCMI-II personality disorders in recent-onset bipolar disorders. *Journal of Clinical Psychology, 48*(3), 320–329.

Tyrer, P., & Alexander, J. (1979). Classification of personality disorder. *British Journal of Psychiatry, 135,* 163–167.

Tyrer, P., Cicchetti, D. V., Casey, P. R., Fitzpatrick, K., Oliver, R., Balter, A., Giller, E., & Harkness, L. (1984). Cross-national reliability study of a Schedule for Assessing Personality Disorders. *Journal of Nervous and Mental Disease, 172*(12), 718–721.

Tyrer, P., Strauss, J., & Cicchetti, D. (1983). Temporal reliability of personality in psychiatric patients. *Psychological Medicine, 13,* 393–398.

Widiger, T. A., Williams, J. B. W., Spitzer, R. L., & Francis, A. (1985). The MCMI as a measure of DSM-III. *Journal of Personality Assessment, 49,* 366–378.

Widiger, T. A., & Frances, A. (1987). Interviews and inventories for the measurement of personality disorders. *Clinical Psychology Review, 7,* 49–75.

Zimmerman, M. (1994). Diagnosing personality disorders. *Archives of General Psychiatry, 51,* 225–245.

Zimmerman, M., & Coryell, W. H. (1990). Diagnosing personality disorders in the community. *Archives of General Psychiatry, 47,* 527–531.

Name index

Subject index